Brewster and Wheatstone
on Vision

Brewster and Wheatstone
on Vision

edited by

Nicholas J. Wade

Department of Psychology
The University of Dundee

1983
Published for
EXPERIMENTAL PSYCHOLOGY SOCIETY
by
ACADEMIC PRESS
London   New York
Paris   San Diego   San Francisco
São Paulo   Sydney   Tokyo   Toronto

ACADEMIC PRESS INC. (LONDON) LTD.
24/28 Oval Road
London NW1

United States Edition published by
ACADEMIC PRESS INC.
111 FIFTH Avenue
New York, New York 10003

Copyright © 1983 by
EXPERIMENTAL PSYCHOLOGY SOCIETY

British Library Cataloguing in Publication Data

Brewster, Sir David
    Brewster and Wheatstone on vision.
    1. Vision   2. Neurophysiology
    3. Optics, Physiological
    I. Title   II. Wheatstone, Sir Charles
    III. Wade, N. J.
    612'.84   QP475
    ISBN 0-12-729550-X

Typeset by Oxford Verbatim Limited, and printed in Great Britain by
St Edmundsbury Press, Bury St Edmunds, Suffolk

Foreword

Although Sir Charles Wheatstone and Sir David Brewster were not the best of friends, we look back at them both with a friendly eye. Nicholas Wade has gone out of his way to journey back in time to meet them and capture their ideas and their words, to bring them back for us to appreciate. And appreciate we do, for both Wheatstone and Brewster made notable contributions over a wide and largely overlapping range. So it is appropriate that now they find themselves locked together within these pages, though in life they were rivals.

There is much here of remaining technical interest for students of visual perception and for historians interested in this most rapid period of technological progress, when single men could perform feats of imagination and development that now require multi-National Corporations. Are the relatively easy insights now used up? I doubt it. Edwin Land is just such a man today, who latches on to phenomena and makes them work for him and the rest of mankind. Though Wheatstone and Brewster did not, as it were by their stereo rivalry, see eye to eye, these carefully collected and annotated papers not only bring them alive, they also strengthen the roots of our thinking and research into these endlessly fascinating questions.

10 March 1983   Richard L. Gregory
Bristol

To

Christine, Rebecca and Helena

Preface

It was in the course of reading some early studies on subjective visual phenomena that I first became aware of the scope of both Brewster's and Wheatstone's researches relating to vision. Many of the phenomena described by Purkinje in the 1820s were also examined by these two natural philosophers. In fact, Wheatstone published, anonymously, a translated summary of Purkinje's first book. I then started collecting the papers of Brewster and Wheatstone on vision. Two things were evident in their early papers – the similarity of the topics they examined and the differences in their interpretations of them. This ambivalence was to pervade their later work on binocular vision, and it provides the basis for presenting their papers together.

I have tried to draw attention to these aspects of Brewster's and Wheatstone's visual researches in my published work, but it was not possible to do justice to the breadth and depth of their observations in this second-hand manner. However, I did not have any specific plans for disseminating their papers more widely until Ross Day suggested republishing them. The idea was very appealing, as it would allow students of vision to appreciate the clarity of their observations and the ingenuity of their interpretations at first hand, rather than being sullied by some intermediary. The idea was given added impetus by Hiroshi Ono, during a sabbatical year he spent in Dundee. Accordingly, I contacted the Experimental Psychology Society to enquire whether it would be willing to support the publication of the collection. This it has done, and I wish to express my gratitude to the Society.

Hiroshi Ono and I had many discussions about Brewster and Wheatstone, often with Mike Swanston and Alan Wilkes. They all read drafts of my commentary, and made many helpful comments. Their sober perspectives on the history of perception have been of great assistance. Many specific points have been clarified by discussion or correspondence with the following authorities: Brian Bowers, George Duncan, Arthur T. Gill, J. R. Levene, Alison Morrison-Low and R. N. Smart.

Historical research is dependent upon ready access to the repositories of our past. I have been fortunate in the assistance I have received from the University Libraries of Dundee, Edinburgh and St. Andrews, and the Scottish National

Library. I wish to express my thanks most particularly to G. D. Hargreaves and R. N. Smart of the Manuscripts and Rare Books Department of the University of St. Andrews for their readiness to search for both literature and portraiture regarding Brewster.

The following societies and publishers have kindly given permission to reproduce the articles and letters by Brewster and Wheatstone:

> Blackwell Scientific Publications Ltd., for article 2.11
> British Association for the Advancement of Science, for articles 2.8, 4.6 and 4.11–4.16
> Taylor and Francis Ltd., for articles 2.15 and 4.7–4.9
> The Royal Photographic Society, for articles 2.13 and 2.14
> The Royal Society, for articles 1.2, 2.4, 2.10 and 4.19
> The Royal Society of Edinburgh, for articles 2.5–2.7, 4.10, 4.17 and 4.18
> Times Newspapers Ltd., for the six letters collected in article 2.12

The sources of the portraits of Brewster and Wheatstone are given with the appropriate illustrations.

December 1982   Nicholas J. Wade
Newport-on-Tay

Contents

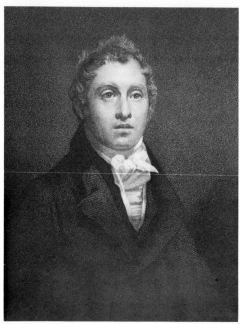

Brewster. An etching by W. Holl of a painting by Henry Raeburn (1815). Reproduced by kind permission of the University of St. Andrews.

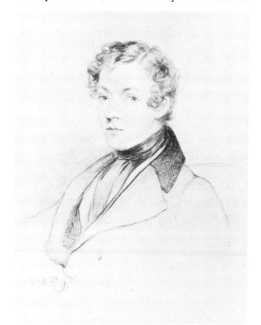

Wheatstone. A chalk drawing by William Brockendon (1837). Reproduced by permission of the National Portrait Gallery.

1. Brewster and Wheatstone

1.1. Introduction

Sir David Brewster (1781–1868) and Sir Charles Wheatstone (1802–1875) are recognized in visual science for their pioneering work on binocular vision. More specifically, they are known for their stereoscopes: Wheatstone devised his reflecting or mirror stereoscope in the early 1830s, and Brewster's refracting or lenticular stereoscope was made in 1849. These instruments have transformed not only our vision of pictures, but also our picture of vision. In Victorian Britain the stereoscope was considered "a piece of domestic apparatus without which no drawing-room is thought complete" (Pepper, 1869, p. 68). It also opened a completely novel area of endeavour for visual scientists – stereoscopic depth perception – and this has proved to be one of the most enduring topics of empirical and theoretical enquiry in vision.

Both Brewster and Wheatstone examined many other phenomena in vision. Neither natural philosopher, however, was primarily concerned with matters visual. Rather, each maintained the tradition of the British scientist as an enquirer into any natural phenomenon, the study of which could benefit from his insights. The phenomena that particularly interested Brewster were optical, whereas Wheatstone was attracted towards electricity. They were both skilful observers and to this they added the mechanical ingenuity that was the hallmark of their era. Thus, in the 1830s, while Wheatstone was conducting experiments with his stereoscope he was also measuring the velocity of electricity and devising the first practical electric telegraph. Brewster had constructed and named the kaleidoscope in 1816, long before the stereoscope was considered, and he was constantly producing improvements to optical instruments as diverse as jewel-lensed microscopes and lighthouse lenses.

It is not, however, in these areas that they are most widely remembered. Wheatstone is known to virtually every high school pupil for his bridge* – the

* Wheatstone (1843) called it "The Differential Resistance Measurer". He did not claim credit for its conception himself, but gave it to S. H. Christie. Posterity has proved less scrupulous than Wheatstone, and his name is now irresistably linked with the device (see Bowers, 1975).

means still employed for measuring the constants in an electric circuit. Brewster is linked eponymously with a more specialized principle in optics. Brewster's angle is the optimal angle of incidence for the polarization of light by reflection. This occurs when the reflected and refracted rays are at right angles, and for glass this is about 57°. Brewster's law states that the refractive index of the material is equal to the tangent of Brewster's angle. A brewster (B) is also a physical unit, used to measure the stress-optical constant when a material shows birefringence under an applied stress. A brewster is the number of angströms per mm path that one component of the light is retarded relative to the other if a stress of 1 bar (atmosphere) is applied. It is equivalent to 10^{-13} cm^2 dyne^{-1} (see Ballentyne and Lovett, 1970).

It is a measure of the men that, despite their preoccupations with physical phenomena, they should have made such major contributions to visual science. Indeed, Brewster and Wheatstone were among the small band of British scientists who consistently studied visual phenomena in the first half of the nineteenth century. The impact of their work has been most profound in the area of binocular vision, but neither commenced their visual enquiries on this topic. In both cases, their initial publications were concerned with subjective visual phenomena. Brewster studied accidental colours (complementary after-images), subjective colours, and the spatial distortions attendant upon viewing geometrical patterns. Wheatstone examined the duration of impressions of light (visual persistence), subjective colours, and the visibility of the retinal blood vessels. Thus, they were well versed in the study of perception when they directed their attention to binocular vision. Moreover, binocular vision was not to be isolated from the perception of space, and so we find that they addressed their observations using the stereoscope to the wider issues of space perception. It is because their work was so interrelated that their papers are presented together. Although they tackled a similar domain of topics, both in binocular vision and in subjective visual phenomena, their interpretations often differed markedly. Brewster sought to relate vision to the pattern of optical projection onto the retina, whereas Wheatstone adopted a more inferential stance. These differences in approach are clearly stated in their papers, and they nurtured in Brewster an antagonism towards Wheatstone that was expressed in a public dispute over the priority of invention of the stereoscope. This dispute was aired in the correspondence columns of *The Times*, in 1856. The letters (reprinted in Article 2.12) say much about the two men, and it will be noted that Brewster does not emerge in too favourable a light.

This book is not intended to be a pair of biographical studies. Rather, its purpose is to place before students of vision the experiments and insights of two pioneers in the field, expressed in their own words. None the less, a little needs to be said about the lives of Brewster and Wheatstone. The skeletons, so to speak, of their endeavours are given in the obituaries below (1.2).

Brewster was trained for the ministry, and he retained close connections with the Kirk throughout his life. From an early age he displayed an interest in astronomy, and he found the pursuit of science more suited to his temperament. As a consequence of making his own astronomical instruments he was led to study optics, starting with interference phenomena and progressing to polarization. He received international recognition for the work on polarization he conducted in the first two decades of the nineteenth century. On his various continental travels Brewster was able to compare the patronage accorded to science and scientists in different countries, and Britain did not fare well from such comparisons. He attributed this to the perniciousness of the Patent laws and the parsimony of the Government, and he sought to change both. In one area he was conspicuously successful. Together with Charles Babbage,* he was instrumental in founding the British Association for the Advancement of Science in 1831 (see Morell and Thackray, 1981). Brewster was knighted in 1832, in recognition for his services to science. Although he urged more financial support for institutionalized science he was not initially supported by it. Brewster's first academic post, at the age of 57, was as Principal of the United College of St. Salvador and St. Leonard at St. Andrews. Prior to that he had made a number of unsuccessful attempts at securing Chairs in Scottish Universities. Unlike many of his English colleagues, he did not have any private means of support and he was often financially insecure. He made his living with his pen – as an editor of scientific journals, as a contributor of reviews, and as an author. Throughout his life he was an active experimenter, but he never had access to a scientific laboratory. It seems likely that all his experimental research was conducted at his home.

Wheatstone, by contrast, was appointed to the Chair of Experimental Philosophy in King's College, London, at the age of 32. Prior to that he had worked in the family business of musical instrument manufacture. His interests in music and acoustics developed early, and during his life he invented a number of novel instruments, the most popular of which is the concertina. However, it was his detailed investigations of the acoustical figures, initially described by Chladni,† that gave him his introduction to a wider scientific audience. The representation of such figures visually, via an instrument of his invention called

---

* Charles Babbage (1792–1871) voiced his deep dissatisfaction over the government of science in his *Reflections on the Decline of Science in England, and on Some of its Causes* (1830). These views, though extremely controversial, were echoed by Brewster (1830) in his review of the book. The seed of the British Association was sown in Babbage's mind following his attendance at a meeting of the *Deutsche Naturforscher* in 1828. He conveyed his idea to Brewster, who used his extensive connections to foster its germination. Despite his attacks on the Government, Babbage received considerable support from it for the development of his calculating machines.

† Ernst Florens Friedrich Chladni (1756–1827) is considered the father of acoustics. By scattering fine sand evenly over a horizontal glass plate, clamped at one end, and then sounding it with a violin bow, he was able to produce symmetrical patterns where the sand gathered. The range of such patterns are called the Chladni figures. Wheatstone was also influenced by Chladni's books on sound.

the kaleidophone, stimulated his interest in vision, generally, and in visual persistence, specifically. He employed the instruments he devised to study visual persistence to good effect, because he used essentially the same techniques in the measurement of the velocity of electricity. All this was achieved before he became an academic, in 1834. His stereoscope was invented before that date, too, although there was a delay of some six years before the paper describing it was published. This delay was occasioned by his electrical diversions, both in terms of his velocity measurements and in the development of the electric telegraph. It was with regard to the latter that Wheatstone's impact on nineteenth-century Britain was most deeply felt. The development of the practical electric telegraph was achieved in partnership with William Cooke,* and both were eventually knighted for this.

These sketches provide the merest outlines of the lives of Brewster and Wheatstone. More detailed considerations of their contributions to vision will be given in the introductions to the following chapters, and also in the final chapter. An excellent biography of Wheatstone is available (Bowers, 1975). Moreover, Wheatstone's scientific papers were collected and published shortly after his death (see Wheatstone, 1879). Had these been complete the need for the present collection would have been reduced. However, three of Wheatstone's papers on vision are not included in the collection, and *The Times* correspondence with Brewster is not given. No adequate account of Brewster's life has been written. The most complete record is by his daughter, Mrs Gordon (1869, 1870), and this is concerned more with domestic than scientific events.

The collection starts with the obituaries of Brewster and Wheatstone, taken from the *Proceedings of the Royal Society*, of which they were both Fellows. Brewster's was written by J. H. Gladstone and Wheatstone's probably by C. Brooks.

1.2. Obituaries

1.2.1. Brewster: *Proceedings of the Royal Society*, 1868–69, **17**, xix–xxiv.

On the 11th of December, 1781, at Jedburgh, was born David Brewster, who, having made a telescope when only 10 years of age, and having entered on his university course at 12, devoted one of the longest of lives to discoveries in optics, and at last, laden with academic and scientific honours, sank peacefully to rest on the 10th February, 1868.

---

* William Fothergill Cooke (1806–1879) was Wheatstone's partner and business associate from 1837, when the first of the patents was taken out in their joint names. Cooke did not only administer the installation of the new telegraphs, but also took part in their development. Precisely how great a part was the cause of later dispute between him and Wheatstone (see Bowers, 1975).

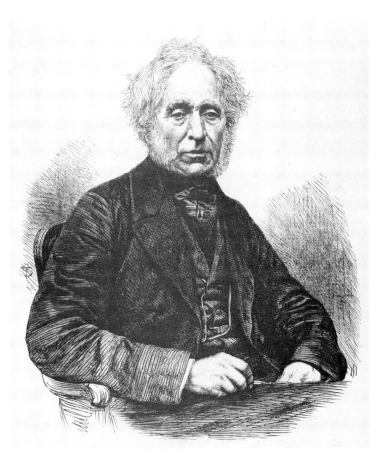

Brewster. An engraving from a photograph by Antoine Claudet, printed in *The Illustrated London News* (1868, 52, p. 189) to mark Brewster's death. Reproduced by permission of *The Illustrated London News Picture Library*.

He was one of four brothers, all educated for the Church of Scotland, and he advanced to the position of a licentiate; but a certain nervousness in speaking and delicacy of health, combined with an overpowering love for scientific pursuits, led him to decline a good presentation, and to abandon the clerical profession for that of an expounder of natural philosophy. Thus he entered on a career of investigation and literary work which for magnitude, as well as importance, has rarely been rivalled.

As an editor, he commenced in 1808 a work so large that it occupied him for twenty-two years – the Edinburgh Encyclopaedia; and in the mean time he began with Professor Jameson the Edinburgh Philosophical Journal, and subsequently the Edinburgh Journal of Science; and from 1832 he was one of the editors of the Philosophical Magazine. Throughout his connexion with these periodicals he was a frequent contributor of original articles to their pages, and he continued to the last to write for the North British and other Reviews in a style so polished and so vigorous, that multitudes learnt from him the actual state of scientific questions who would never have read a merely learned dissertation.

But his fame rests not so much on this literary work as on his original researches, which were so numerous that the 'Catalogue of Scientific Papers' now being published by the Royal Society contains the titles of 299 papers by him, besides five in which his name is conjoined with those of other investigators. And these researches, though principally connected with the phenomena of light, spread over many other departments of human knowledge.

Nor were Brewster's labours for the advancement of science confined to the laboratory and the desk. In 1821 he founded the Scottish Society of Arts, and in 1831 he was one of the small party of friends who instituted the British Association, in the meetings of which he usually took a prominent part.

During this time honours steadily flowed in upon him. He was made an honorary M.A. of Edinburgh in 1800, and seven years afterwards an honorary LL.D. of Aberdeen. From 1838 to 1859 he was Principal of the United Colleges of St. Salvador and St. Leonard's at the University of St. Andrews; and for the last eight years of his life he held the same important office in the leading University of Scotland.

Having been chosen a Fellow of the Royal Society of Edinburgh in 1808, Sir David acted for a long time as its Secretary, and he was President at the time of his death. In 1815 he obtained both the Copley Medal and the Fellowship of our Society; and this was followed three years afterwards by the Rumford Medal, and subsequently by one of the Royal Medals; and, singularly enough, in each case for discoveries concerning the Polarization of Light. In 1816 the French Institute awarded him a pecuniary prize, and nine years afterwards he became a Corresponding Member of that body; while in 1849 there was conferred upon him the distinguished honour of being chosen one of the eight Foreign Associates of the Academy of Sciences.

It would be tedious to enumerate his other honours from learned bodies at home and abroad; suffice it to add that he was made a Chevalier of the Prussian Order of Merit, and was knighted by his sovereign in 1832.

Sir David was twice married: first to the daughter of James Macpherson, M.P., of Belleville, the translator of Ossian, and afterwards to Jane Kirk, second daughter of the late Thomas Purnell, Esq., of Scarborough.

To give any adequate idea of the discoveries made known in those scientific papers which Sir David Brewster published every two or three months for sixty years, would be a task of gigantic magnitude. There seem to be thirty papers by him in our Transactions, principally in the earlier part of his career, and, with two exceptions, they are all on optical subjects. In 1813 he commenced with a communication "On some Properties of Light," and in the two succeeding years our Society published for him no less than nine papers – on the polarization of light by oblique transmission, by its passage through unannealed glass, by simple pressure, or by reflection, and on the optical properties of mother-o'-pearl, on calcareous spar. The phenomena of double refraction were indeed treated of in several subsequent papers; but there is a gap between 1819 and 1829, when he wrote on the periodical colours produced by grooved surfaces, investigated elliptic polarization by metals, and reverted to the optical nature of the crystalline lens. Two papers, one on the Diamond and the other on the Colours of Thin Plates, terminate this series in 1841; and the only paper he afterwards sent to our Transactions was one in conjunction with Dr. Gladstone on the Lines of the Solar Spectrum. But there seems never to have been any long intermission in his researches on light; for he was constantly sending communications on this subject to the Royal Society of Edinburgh or some other learned body, or to the various scientific serials with which he was connected. Thus in the first Number of the Edinburgh Philosophical Journal we find two papers from his pen, the first on new optical and mineralogical structure exhibited in certain specimens of Apophyllite and other minerals, the second on the Phosphorescence of Minerals.

It was as a laborious observer and ingenious experimenter that he excelled; he cared rather to collect a multitude of facts than to deduce from them general laws. Wonderful proofs of perseverance are his Tables of refractive indices, of dispersive powers, and of the polarizing angles of various reflecting bodies; and he seems to have submitted to optical examination every mineral that came in his way. Frequently one of these substances would form the subject of a monograph, as diamond, or amber, the double cyanide of platinum and magnesium, the felspar of Labrador with its changeable tints, or Glauberite with its one axis of double refraction for the violet, and two axes for the red ray. The prismatic spectrum arrested his attention, and in 1834 he announced the absorption of certain rays by the earth's atmosphere, and by nitrous gas; while eight years afterwards he pointed out the existence of luminous lines in certain flames corresponding to those defective in the light of the sun; but he missed the beautiful explanation of Kirchhoff. He also investigated the phenomena of diffraction and dichroism, and of late years exhibited to the British Association the tints of a soap-bubble, or of decomposing glass rendered still more lively by being viewed through a microscope. Indeed his last legacy to science was a paper on Film forms.

The best monument to his fame is perhaps his investigation of polarized light. Malus had first set foot on this domain, but his premature death left it open to the entrance of Brewster, and what wonderful regions did he explore! It not unfrequently happened that some other philosopher, with perhaps a profounder knowledge of mathematics, stepped in and deduced important laws; but sometimes he himself arrived at the higher generalizations; as, for instance, may be cited that of the refractive index of a substance being the tangent of its polarizing angle. But he was not always fortunate in his theories; thus his ingenious views of solar light, as composed of three primary colours (red, yellow, and blue) forming coincident spectra of equal length, has been shown to be completely fallacious. Yet he never abandoned his theory; a fact which we are disposed to attribute, not to a want of conscientious truthfulness, but rather to an inability to appreciate the real bearing of an argument, and to an over confidence in his own memory and the testimony of his senses.

During his optical investigations Sir David often turned from the phenomena seen to the organ of sight, and experimented on that wonderful eye which saw bands in the red rays less refrangible than Fraunhofer's A. Of late years especially he examined the functions of the retina, the *foramen centrale*, and the choroid coat of the eye of animals; he wrote several papers on the *muscae volitantes*, and explained many peculiarities of single and binocular vision, and not a few optical illusions.

While pursuing these researches on light, he made frequent excursions into other regions of science; he discovered fluids in the cavities of some of the minerals he was examining, and these must be investigated; he wrote much on the mean temperature of the globe; his attention was attracted at one time to fossil bones from Ava, at another to the varnish-trees of India; while systems of double stars, and the pyro-electricity of minerals shared the notice of his comprehensive mind.

As an inventor of new apparatus Brewster also acquired no little renown. His first paper on this subject appears to have been "Some remarks on Achromatic Eyepieces" in Nicholson's Journal for 1806; and seven years afterwards he published a separate "Treatise on new Philosophical Instruments for various purposes in the Arts and Sciences." In 1816, while repeating some experiments of Biot with a glass trough, he noticed that peculiar method of reflection which is the principle of the Kaleidoscope; and no sooner was this pretty instrument before the public than it became marvellously popular, and that not only as a toy for old and young, but large expectations were raised of its usefulness to the artist and designer of patterns. We are also indebted to him for many other ingenious contrivances for micrometers, burning-glasses, &c., and his writings frequently contained the germs of future inventions. Hence it is not easy to determine his precise share of merit in such appliances as the lenticular stereoscope, or the polyzonal lenses used in lighthouses. In regard to the latter, however, it may be safely maintained that while the chief credit of elaborating the dioptric system of illumination must be given to Fresnel, the persistent advocacy of Brewster materially contributed to its adoption on the shores of our own island.

In addition to the treatises already mentioned he wrote several distinct works of a biographical character: – the Memoirs of Sir Isaac Newton, Euler's Letters and Life, and the Martyrs of Science, viz. Galileo, Tycho Brahe, and Kepler. Nor must be omitted his letters on Natural Magic, and his 'More Worlds than One, the Creed of the Philosopher, and the Hope of the Christian.'

Sir David's anonymous writings were nearly as numerous as those to which his name was attached, and they spread over a wider range of subjects. The elaborate treatises on Optics in the Edinburgh Encyclopaedia and in the recent editions of the Encyclopaedia Britannica are both from his pen, and to each he contributed the articles on Hydrodynamics and Electricity. In the older work he also wrote on Astronomy, Mechanics, Microscopy, and Burning instruments, while in the later work he turned his attention among other subjects to that of photography.

To the Edinburgh Review he contributed twenty-eight articles, which are comprised between the Nos. LVII. and LXXXI. They include biographical notices of such men as Davy and Watt; reviews of such philosophical works as Whewell's 'History and Philosophy of the Inductive Sciences,' Mrs. Somerville's 'Connexion of the Physical Sciences,' Lord Brougham's 'Discourse on the Study of Natural Philosophy,' and even Compte's 'Philosophie Positive:' they pass from Buckland's Geology or Daguerre's photogenic drawings to the lighter subjects of deer-stalking or salmon-fishing; they follow Sir James Ross or Sir George Back in their arctic researches, and describe the British lighthouse system or the phenomena of thunder-storms.

To the Quarterly Review he seems to have contributed five articles, and in them he gives his estimate of works by Babbage, Herschel, and Abercrombie; while the subjects he treats are as wide apart as the production of sound, and the analysis of the intellectual powers, the supposed decline of science in England, and the philosophy of apparitions.

'Meliora' and the Foreign Review each contain two articles from his pen; one in the latter being a notice of Dutrochet's 'Observations sur Endosmose et Exosmose.'

But it was in the North British Review that the longest series of articles appeared. We have a list before us of seventy-six in the first thirty-nine parts of that quarterly serial, and we doubt whether the enumeration is complete. This shows that, on an average, Sir David wrote two of these literary productions for each part, and suggests the idea that he must have reviewed every book of note that he read. The first Number of the North British commences with an article by him, on Fluorens's 'Eloge Historique de Cuvier:' and further on in the same part he discusses the 'Lettres Provinciales' and other writings of Blaise Pascal. In the second Number he describes the Earl of Rosse's great reflecting telescope; and shortly we find him engaged with such serious works as Humboldt's 'Cosmos' or Murchison's 'Siluria:' the rival claimants for the honour of having discovered Neptune divide his attention with Macaulay's 'History of England,' or the 'Vestiges of the Natural History of Creation.' With Layard he takes his readers to Nineveh, with Lyell he visits North America, and with Richardson he searches the Polar seas. The Exhibition of 1851, the Peace Congress, and the British Association, come in turn under his descriptive notice; or turning from large assemblies to individual philosophers, he sketches Arago, Young, or Dalton. In one Number we have "The Weather and its Prognostics," and "The Microscope and its Revelations:" elsewhere he describes the Atlantic telegraph, whilst in a single article he groups together "the life-boat, the lightning-conductor, and the light-house." He reviews in turn Mary Somerville's 'Physical Geography,' and Keith Johnston's 'Physical Atlas;' the History of Photography engages him at one time, and at another Weld's History of our Society. Under the guidance of Sir Henry Holland he investigates the curious mental phenomena of mesmerism and electro-biology, and under that of George Wilson he inquires into colour-blindness. He criticises Goethe's scientific works, expounds De la Rive's 'Treatise on Electricity,' and Arago's on Comets; or turning from these severer studies, he allows Humboldt to exhibit the 'Aspects of Nature' in different lands to the multifarious readers of the Review.

In addition to all this Sir David issued some pamphlets of a personal nature – controversial writings which some objected to as unnecessarily persistent, though it should be recorded to his honour that he was ready to profit by friendly remonstrance.

Few of his living companions will remember this Nestor in science otherwise than as a venerable form full of vivacity and intelligence, keenly alive not to physical questions alone, but to the various social, political, and ecclesiastical interests of his time, and giving frequent indications of that humble faith in God which was the foundation of his character, and which brightened his declining years and the closing scenes of his earthly life. His many personal friends will retain his memory in their warm affection. Posterity will know him mainly for having opened up new regions in our knowledge of optical phenomena, and for having given a mighty impulse to science during two-thirds of the nineteenth century.

J. H. G.

1.2.2. Wheatstone: *Proceedings of the Royal Society*, 1875–76, **24**, xvi–xxvii.

Charles Wheatstone was born in February 1802, in the vicinity of Gloucester, and was educated at a private school in his native city, at which he evinced his predilection for Mathematics and Physics. In 1823, at the age of 21, we find him, in conjunction with his brother, long since deceased, engaged in the manufacture and sale of musical instruments in London. But his genius was not long in finding opportunities of development; for in the same year he made his first contribution to science in a paper published in Thomson's 'Annals of Philosophy,' entitled "New experiments on Sound," containing the results of his earlier experiments on the vibrations of chords, rods, and surfaces, which excited so much attention among physicists, that it was reproduced the same year in the 'Annales de Chimie,' and in the following year in 'Schweigger's Jahrbuch.' His next papers, also on Acoustics, were published in the 'Quarterly Journal of Science,' on "New experiments on Audition," in 1827, and on "the Kaleidophone," in the following year. This elegant philosophical toy consists of a steel wire fixed vertically in a heavy base, or in a vice, and surmounted by a silvered glass bead. If this, by an appropriate displacement, be thrown into a compound vibration, consisting of the simple vibration of its entire length accompanied by that of the first harmonic subdivision, a series of beautiful circular or elliptic epicycloidal curves are revealed by the persistence on the retina of the reflection of a fixed light from the glass bead; and if a rectangular wire be employed, the dimensions of which are such that its periods of vibration in two planes at right angles to each other are in the simple harmonic ratios of $1:2$, $2:3$, or $3:4$, the curves formed respectively by the superposition of these two modes of vibration will be beautifully exhibited. Subsequently, by an aptly contrived mechanism, Wheatstone succeeded in obtaining a visual combination of rectangular vibrations in any given ratio to each other. The principle of the kaleidophone was subsequently applied in the construction of a photometer. In this instrument a silvered bead is made to describe rapidly a narrow ellipse, or to oscillate in a straight line by means of an epicyclic train of the simplest construction; the relative brightness of two lines, formed by the reflections of two lights to be compared, may be very readily estimated.

At this period of his life Acoustics (doubtless in relation to his business) engrossed the chief part of Wheatstone's attention. He was especially interested in the application of the free reed to musical instruments; and the elegant little Symphonion, which, from the many objections to the needless employment of the breath, soon gave place to the bellows of the Accordion, offered ample evidence of the success of his labours in this direction. In the construction of these instruments, the admirable mode of fingering, in which the successive notes are

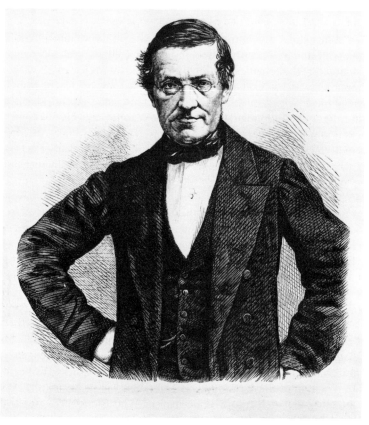

Wheatstone. An engraving from a photograph by Hills and Saunders, printed in the same volume of *The Illustrated London News* (1868, 52, p. 145) to mark Wheatstone's knighthood. Reproduced by permission of *The Illustrated London News Picture Library*.

placed in double rows alternately on opposite sides of the instrument, so that consecutive notes on either side, which may be touched by the same finger, always belong to the same chord, must not remain unnoticed.

In 1828 Wheatstone wrote on the resonance of columns of air, and in 1831 on the transmission of musical sounds through rigid linear conductors, a subject which was subsequently well illustrated at the Polytechnic Institution by the transference to an upper room of music played in the basement. In the same year he contributed to the British Association an experimental proof of Bernouilli's theory of the vibrations of air in wind instruments. His principal contribution to Acoustics is a memoir on the so-called Chladni's figures, produced by strewing sand on elastic planes, and throwing them into vibration by means of a violin-bow drawn across the edge; this was presented to the Royal Society in 1833, and subsequently published in their Transactions, and is probably the most remarkable of his early scientific labours; for he showed that, in square or rectangular plates, every figure however complicated was the resultant of two or more sets of isochronous parallel vibrations; and by means of some simple geometrical relations he carried out the principle of the "superposition of small motions" without the aid of any profound mathematical analysis, and succeeded in predicting the curves that given modes of vibration should produce.

In 1834 Wheatstone was appointed to the chair of Experimental Physics at King's College, London. In fulfilment of the duties of his office he delivered a course of eight lectures on Sound in the early part of the following year; but his habitual though unreasonable distrust of his own powers of utterance proved to be an invincible obstacle, and he soon afterwards discontinued his lectures, but retained the professorship for many years. Although any one would be charmed by his able and lucid exposition of any scientific fact or principle *in private*, yet his attempt to repeat the same process *in public* invariably proved unsatisfactory. An anecdote may here be mentioned in confirmation of this his peculiar idiosyncracy. Wheatstone and the writer of this memoir were for several years members of a small private debating society, comprising several familiar names in science, art, or literature, that met periodically at one another's houses to discuss some extemporized subject, and every member present was expected to speak: Wheatstone could never be induced to open his lips, even on subjects on which he was brimful of information. Several of his more important investigations were for the same reasons from time to time brought before the public by Faraday in the theatre of the Royal Institution.

In 1835 Wheatstone communicated to the British Association a paper "On the Attempts which have been made to imitate Human Speech by Mechanical Means;" and he produced a much improved edition of De Kempelen's speaking-machine; but his researches in this direction were not long continued, and have since been far surpassed by others.

The analogies of vibratory motion led the philosophic mind of Wheatstone from the subject of sound to that of light. In 1838 he communicated to the Royal Society an account of some remarkable and hitherto unobserved phenomena of binocular vision, with a description of the reflecting stereoscope, an instrument by which these phenomena were first illustrated. The conception that the idea of solidity is derived from the mental combination of two pictures of the same object in dissimilar perspective, as seen by the two eyes respectively, is undoubtedly and solely due to Wheatstone. In demonstration of this principle he drew two outlines of the same geometrical figure or other object, just as they would be seen in perspective by either eye respectively; and these outlines were so placed that they might be seen each by one eye, but visually superposed, either by reflection or by refraction; this he effected by a combination of lenses either with plane reflectors or with prisms. All that is really due to Brewster in relation to the stereoscope is the use of wedgeshaped segments of larger lenses, in which the lens and prism of Wheatstone are combined; the construction now universally adopted, and popularized by the application of photography.

In 1852 Wheatstone presented a second memoir on Binocular Vision to the Royal Society, in which he produced a striking confirmation of his former views by the invention of the Pseudoscope, an instrument in which the perspective pictures of a given object as seen by the two eyes respectively are reversed by internal reflection from the bases of two right-angled prisms, and convex objects appear to be concave, or *vice versâ*; thus a globe on which figures are traced will appear to be concave, and the inside of a painted basin or saucer to be convex, or the object as it were turned inside out.

The use of this instrument has produced some curious illustrations of mental phenomena: with most persons an object, of which the convexity or concavity is unknown, will at once appear inverted; but when the real form is known, with some persons experience appears to overrule visual perception, and they cannot succeed in seeing the inversion of the object; with others the appearance derived from previous knowledge persists for a shorter or longer period, and then suddenly gives way to the visual impression, and the object appears to be suddenly turned inside out; while with others, again, the change is more or less gradual, and during the period of transition the visual impression is uncertain and indistinct. In this memoir the idea of the mental character of binocular vision was still further supported by experimental evidence that the *apparent* magnitude of objects is governed by the relative position as well as the size of the visual pictures. In fact the whole of these investigations may be viewed in their relation to mental conditions; and when thus regarded, they possessed a higher interest than that which arose from their great value as contributions to physiological optics.

At one period, indeed, Wheatstone's attention was for a time directed to problems of mental philosophy, and especially to the *quasi*-mechanical solution of some of them, which was hoped for by the followers of Gall and Spurzheim; he was an active member of the London Phrenological Society, then presided over by Dr. Elliotson; and in January 1832 he read at one of the meetings a paper on Dreaming and Somnambulism, which was published *in extenso* in the 'Lancet' of that date. This paper is remarkable, like all his writings, for the extreme clearness with which known facts are stated, and the deductions based upon them.

Amongst Wheatstone's many ingenious inventions may be mentioned his automatic apparatus for recording periodically the height of the barometer, and the temperatures of the dry- and wet-bulb thermometers, by means of wires descending vertically in the open tubes, a circuit closed by the contact of the wire with either column of mercury indicating by electro-magnetic action the moment at which the contact takes place, and by inference the position of the point of contact. Precisely the same principle, with minor modifications, has of late years been practically applied by Padre Secchi, and more recently by M. van Rysselberghe.

Another is the electro-magnetic counter, by which the number of any given repeated mechanical actions is readily and certainly recorded; and the electric chronoscope, by which very small intervals of time may be determined (as, for example, in estimating the velocity of projectiles), must also be mentioned.

Cryptography, or the art of writing in ciphers, is indebted to him for a compendious apparatus, by which the characters representing the successive letters of the written communication are periodically changed by the machine, so as to defy the ordinary well-known methods of deciphering. The receiver, possessing a machine set by agreement in the same manner as that of the sender, can immediately decipher the dispatch by reversing the process by which the cipher was constructed.

The fact, discovered by Brewster, that the plane of polarization of the sky is always 90° from the sun, gave rise to Wheatstone's "Polar Clock," which consists of a double-image prism and a thin plate of selenite enclosed in a tube placed parallel to the earth's axis. When the prism, which carries an index traversing a circular arc marked with the hours, is turned round until no colour is perceived, the index, when once adjusted, will mark the hour of the day; this is a pleasing philosophical toy, but of little practical utility.

The name of Wheatstone is intimately connected with the earliest development of spectrum-analysis. In a paper on "The Prismatic Analysis of Electric Light," read before the Meeting of the British Association at Dublin in 1835, he announced the existence of bright lines in the spectrum, emitted by the incandescent vapour of metals volatilized by the heat of an electric discharge. He was then the first to demonstrate the fact that the spectrum of the electric spark from different metals presented respectively more or less numerous rays of definite refrangibility, producing each a series of lines differing in position and colour from each other, and that thus the presence of a very minute portion of any given metal might be determined. "We have here," he adds, "a mode of discriminating metallic bodies more readily than that of chemical examination, and which may hereafter be employed for useful purposes." This remark has been abundantly verified by the many important recent investigations that have been based on spectrum-analysis – such, for example, as the discovery and isolation of thallium by Mr. Crookes.

It would occupy too much space to enumerate all Wheatstone's ingenious contrivances; but his most important contribution to the wants or conveniences of civilization, the *practical* electric telegraph, must now be considered. On this point it has been justly remarked by De la Rive* that "the philosopher who was the first to contribute by his labours, as ingenious as they were persevering, in giving to electric telegraphy the practical character that it now possesses, is undoubtedly Mr. Wheatstone." He has no more claim to the title of "inventor" of the electric telegraph than any one of those who have long preceded him in proposing unpractical schemes for transmitting signals to a distant station, first by frank-linic, and subsequently by voltaic electricity. The earliest of these appears to be Stephen Gray, who in 1727 suspended by silk threads a wire 700 feet long; and on applying an excited glass tube to one end of the wire electrification was observed by an assistant to occur at the other end. Similar experiments were made by Dufay a few years subsequently, and by Winckler of Leipsic, by Lemonnier of Paris in 1746, and by Dr. Watson, Bishop of Llandaff, in 1747, one of whose experiments had a remarkable (but then unnoticed) bearing on electro-telegraphy, namely, the employment of the earth to conduct the return current: he stretched a wire across the Thames, one end of which was attached to the exterior coating of a Leyden jar, while the interior coating was connected to earth through the body of the experimenter, and the other end was held by an assistant, who grasped an iron rod; the moment the latter dipped the rod in the river both felt a shock. He subsequently experimented on much longer circuits, one of which was 10,600 feet in length, suspended from wooden poles erected on Shooter's Hill. Franklin made similar experiments across the Schuykill at Philadelphia in 1748, and De Luc about the same time across the Lake of Geneva.

The earliest definite scheme for the employment of franklinic electricity for telegraphic purposes was propounded by "C. M.," an anonymous writer in the 'Scot's Magazine' for 1753; this required a separate insulated conductor for each letter; and a very similar idea was subsequently carried out at Geneva by Lesage in 1774. Lomond was the first to propose in 1787 the transmission of various signals through a single line-wire; this he effected by the varied movement of the pith balls of a delicate electroscope; and Cavallo in 1795 proposed to effect the same object by varied combinations of sparks and pauses. In 1816 Francis Ronalds proposed the hopeless scheme of employing two *perfectly isochronous* clocks to indicate continuously the same letters or numerals at the two stations,

* 'Treatise on Electricity,' pt. vii, ch. 1.

the signal intended being indicated by simultaneous sparks at both. This telegraph was offered to the Government by the inventor, who received an official reply from the then Secretary of the Admiralty, that "telegraphs of any kind are now wholly useless, and no other than the one now in use will be adopted" – a conspicuous example of the slow progress proverbially due to the inertia of great bodies.

The first proposal to employ voltaic electricity for telegraphic purposes appears to have been made by S. T. Sömmering, a surgeon, to the Academy of Sciences at Munich in 1808; this involved a separate insulated conductor for each letter and numeral, any two of which might be indicated by a small evolution of gas from two corresponding gold points immersed in a common fluid. A very similar system was suggested by Prof. Coxe of Philadelphia in 1810, who proposed to indicate the signals by the decomposition of some metallic salt. Prof. Schweigger of Erlangen proposed to reduce the number of conductors in Sömmering's telegraph to two, and to employ an electric pistol to call attention at the receiving station.

In relation to the dawn of practical electro-telegraphy, the names of Froment in France, of Gauss, Weber, and Steinheil in Germany, and of Morse in America, will immediately suggest themselves, but to Charles Wheatstone is undoubtedly due the merit of having been the first to render the electric telegraph practically available. In 1834, the year of his appointment to the Professorship, he devised an experiment which at once attracted the attention of scientific minds throughout Europe, and ultimately had a large influence in determining the direction of his future labours. His object was to ascertain the rate at which an electric wave travels through a metallic conductor. For this purpose about half a mile of copper wire was insulated by suspension in the vaults under King's College; and three interruptions of this circuit were made by three pairs of small brass knobs, with a small interval between them, placed in a horizontal line at a few inches distance from each other, one being near each end of the conductor, and the other one at its middle point. It was presumable that the positive and negative terminal sparks produced by the discharge of a Leyden jar through the insulated wire would be absolutely simultaneous, but if any perceptible time were occupied by the passage of the wave, the middle spark would occur *later* than the terminal ones. To determine this a small plane mirror mounted on an axis parallel to the line of sparks was made to revolve with great rapidity by a train of clockwork. If any sensible angle were described by the mirror during the passage of the wave, the middle spark would be seen either above or below the line joining the other two, according to the direction of rotation of the mirror. This in fact proved to be the case; and from the estimated amount of displacement and rate of rotation, the velocity of transmission was inferred to be over 250,000 miles in one second; but from the nature of the observation the limits of error are necessarily very wide. This experiment was subsequently repeated with an extended circuit of nearly four miles, which was further utilized in the transmission of electric signals by the deflections of a galvanometer-needle.

In 1836 Mr. W. F. Cooke having been struck, during a visit to Germany, by the applicability of an electric telegraph devised by Baron Schilling to practical and especially to railway purposes, brought back with him on his return to London a working model of Schilling's apparatus, to which he directed the attention of Faraday and of the then Secretary of the Royal Society, Dr. Roget, by whom he was informed that Wheatstone has been for some time engaged in analogous investigations. An introduction followed, and shortly afterwards Wheatstone entered into partnership with Mr. Cooke, and a patent for a five-needle telegraph (which from the number of insulated conductors was deemed too expensive for general use), and subsequently another patent for the two-needle telegraph, the first that came into general use, were taken out in their joint names.

To Mr. (now Sir W. F.) Cooke much credit is undoubtedly due for the tact and ability he evinced in directing public attention to the importance of the electric telegraph, and in conducting the joint enterprise to a most successful commercial issue; but to Wheatstone alone must be ascribed the inventive genius and fertility of scientific resource which led to the many successive developments of the electric telegraph – the letter-showing dial telegraph in 1840, the type-printing telegraph in 1841, the magneto-electric dial telegraph, a subsequent extension of the same to type-embossing, and lastly the automatic telegraph, by which messages are transmitted with such unprecedented rapidity. It must also be borne in mind that the idea of subaqueous telegraphy was first developed by Wheatstone. It appears from his manuscripts that in 1837 he devoted a good deal of time and attention to this subject; and in the Bulletin de l'Académie Royale de Bruxelles for October 7, 1840, in a notice by Prof. Quetelet of his telegraph instruments, it is remarked: – "On sera sans doute charmé d'apprendre que l'auteur a trouvé le moyen de transmettre les signaux entre l'Angleterre et la Belgique, malgré l'obstacle de la mer." But it appears that his first practical essays at submarine telegraphy were made in the autumn of 1844 in Swansea Bay, with the assistance of Mr. J. D. Llewellyn.

More recently the Society of Arts, in tendering precisely the same award for public services to the two former partners, failed to discriminate between very successful commercial tact and ability, and both inventive and constructive genius of an exceptionally high order; under these circumstances it is not surprising that Wheatstone should have declined the proffered distinction, considering that he could present no claim to that commercial merit which it must be, from its title, the special function of that Society to foster. But scientific honours were profusely bestowed on the great physicist; he was elected a Fellow of the Royal Society in 1836, a Chevalier of the Legion of Honour in 1855, and a foreign Associate of the Academy of Sciences of France in 1873; he moreover possessed thirty-four distinctions or diplomas conferred upon him by various governments, universities, and learned societies, of which eight are German, six French, five English, three Swiss, two Scotch, two Italian, two American, and of Irish, Belgian, Russian, Swedish, Dutch, and Brazilian each one. In 1868 the Government of Lord Derby conferred on him the honour of knighthood, an honour so variously bestowed that it can only be viewed as a bare recognition of scientific labours which have rarely been equalled in their extent, their variety, and their fruitfulness.

Charles Wheatstone was not less conspicuous for his sagacity in perceiving the practical bearings of ascertained scientific principles, than for his ingenuity in devising suitable mechanical means for their application to useful purposes. He was one of the first, if not the very first, in this country, to appreciate the importance of Ohm's beautiful and simple law of the relation between electro-motive force, resistance of conductors, and resulting current; he thence rightly inferred that in establishing electric intercommunication between two distant stations by means of the deflections of a galvanometer-needle, or the attraction of an iron keeper by an electromagnet, the coil of which is actuated by a current sent from the other station, the resistance of the coil must necessarily be small compared with that of the intervening conductor, and hence that a coil of much larger resistance than was at first contemplated might be beneficially employed: Ohm's law in fact affords the means of determining in any given circuit the quality of coil by which the largest amount of dynamic energy may be imparted to the moving mechanism.

Very early in his electrical researches Wheatstone perceived the necessity of some more accurate means of measuring resistances and the strength of currents than even the most sensitive tangent-galvanometer presented; it occurred to him that small differences between two currents might be much more accurately determined by sending them in *opposite directions* through the coil of a sensitive sine-galvanometer, the needle of which will then be affected only by their *difference*, than by estimating the small differences of displacement of the needle due to small differences in a single current. Accordingly he devised the well-known "Bridge," which has been, and must ever continue to be, the basis of all accurate quantitative determinations in electricity. In this instrument the two portions of a divided current are conducted in opposite directions through the galvanometer-coil and again reunited; and the resistance sought is interposed in one circuit, and "balanced" by known resistance interposed in the other circuit until the needle is brought to zero. The form of this instrument has varied considerably from that originally proposed, but the principle is precisely the same.

As necessary adjuncts to this instrument, Wheatstone proposed as a unit of resistance one foot in length of soft pure copper wire, weighing 100 grains, and constructed a series of "resistance-coils," each coil containing some decimal multiple of the proposed unit; he also devised the "rheostat," consisting of a fine wire wound in the thread of a screw cut on the surface of a cylinder of non-conducting material, any portion of which wire may be put into or taken out of the circuit by merely turning the cylinder on its axis by a handle. But several circumstances rendered Wheatstone's proposed unit unavailable, viz. the difficulty of maintaining uniformity in the size and quality of the wire, the variation of resistance produced by any molecular disturbance, such as change of temperature, stretching or bending, and the instability of resistance, even when the wire is protected from mechanical disturbance; and the British Association unit is now generally adopted.

Wheatstone was the first to appreciate the importance of reducing to a minimum the amount of work to be done by the current at the receiving station, by diminishing as far as practicable the mass and therefore the inertia of the moving parts; this was beautifully exemplified in that marvel of ingenuity the magneto-electric letter-showing telegraph, now generally adopted for private telegraphic communication, in which the wheel attached to the index is as delicate as the scape-wheel of a small Geneva watch. And there are one or two more points of construction in this admirable instrument which, as exemplars of the mind of the inventor, should not escape notice. Faraday had discovered that if a soft iron keeper furnished with armatures revolve in front of the poles of a permanent magnet, instantaneous currents in opposite directions are developed as the revolving keeper approaches to and recedes from the position of maximum induction; accordingly Wheatstone placed four fixed armatures coiled alternately in opposite directions in front of the poles of a small but powerful permanent magnet, and made the keeper alone to rotate in close proximity to the iron cores of the armatures; as therefore the extra currents induced by the keeper in *receding* from one and *approaching* the other pair of armatures coincide in direction and reinforce each other, four equal currents, alternately positive and negative, will be developed by each revolution of the iron keeper; and these, by causing a pair of magnetic needles, moving on an axis passing through their common centre of gravity, to oscillate between a pair of small electro-magnets, actuate the index of the receiving instrument.

Another peculiarly happy and simple contrivance in this apparatus must also be mentioned. The letters of the alphabet surround the transmitting-dial; and opposite each of these is a stud at the end of a radial lever, the depression of which closes a short circuit, which intercepts all currents when the index arrives at the corresponding letter, and the indicator of the receiving instrument consequently stops at the same letter, it having been first ascertained that they start in unison. It then became necessary that the depression of any other lever should raise the one previously depressed; and for this purpose some very complicated arrangements of interacting levers were first devised, but the plan adopted is remarkable for its simplicity: a circular endless chain lies in a groove beneath all the levers, in which there is just "slack" enough to allow of the depression of *one* lever; consequently the depression of any other pulls up the former, and opens the short circuit previously closed.

The catalogue of Wheatstone's valuable labours is still far from being exhausted; but it must now suffice only to mention some of his unpublished and incomplete researches, of which many exist, and will be, it is hoped, by some means made public. At the early part of his career, when his thoughts were mainly directed to Acoustics, he endeavoured to investigate the causes of the differences of "timbre" or *quality* of tone in different musical instruments, presuming it to depend on the nature of superposed secondary vibrations, and of the material by which they are affected. This the writer has frequently, but in vain, urged him to complete and publish; but such was the fecundity of his imagination that he would frequently work steadily for a time at a given subject, and then entirely put it aside in pursuit, it may be, of some more important or more practical idea that had presented itself to his mind. A short treatise is in existence on the capabilities of his well-known wave-machine, in which rows of white balls, mounted on rods, are actuated in two directions perpendicular to each other by guides or templets with suitable curved outlines; by means of this machine many combinations of plane and helical waves may be demonstrated, and especially those related to the theory of polarized light.

In furtherance of this subject he devised a new form or mode of geometrical analysis, to which he gave the title of Bifarial Algebra, in which both the magnitude and the relative position of lines on a plane surface are designed to be represented by the introduction of two new symbols to represent positive and negative perpendicular directions. The same principle has also been extended to three dimensions, with a further proposal of new symbols, under the name of Trifarial Algebra. On this subject a brief treatise exists in manuscript.

Amongst the subjects of his more recent but still incomplete investigations in Light and Electricity the following may be mentioned: –

Colours of transparent and opaque bodies.
Colours obtained by transmission and reflection.
Absorption-bands in coloured liquids.
Spectroscopic examination of light reflected from opaque and dichroic bodies.
Electromotive forces of various combinations.
Inductive capacities of various bodies.
Experiments on electro-capillarity.
Telegraph construction.
Construction of relays.

Such of these as may be found sufficiently advanced to be of any scientific value will probably be made public in a collective form.

Charles Wheatstone was married on the 12th of February, 1847, and had a family of five children, who survive him, Mrs. Wheatstone having deceased many years. He died in Paris on the 19th of October, 1875, whence his remains were removed to his residence in Park Crescent, and were followed to their last resting-place in the cemetery at Kensal Green by a numerous assemblage of attached friends, with some of whom he had maintained an uninterrupted intimacy from his early manhood, and by several leading members of the scientific world, who felt it due to his great merit to pay this last tribute of regard to his memory.

This memoir cannot be more suitably concluded than by the expressions of M. Dumas, perpetual Secretary of the French Academy of Sciences, uttered on the occasion of the removal of the remains from Paris: –

> To render to genius the homage which is its due, without regard to country or origin, is to honour one's self. The Paris Academy of Sciences, always sympathizing with English science, did not hesitate, during the troubled time of the wars of the Empire, to decree a 'grand prix' to Sir Humphry Davy. Now in a time of peace it comes to fulfil with grief a duty of affection to one of his noblest successors, by gathering round his coffin to offer him a last homage. A foreign Associate of the Academy of Sciences, exercising by a rare privilege in virtue of that title all the rights of its members during his life, we are bound to render to his mortal remains the same tribute which we render to fellow-countrymen who are our colleagues. The memory of Sir C. Wheatstone will live among us not only for his discoveries and for the methods of investigation with which he has endowed science, but also by the recollection of his rare qualities of heart, the uprightness of his character, and the agreeable charm of his personal demeanour. The friends that he has left among us, unable to avert destiny, hope that they were at least able to soothe the last hours of his life – of that life which, alas! was closed away from his beloved home, from that family circle the sweet recollection of which animated his last hours, and to which the eye of the dying one turned once more, before his soul, quitting its earthly tenement, took its flight to a better world.

1.3. Outline of Papers Selected

This collection of papers is concerned with one aspect of Brewster's and Wheatstone's work – that relating to vision. As is evident from the obituaries above, this was considered by their contemporaries to be but a small fragment of their lifes' work. It is, however, probably the most enduring aspect of their experimental enquiries. While their contributions to physics have an historical relevance, those to vision retain a contemporary significance in terms both of their observations and of their insights. It is also instructive for us to appreciate how much they achieved theoretically with recourse to relatively simple equipment. This appreciation can only be achieved by consulting the original sources, and it is convenient to have them available together.

The quantity of Wheatstone's writing was, relative to Brewster's, meagre, but

a stereos...
no... single instead.
...as not till a year after...
...it was exhibited in England. The th...
...Philosophical ir... ...iich M. Dub...
...told to recommend t... ...ne, and for...
...theoretical and... ...he placed a lens...
...concern, with a... ...ular Daguerreo...
...This instrument attracted the particular attention of...
...and before the closing of the Crystal Palace...
...executed beautiful stereoscope, which I pres...
...Majesty in... ...consequence of this...
...tion of the instrument, M... bu...q received...
...from England, and a large number of...
...introduced into... ...ountry. The dem...
...so great, that opticians of all kin...
to the manufacture of the instrument...
...ners, both in Daguerreo... and Talbota...
...most lucrative branch of their profession, to...
portraits of views to be thrown into rel...
scope. Its application to sculpture, whic...
out, was first made in France, and an artist in...
copied a statue from the *relie...* produced by the stere...

Three years after I had published a description of
lenticular stereoscope, and after it had been in general u...
in France and England, and the reflecting stereoscope forgotten,[1] Mr. Wheatstone printed, in the *Philosophical
Transactions* for 1852, a paper on Vision, in which he says

Brewster's face embedded in text from *The Stereoscope* (1856, p. 31).

...may pres...
...y be asked, that person...
...correct notions of solid objec...
...pictures? and how happen it...
...g the perfect use of th... ...areou...
...jects... ...ng of...
...an this... ...ust the...
...but althou... ...of two...
...res sugges... ...he may...
...there ap... ...the g...
...d, which, though... ambiguo... ...than...
...re less liable to... ...ad... ...n... ...e...
...ten... ...ue... ...a...
...tron... ...o...
...g, the... ...s a... ...th...
...th... ...c... ...e the...
...th... ...e optic... ...p... ...th...
...on... ...u... ...beyon...
...s... ...ep... ...in a single ey...
...re the res... ...even exactly similar, a...
...nates no difference whether two identical pictures...
...corresponding parts of the two retina, or whether...
...ye is impressed with only one... these pictures. A
person deprived of the sight of... s, therefore, all external objects, ne... ...on with both eyes
sees remote object... ...t effect arising from
the binocular vis... ...not perceived by the
former, to suppl... ...has recourse throug...

Wheatstone's face in text from his first memoir on binocular vision.

its quality and influence have far exceeded Brewster's. Wheatstone's writing style is an example of clarity. The same cannot be said of Brewster. Moreover, a number of careless errors have been found in Brewster's papers, and these have been corrected in the text.

To the best of my knowledge, all the papers by Wheatstone on vision are reprinted here. He did write some additional papers on optics – concerning the spectrum of electric light (1835) and on polarization (1848, 1871) – but these have not been included.

The sheer volume of Brewster's writing has necessitated some selectivity regarding the material reprinted. The selection was relatively easy where multiple copies of given articles had been published. It was not uncommon in the nineteenth century for articles published in one journal, or in the proceedings of some society, to be reprinted in another journal. Brewster took frequent advantage of this tradition in the journals he edited, particularly for his own work. In choosing between the duplicate reports I have tried to use the original, unless there was some addition to the later one. The selection was more difficult for some articles that were clearly concerned with vision, but were addressed to either a specific theory, like Plateau's theory of after-images (Brewster, 1839), or a specific observation, like Haidinger's brushes (Brewster, 1850). Furthermore, these were areas in which there is no counterpoint in Wheatstone's work. I decided to exclude Brewster's papers on the nature of light, particularly with regard to his theory of the triple spectrum (1831c, 1847, 1855b). None the less, these issues will be raised again in the final chapter. There remain many articles and abstracts by Brewster on vision that are not reprinted here. These tend to repeat or extend observations made in the papers selected, which I believe adequately reflect his views on vision.

In addition to his scientific papers, Brewster wrote a number of books, anonymous reviews, and encyclopaedia articles dealing in whole or part with visual phenomena. Amongst his books were *A Treatise on the Kaleidoscope* (1819, 1858), *A Treatise on Optics* (1831, 1853), *Letters on Natural Magic Addressed to Sir Walter Scott, Bart* (1832) and *The Stereoscope. Its History, Theory and Construction* (1856). Fortunately, most of the relevant material in these books can also be found in the articles reprinted here. The plethora of Brewster's papers and books has, I believe, operated against him: his contemporaries would have felt overwhelmed by the quantity and scope of his work, and now it has become relatively inaccessible to present-day students of vision.

The aim of this collection is more than to remedy this last mentioned state of affairs. The scientific study of visual perception proceeds at a more leisurely pace than in other branches of natural science. Brewster's and Wheatstone's observations and theories have more than historical significance, they have a contemporary relevance too. Close parallels can be found in the theoretical stances taken today and those expressed well over a century ago by Brewster and Wheatstone.

We have a similar division between theories based upon an analysis of the visual projection (as Brewster proposed) and those giving more weight to inferential or cognitive processes (as Wheatstone argued). Hence, their theories have been rephrased rather than replaced. This is a statement of my belief. It is left to the readers to determine its validity, and the articles here reprinted will allow them to do so.

The papers are grouped into three chapters – on binocular vision and space perception, on inventions relating to vision, and on subjective visual phenomena. Within each chapter the papers are presented chronologically, irrespective of the author. It is hoped that this arrangement will assist the reader both in assessing the influence of one writer on the other and in charting the development in their ideas.

Each chapter commences with an introduction in which the salient features of the papers are summarized, and additional background information is given. The final chapter provides an assessment of the contributions of and conflicts between Brewster and Wheatstone.

The references cited in the individual papers and in the introductory sections are given in the Bibliography rather than following each paper, because the same sources are cited many times. Wherever possible I have given the full references cited by Brewster and Wheatstone, but in some cases insufficient evidence is provided in the text to trace the source. The figures are placed near the text to which they apply rather than in accompanying plates, as was the practice for a number of the original articles.

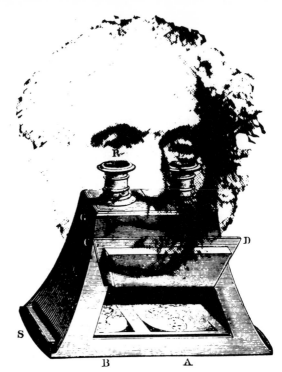

Brewster and his lenticular stereoscope.

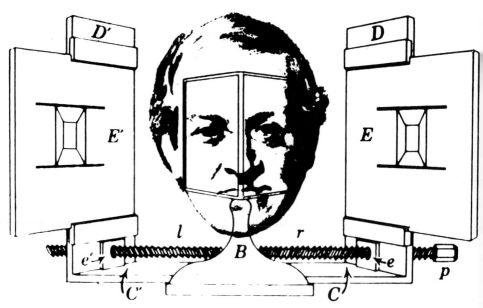

Wheatstone and his mirror stereoscope.

2. Binocular Vision and Space Perception

2.1. Introduction

Of the fourteen articles in this chapter, one will be better known than all the others – Wheatstone's description of the reflecting stereoscope (2.4). Despite the frequency with which it is cited, few writers go beyond the instrument, the stereoscope, to consider the use Wheatstone made of it – that is, to examine the theoretical views he proposed on the basis of his experiments with the stereoscope. Wheatstone's interpretation was that of an empiricist, with explicit appeal to the notion of unconscious inference, long before this was espoused by Helmholtz (1866, 1924, 1925). Indeed, Helmholtz's theories of perception owed much to Wheatstone, as Helmholtz himself readily acknowledged. Of the many articles describing some new contrivance to assist in the study of perception few can have had such an influence as the stereoscope. None are likely to have been used so extensively and with such ingenuity in the original publication: "Part the first" of Wheatstone's memoir was published in 1838 and this was followed, some fourteen years later, by "Part the second". Taken together, these two papers address almost all the major issues in binocular vision, in addition to some central themes in space perception.

Brewster's work in this area has been concerned primarily with space perception, and his stereoscopic observations are moulded into the same framework. The central concept employed in the analysis of space perception was visible direction, and this was elevated to the status of a law. Brewster defined the law in the article on optics in the *Edinburgh Encyclopaedia*: ". . . we know nothing more than that the mind, residing, as it were, in every point on the retina, refers the impression made upon it at each point to a direction coinciding with the last portion of the ray which conveys the impression" (1830b, p. 615). This definition also illuminates another fundamental belief of Brewster's – that the "seat of vision" resided in the retina. Accordingly, we find that his interpretations of visual phenomena were referred consistently to the analysis of the retinal projection and visible direction. In modern parlance, Brewster's visible direction would be referred to as oculocentric direction; that is, the specification of direction with respect to the centre of the eye rather than the head (see Howard, 1982).

It is not surprising, therefore, that in the first article reprinted (2.2) Brewster launched a vitriolic attack on his fellow countryman, Charles Bell,* for suggesting that visible direction was not determined solely by the projection onto the retina. Bell (1823) observed that an after-image appeared to move when the eye was moved voluntarily, but remained stationary during passive displacements of the eye. From these observations Bell gave a description of what would now be termed "outflow" theory (see Wade, 1978a). Brewster did not deny the phenomenon that was so damaging to his conception of visible direction, rather he presented additional observations that were considered difficult for Bell to encompass within his theory. Brewster was probably incensed by the manner in which Bell referred to his work: Bell stated: "These experiments and this explanation of the effect of the associated action of the voluntary muscles of the eye-ball, appear to remove an obscurity in which this subject has been left by the latest writers" (1823, p. 180). There followed Brewster's definition of visible direction, given above, without citing its source. Such was Brewster's antagonism that he returned to the issue in an anonymous report in his *Edinburgh Journal of Science* (1826b). Here there is reference "to the optical and physiological phantasies of Mr. Charles Bell". In addition to repeating the points raised in Article 2.2, Brewster drew attention to the similar experiments conducted by Dr. Wells,† in the previous century. Wells (1792) had conducted some ingenious experiments with binocular after-images. For example, he projected binocular after-images onto a piece of paper and then moved one eye with his finger: the edges of the paper appeared double, but the after-image remained single. In order to exclude the possibility that the passively moved eye suppressed its after-image he repeated the experiment, but with an after-image in only one eye, and obtained the same result. Brewster used these experiments to belittle Bell.

* Charles Bell (1774–1842) wrote, with his surgeon brother John, a textbook *The Anatomy of the Human Body* (1803) in which a considerable portion of the third volume (written by Charles) was addressed to vision. Essentially, Bell summarized the state of knowledge of visual phenomena and physiology at the beginning of the century. In 1811 he published, privately, his *Idea of a New Anatomy of the Brain*, which described the separate functions of the dorsal and ventral spinal nerve roots, as well as the principle of specific sensory nerve energies. Bell's religious convictions were close to Brewster's, and Bell wrote one of the celebrated Bridgewater Treatises *On the Power, Wisdom, and Goodness of God, as manifested in the Creation*. Bell's contribution was on *The Hand, Its Mechanism and Vital Endowments, as evincing Design* (1834). Two other associates of Brewster and Wheatstone – Whewell and Roget – also contributed to the eight Treatises. Babbage wrote an irreverent and unrequested ninth Treatise! Bell was knighted, along with Brewster, in 1832.

† William Charles Wells (1757–1817) was born in America of Scottish parents, and received his education in Scotland. Most of his medical career was spent in London. He was attracted to problems of visible direction with two eyes, and devised some novel demonstrations of singleness of vision. These were embodied in three propositions that were rediscovered nearly a century later by Hering (see Ono, 1981). Wells also provided the appropriate theory for the formation of dew, and anticipated Darwin in proposing a theory of evolution by natural selection.

Brewster attempted to account for the observations by arguing that the passive motions of the eye were translations rather than rotations, and that the former were small in comparison to the rotations that normally occur. If this was indeed the case, Wells's binocular after-images should have moved as much as the pages upon which they were projected, but he did not report any such shift. The acrimonious attack on Bell, and indirectly on Wells, reflected the significance of the "law" of visible direction to Brewster, and his defense of this concept was a constant theme of his work on vision.

In the second, anonymous, article (2.3) Brewster addressed a problem of recurrent interest to him – that of reversals in depth of depressed or elevated forms. He interpreted the phenomenon in terms of the learned directions of light sources and shadows, and discussed the influence that information from other senses, like touch, can have on dispelling illusory impressions of depth. It is noteworthy that the final paragraph of the article drew attention to the protuberant appearance of a hollow mask of a human face. This demonstration has a remarkably contemporary ring to it (see Gregory, 1981b).

Wheatstone also discussed the conversion of relief in his memoir on the stereoscope (2.4, § 11), but he differed from Brewster in his interpretation: the monocular projection of an evenly illuminated cameo corresponds to that of an intaglio, and the ambiguity could result in reversals of relief (see Day and Power (1965) for a modern application of the same principle to depth reversals during rotation). Wheatstone noted that a skeleton cube reversed in depth very readily when viewed with one eye. The reversals of an outline rhomboid, of the type described by Louis Necker (1832), are discussed in section 10 of the article. Perhaps we should cite the Wheatstone cube and the Necker rhomboid when referring to the familiar oscillating forms!

The "hitherto unobserved phenomena" with which the article is concerned are, of course, stereoscopic. Wheatstone commenced by describing the differences in the projections of three-dimensional objects to each eye. He then considered the perceptual consequences of presenting two flat projections, one to each eye. Such combination could not readily be achieved: he described the means available for binocular superimposition like varying convergence, but found them all wanting. To overcome these difficulties a new instrument, the stereoscope, was described and illustrated as were a variety of paired outline drawings. Outlines were employed in order to exclude, as far as possible, any monocular cues to depth (cf. Julesz, 1971). The combination of dissimilar pictures in the stereoscope led to the remarkable impression of relief, which could itself be reversed by transposing the left and right pictures.

These observations were taken as evidence that the singleness of vision can follow from the stimulation of non-corresponding retinal points. The converse was also shown to be the case – the stimulation of corresponding points can result in double vision. Images of different retinal magnitude could be combined, as long as the difference was not too great, but radically different forms did not combine – they alternated in visibility. The combination of dissimilar pictures to be seen singly and in relief posed problems for the extant views of visible direction, like Brewster's, and of the horopter, as Wheatstone discussed in section 15 of his article. In the same section Wheatstone made reference to Wells's (1792) much neglected essay on single vision, in which what are generally called "Hering's principles of visual direction" were clearly formulated (see Ono, 1981).

The final section of the article contains Wheatstone's disclaimer concerning any complete explanation of the means whereby dissimilar pictures can be perceived as objects in relief. Perhaps it is this statement that has led some to consider his approach as atheoretical. What Wheatstone did in fact provide were the empirical grounds for rejecting the then prevalent notions of binocular combination.

It was during the 14 years which elapsed between Wheatstone's first and second memoirs on stereoscopic vision that Brewster's attention was drawn to the problems of binocular vision. Brewster's lenticular stereoscope was not made until 1849 (see 2.8), and so his experiments before that date would have been conducted using an instrument of Wheatstone's design. Indeed, Brewster had purchased a reflecting stereoscope from Andrew Ross, the London optical instrument maker, after seeing Wheatstone's demonstration of his device at the British Association meeting in 1838 (see Brewster, 1856, p. 34; Wheatstone, 1838).

Brewster's reception of Wheatstone's address to the Newcastle meeting was very enthusiastic, as is evident from the report in *The Athenaeum*:

> Sir David Brewster was afraid that the members could scarcely judge, from the very brief and modest account given of this principle, and the instrument devised for illustrating it, by Professor Wheatstone, of its extreme beauty and generality. He considered it as one of the most valuable optical papers which had been presented to the Section. He observed, that when taken in conjunction with the law of visible direction in monocular vision (or vision with one eye), it explains all those phenomena of vision by which philosophers had been so long perplexed (*Athenaeum*, 1838, p. 650).

One of the reasons for this rapturous reception was that Wheatstone had been circumspect in his choice of words. His paper to the Royal Society (2.4) had been presented but not published at the time of the British Association meeting. Moreover, "He did not, he said, on the present occasion, intend to enter on the consideration of any of the views and conclusions of that paper, for they related rather to mental than to physical philosophy" (*Athenaeum*, 1838, p. 650). Wheatstone's concluding remarks would have been music to Brewster's ears:

> The law of visible direction, which is universally true for all cases of monocular vision, may, Professor Wheatstone stated, be extended to binocular vision by the

following rule: that every point of an object of three dimensions is seen at the intersection of the two lines of visible direction, in which that point is seen by each eye singly (*Athenaeum*, 1838, p. 650; Wheatstone, 1838, p. 17).

By referring to this interpretation as relating to physical rather than mental philosophy, Wheatstone was distinguishing, albeit obliquely, between the analysis of the optical projection and that of the resulting perception. Brewster did not entertain such a distinction, and so his interpretation corresponded almost exactly with that stated by Wheatstone at Newcastle. Brewster's analysis of stereoscopic depth perception is given in Article 2.5, together with some additional observations. One of the latter concerned the distinction between the centre of ocular rotation and the optical centre – ocular parallax – and a simple demonstration of it. Here Brewster was essentially repeating the views he had stated previously to the British Association (Brewster, 1838). The first paragraph of his treatment of visible direction in binocular vision gives one of the clearest and most explicit statements of his views: the laws of binocular vision must conform with those for vision with each eye alone, and visible direction with two eyes can only be reconciled at the points of convergence of the two monocular directions.

Many problems of interpretation regarding Brewster's ideas derive from the constant reference to "convergence", and these are due, in part, to his own loose use of the term. In the same paragraph Brewster referred to the "rapid survey which the eye takes of every part of the object". If this rapid survey was taken as scanning eye movements then he is clearly in error, as Wheatstone had demonstrated the occurrence of stereoscopic depth with binocularly disparate after-images. However, it must be remembered that to Brewster the eye was the "seat of vision", and hence the phrase need not refer to eye movements, but to some "scanning" of the convergences of monocular visible directions. If this point is accepted then Brewster's views differed less from Wheatstone's than is generally supposed. Brewster gave a redescription of stereoscopic phenomena in terms of geometrical optics. Wheatstone wished to transcend such redescriptions, in order to establish the general principle that the perception of depth is determined by retinal dissimilarities, no matter how these are produced. Indeed, that this interpretation of Brewster's thinking might be correct is indicated by two other features of his writing. First, Brewster referred constantly to the three-dimensional objects that could yield the dissimilar pictures on the eyes. In Article 2.7, he stated that the perception of relief was an unavoidable accompaniment of binocular vision. Secondly, Brewster took issue with Wheatstone over those few demonstrations for which the interpretation in terms of monocular directions has difficulty. One of these was the claim that stimulation of corresponding points could lead to double vision. Wheatstone had argued that in his Fig. 23 (p. 83) the thick vertical line in the right eye combined with the thick inclined one rather than the thin vertical in the left. This was disputed by Brewster (see Article 2.5, section 4(1)), who presented various other stimulus configurations to support his view that the apparent combination of corresponding images results from the disappearance of one of them. That is, what might appear as the combination of two similar images could be the single visibility of one of them, due to ocular equivocation (binocular rivalry). There is a very real sense in which Wheatstone's Fig. 23 can be considered as an impossible representation of a three-dimensional scene: if the thicker line appears inclined and nearer in the upper half it would obscure the thin vertical, but should in turn be partially obscured by the latter in the lower half.* Brewster, unlike most others, seemed to have appreciated this problem, and he gave an illustration (Fig. 8, p. 104) which could represent two solid triangles "united at their apex".

Brewster also took issue with Wheatstone's suggestion that images of different magnitude could be combined binocularly. This seemed to contravene his law of visible direction so fundamentally that he entertained the possibility that the refractive states of each eye were modified in order to equate the image sizes.

In the fifth section of the article, Brewster presented his optical analysis of the projection from the frustum of a cone, together with the corresponding two-dimensional pictures that would yield the same retinal projections. It may have been this illustration that led Helmholtz (1925) and Boring (1942) to conclude, incorrectly, that Brewster gave the principles of his refracting or lenticular stereoscope in 1843 (the date the paper was delivered to a meeting of the Royal Society of Edinburgh). This error was compounded by Brewster's own statement that "in the *Edinburgh Transactions* for 1843 I have given the true and demonstrable theory of the stereoscope" (see Article 2.12). Brewster's lenticular stereoscope was not described until 1849.

In the last two sections of the article, Brewster returned to conversions of relief in cameos and intaglios, as well as in outline drawings like Necker's rhomboid. In both instances, Brewster's interpretations were at variance with Wheatstone's.

The next article (2.6) is taken from the same volume of the *Edinburgh Transactions*, and treats, in a less polemical manner, the issue of conversion of relief when using inverting glasses. Brewster did return to binocular vision in yet another article (2.7) in Volume 15 of that august journal. The article commences with a detailed description of what is now called the wallpaper illusion: viewing a large, repetitively patterned surface can lead to the false judgement of its distance, so that the surface usually appears closer than it is. Brewster analysed this phenomenon in terms of convergence both of the eyes and the two monocular visible directions. With regularly patterned wallpaper, equivalently shaped but displaced elements can be combined binocularly when the eyes are converged to a plane other than that of the wall. Many aspects of the phenomenon were

---

* I am very grateful to Hiroshi Ono for this analysis of Wheatstone's figure.

discussed and a formula was provided for calculating the apparent distance of the surface from the eyes. Brewster then considered the binocular combination of two lines meeting at a point (like a V-shape with its open end towards the eyes) and observed from different elevations. The two lines united when their ends were fixated, but they appeared different in depth and extent by amounts calculable from the same general formula applied to the wallpaper phenomenon. These observations were related to Robert Smith's (1738) celebrated demonstration with extended compass legs (see Gulick and Lawson, 1976) and Wells's (1792) experiments on visual direction. It is, perhaps, Brewster's consideration of convergent eye movements in these phenomena that has resulted in him being cast as an eye movement theorist in the context of stereoscopic vision (see Gulick and Lawson, 1976). Brewster concluded the article by describing and representing the general case of the wallpaper phenomenon for transparent repetitive patterns. In so doing, he drew attention to the observation that the sense of touch is brought into conformity with that of vision, even when the latter is in error (this would now be called "visual capture"). He also described the changes in apparent size that accompany those for apparent distance, and gave a formula for relating apparent size and apparent distance.

Brewster announced the invention of the lenticular stereoscope at the Birmingham meeting of the British Association in 1849, and he described a variety of alternative means for the binocular combination of dissimilar pictures in a subsequent article. In the first of these (Article 2.8), a number of other issues were touched upon, such as the simultaneous visibility of elevation and depression due to the combination of stereopairs of three figures, an interpretation of the moon illusion, and a refutation of Bishop Berkeley's theory that sight is secondary to touch. The second article (2.9) essentially reprinted the British Association report, and then provided details of other simple stereoscopes using mirrors and prisms, together with directions for their construction. Illustrations of the lenticular stereoscope and its optical principles are given in Fig. 1, taken from Brewster's *The Stereoscope* (1856, p. 67 and p. 74), because they do not appear clearly in any of the articles reprinted.

Brewster's first lenticular stereoscope was made by George Lowdon, an optical instrument maker in Dundee. Lowdon considered that the lenses in Brewster's design were too small and he found that stereoscopes made with larger lenses generally more convenient for use. He suggested this improvement to Brewster, who did not receive the advice favourably, and relations between the two soured thereafter (see Millar, 1925).

The lenticular stereoscope was ingenious because the semilenses acted both as prisms and as magnifiers. Moreover, a single lens could be used for the separation into two halves, thus equating the optical characteristics of the two channels in a manner that would have been difficult to achieve otherwise. It was also inexpensive, which appealed to Brewster's native sentiments. As a popular

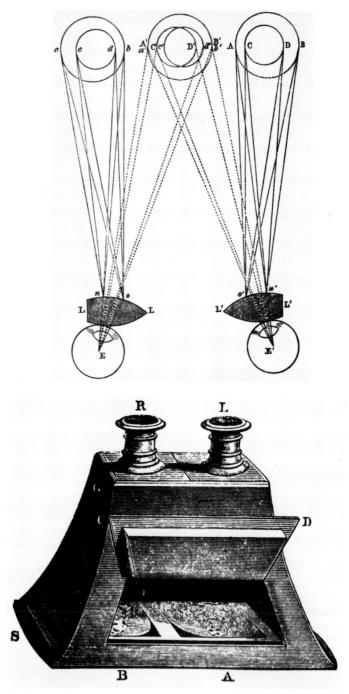

Fig. 1. Brewster's lenticular stereoscope and the optical principles of its operation.

instrument it surpassed Wheatstone's reflecting stereoscope, due largely to its portability and cost. Another important factor was its potential for use with stereoscopic pairs of photographs, which were slowly gaining in popularity.

Despite these advantages, Brewster was unable to persuade any of the leading optical instrument makers in Britain to manufacture his stereoscope, even though it had been demonstrated at two successive meetings of the British Association (1849 and 1850). Consequently, in 1850 he took "a very fine instrument", made by Lowdon, to Paris along with stereoscopic photographs and drawings. These impressed the Parisian opticians and arrangements were made for Duboscq* to produce lenticular stereoscopes and photographs to go with them.

Duboscq displayed a large range of his optical instruments at the Great Exhibition of 1851, and among them was a lenticular stereoscope with sets of stereoscopic photographs. These last attracted the attention of Queen Victoria and, before the closing of the Crystal Palace, Brewster presented her with one of Duboscq's stereoscopes and the accompanying photographs. Thus, the craze for stereoscopic photography was started. Most of the photographs were still taken with single or paired normal cameras, although many different designs of binocular camera were to appear subsequently (see Coe, 1978).

Both Brewster and Wheatstone were quick to appreciate the application of the camera to the stereoscope. Not only would the tedium of making precise perspective drawings be removed, with all the errors attendant thereupon, but more realistic images could be paired – portraits even. In section 19 of his second memoir (2.10), Wheatstone mentioned that Mr. Talbot† and Mr. Collen‡

---

*Louis Jules Duboscq (1817–1886) took out a patent for his stereoscope in 1852, and produced them in large numbers. He modified Brewster's design slightly, replacing the wooden end by a plate of ground glass, so that transparencies could be viewed, as well as printed photographs. In 1852 he also constructed an apparatus for synthesizing motion from a series of stereoscopic photographs presented successively.

† William Henry Fox Talbot (1800–1877) was a gentleman scientist having interests in mathematics, chemistry and optics. His measurements of the brightness of lights having different intensities and intermittencies were published in Brewster's *Philosophical Magazine* (1834) and form the basis for the Talbot-Plateau law. Talbot was also a keen artist, but his frustrations in attempting to represent landscapes led him to try fixing images, formed in a camera obscura, chemically. He worked on the problems associated with forming and fixing images from the mid-1830s, but did not make public his endeavours until 1839, following the report in France of Daguerre's experiments. Talbot had shown interest in Wheatstone's experiments on electricity from the early 1830s, but he improperly anticipated Wheatstone in reporting them (Talbot, 1833). Wheatstone (1833) corrected the reported errors in a letter to the Editor of the *Philosophical Magazine* and lamented the fact that his measurements should have been made public when he was not sufficiently satisfied with their precision. He may still have completed his report to the Royal Society on the velocity of electricity (Wheatstone, 1834) with more haste than he desired (see Bowers, 1975). Talbot had developed an early interest in ancient languages, and shared with Wheatstone considerable expertise in cryptography (see Arnold, 1977).

‡ Henry Collen (1800–1875) was the first professional calotypist, and he worked closely with Talbot. Collen had formerly been a painter of miniatures, and applied his artistic skills to retouching

produced stereoscopic Talbotypes (photographs from paper negatives) for him in 1839. Collen (1854) gave the date as 1841, and the sitter was Charles Babbage. Two photographs were taken at different positions and times using the same camera, as "*two* cameras were not to be had equally good" (Collen, 1854, p. 200). Wheatstone gave directions and tables for the preparation of photographs for use with the stereoscope in his second memoir (2.10). The inconvenience of using two cameras or moving one to different positions was overcome with Brewster's invention of the binocular camera (see Article 3.5).

Collen's letter to the Photographic Society on the earliest stereoscopic portraits corrected an error made by Antoine Claudet,* that "no person had the idea of making stereoscopic portraits: nor was this the case until in 1849 Sir David Brewster read his paper on what he called the lenticular stereoscope" (see Collen, 1854, p. 200; Claudet, 1853). Ironically, the only stereoscopic photograph of Wheatstone that I have been able to trace was taken by Claudet (Fig. 2).

It is clear that Brewster and Wheatstone had keen interests in the emergent art of photography, as well as close associations with two of its pioneers, Talbot and Herschel.† They would have been aware of Talbot's process long before its details were made public in 1839, as they had been his guests at Laycock Abbey prior to the Bristol meeting of the British Association in 1836. Talbot was engaged in his photographic experiments at that time, and subsequently corresponded with Brewster about them. When the process was published and patented, Brewster advised Talbot against the profitability of taking out a Scottish patent for it, although he did encourage its introduction in Scotland. More

---

photographic portraits. Brewster was impressed by Collen's work, as is indicated in his correspondence with Talbot: "Mr. Collen has been so kind as to send me one of his calotypes which has astonished me and all who have seen it" (see Thomas, 1964).

* Antoine François Jean Claudet (1797–1867) was a scientist as well as a photographer. He established one of the first photographic studios in London, and he shared Daguerre's licence in England. Claudet patented a number of novel stereoscopic instruments, including the stereomonoscope. This projected two stereo images at an angle onto a ground glass screen so that they virtually coincided; when viewed from the appropriate distance with a large magnifying glass the different images were projected to each eye (see Gill, 1967). Claudet collaborated with Brewster in producing a small topaz camera lens, because Brewster held that the ideal photographic instrument would use a single lens of least dispersion, aberration and thickness.

† John Frederick William Herschel (1792–1871) was the son of Sir William Herschel, the discoverer of Uranus. John Herschel was also an eminent astronomer. Among his many contributions to photography was the discovery of the fixing properties of sodium hyposulphite. He introduced many novel terms, like positive and negative, and he is usually attributed with the first use of the word "photography", although Wheatstone used the term "photographic" for the first time (see Arnold, 1977). The young Wheatstone was introduced to Herschel by the Danish physicist, Oersted, who had conducted similar acoustical experiments to Wheatstone. Herschel was an acquaintance of Brewster's for much of his life, and he contributed articles for Brewster's *Edinburgh Encyclopaedia*. It was Herschel who provided a fitting epitaph for the dispute between Brewster and Wheatstone over the stereoscope: Wheatstone was the inventor of the stereoscope; Brewster invented a way of looking at stereoscopic pictures.

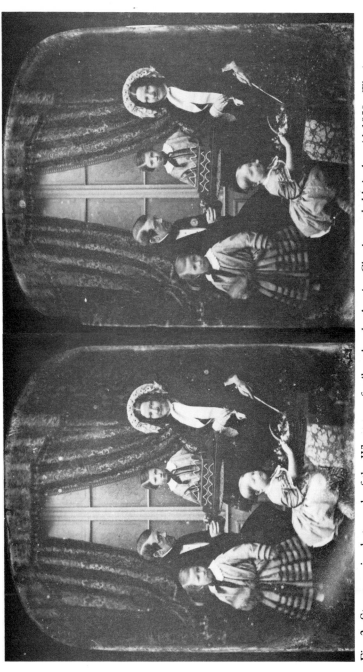

Fig. 2. Stereoscopic photograph of the Wheatstone family, taken by Antoine Claudet probably in the mid-1850s. The instrument which Wheatstone is manipulating is his wave machine. Reproduced by permission of the National Portrait Gallery.

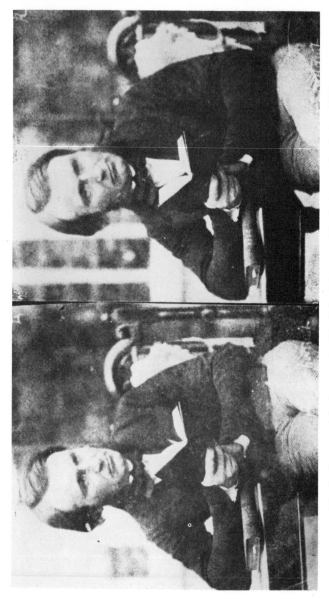

Fig. 3. Stereoscopic photograph of Dr. John Adamson of St. Andrews, taken before 1850. Reproduced by kind permission of the University of St. Andrews.

particularly, Brewster (assisted by detailed correspondence with Talbot) instructed Dr. John Adamson, of St. Andrews, in the art of making Talbotypes (or calotypes, as Talbot preferred them to be called). Under Brewster's direction, the following stereoscopic photographs of Dr. Adamson were taken (Fig. 3). According to Gill (1969), these could be amongst the oldest stereoscopic photographs still extant. Dr. Adamson, in turn, passed on the techniques of photography to his brother Robert, who started in business as a calotypist in Edinburgh in 1843. Brewster introduced Robert Adamson to the painter, David Octavius Hill. Their collaboration between 1843 and 1847 resulted in the celebrated "sun pictures", which are regarded as amongst the finest examples of early photographic art (see Bruce, 1973). The Hill-Adamson portrait of Brewster is shown in Fig. 4.

Brewster also championed the calotype against its competitor, the metal-plated Daguerreotype, even though the latter then produced far more sharply defined images. Comparing the two processes in an *Edinburgh Review* article, Brewster (1843) made the astute prediction that the production of multiple copies from a paper negative would act to the advantage of the calotype, together with the fact that it "will not cost as many pence" as a Daguerreotype.

The marriage between the photograph and the stereoscope took place after receiving the Queen's approval at the Great Exhibition. From 1854, both stereoscopes and stereoscopic photographs were produced in large quantities by the London Stereoscopic Company. Brewster's history of *The Stereoscope* (1856) contains an Appendix in which a catalogue of their binocular pictures is given. The Appendix also gives a "Description and Prices of Sir David Brewster's Lenticular Stereoscopes". These range from the "Japanned Tin Stereoscope, open at sides, front and bottom" for half a crown, to the "Very superior Rosewood or Mahogany, with patent adjusting screw and rack work, sliding eye pieces, beautifully carved, in polished ebony, ivory patent screw, &c." for 50 shillings. It is said that the London Stereoscopic Company made a million stereoscopes (see Gill, 1969).

None the less, the union between the photograph and the stereoscope was a turbulent one. When the wonders of the world had been suitably captured by the twin lenses of the binocular camera, subjects of a more domestic nature were selected. The public appetite for these was rapidly sated, and the demise of stereoscopic photographs was occasioned by the depiction of subjects of questionable taste to right-minded Victorians (see Clay, 1928).

Returning to the narrower confines of stereoscopic vision, Wheatstone published his second memoir in 1852 (2.10). He commenced with an analysis of the changes produced by approaching objects – increases in retinal image sizes, convergence, adaptation (accommodation) and retinal disparity. He then applied the physicists experimental rigour to determining their separate influences. This he achieved with a modified reflecting stereoscope, having arms that could rotate

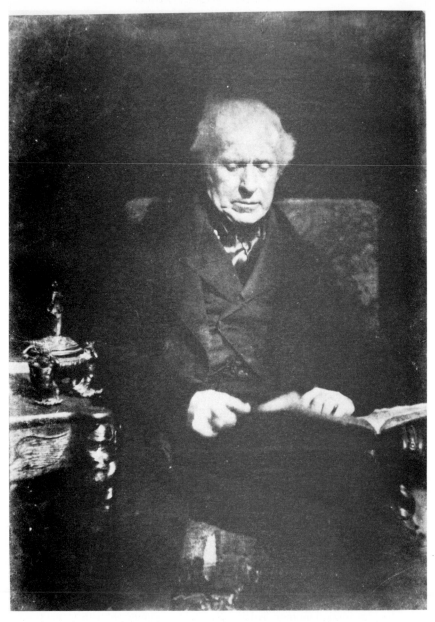

Fig. 4. The Hill-Adamson portrait of Brewster, taken in the mid-1840s. Reproduced by kind permission of the University of St. Andrews.

about a common centre, and sliding panels as in the original design. By dissociating accommodation from convergence, Wheatstone noted the variations in perceived size and distance. The dissociation of disparity from convergence and accommodation was discussed in Article 2.10, sections 20 and 21: stereoscopic photographs taken from different separations were compared for the same settings of the stereoscope. When analysing size perception he found it necessary to distinguish between the real, retinal and perceived magnitudes of objects. In section 18 Wheatstone described several new forms of the stereoscope, including a portable reflecting model and a prism (refracting) stereoscope, and discussed their relative merits for viewing paired photographs. The depth seen in stereoscopic pictures can be reversed in a number of ways, as Wheatstone listed in section 22. In so doing, he specified the depth seen with crossed and uncrossed disparities (although he did not use these terms). Such conversion of relief was readily achieved for solid objects rather than stereoscopic pictures using another novel instrument of Wheatstone's invention – the pseudoscope. "With the pseudoscope we have a glance, as it were, into another visible world, in which external objects and our internal perceptions have no longer their habitual relation with each other", because increased convergence was accompanied by decreasing retinal image size. The conversion of relief with objects was not always easy to perceive, however, particularly when monocular and binocular cues to depth were in conflict; the impressions could then alternate between hollow and protuberant. Approaching objects were said to appear both approaching (from the increasing retinal size) and receding (from the decreasing convergence) at one and the same time! Wheatstone returned, finally and briefly, to the issue of conversion of relief without the intervention of any optical device. He noted the ease with which drawings or photographs of objects in low relief reversed, but the impossibility of conversion with solid objects viewed binocularly.

One area in which the precise solidity of objects was notoriously difficult to ascertain visually was that of the minute, when observed microscopically. Wheatstone's next article (2.11) was addressed to this problem. He reported that he had approached Messrs. Ross, Powell and Beck (London's leading microscope manufacturers) to make a binocular microscope, soon after the publication of his first article on the stereoscope, because the advantages associated with such an instrument would be considerable. Unfortunately, no such instrument was made to his design. The communication to the Microscopical Society of London (which is not included in Wheatstone's collected papers) was a consequence of a report by an American, J. L. Riddell (1853), describing a binocular microscope similar in design to the one proposed by Wheatstone. An improved design was promised in a second communication to the Microscopical Society, but the promise was unfulfilled – no further article on the subject was written by him. The probable reason for this is that he was pre-empted by Wenham's (1854)

elegant binocular microscope, which was described in the very next communication to the Microscopical Society (although it did not appear until the following
issue of the Society's Transactions).

In prosecuting his research into the history of binocular microscopes, Wheatstone found a description of one such by a French friar, le Père Cherubin
d'Orleans, published in 1677. Wheatstone argued that the real advantages of the
instrument were lost on Père Cherubin, because the significance of presenting
dissimilar pictures to each eye was not appreciated. Moreover, because the
images produced by the early microscope were inverted they would have produced pseudoscopic rather than stereoscopic effects.

Considerable significance has recently been attached to this seventeenth
century binocular instrument by Gregory (1980, 1981a), who has argued that
"contrary to accepted belief, Sir Charles Wheatstone was not the inventor,
around 1832, of the first stereoscopic instrument for revealing the third dimension by stereopsis" (1981a, p. 1). Furthermore, he stated that "There is no
evidence that Wheatstone knew of seventeenth century stereo"! (1980, p. 615).
This is an understandable oversight for two reasons. First, Wheatstone's collected papers were, in fact, incomplete and this article (2.11) is one of several that
are neither reprinted nor listed. Secondly, Gregory has relied on the two major
texts on microscopy of the late nineteenth century – Hogg (1854) and Carpenter
(1856) – both of which ran into many editions. Le Père Cherubin's binocular
microscope was not mentioned until later editions of Carpenter's text, but it was
discussed briefly by Jabez Hogg in 1854. Hogg gave the date and the name of the
inventor and then reprinted the first of Wheatstone's brief translations, without
citing either the primary or secondary source. Hogg continued with the following
passage:

> This appears to have slumbered long and been forgotten, and nothing more was
> heard of the subject until Professor Wheatstone's very surprising invention of the
> stereoscope, when it again attracted the attention of the above philosopher, who
> applied to both Ross and Powell to make him an instrument (1854, p. 113).

Suffice it to say that Wheatstone was neither convinced that the earlier binocular
microscope was stereoscopic nor did he believe that the stereoscopic principles,
with which a binocular microscope could be used to advantage, were appreciated
by le Père Cherubin.

Issues of priority concerning the stereoscope are by no means new. In 1856
Brewster published *The Stereoscope*, with accounts of its history, theory and
applications. The historical section appears aimed at wresting from Wheatstone
any credit for demonstrating that binocular depth perception is dependent upon
the dissimilar images in each eye: "It is, therefore, a fact well known to every
person of common sagacity that *the pictures of bodies seen by both eyes are formed by
the union of two dissimilar pictures formed by each*" (Brewster, 1856, p. 6). The list of

those aware of "this palpable truth" included Euclid, Galen, Porta, Leonardo da Vinci, Aguilonius and Joseph Harris. Again we can cite Brewster:

> What student of perspective is there – master or pupil, male or female – who does not know, as certainly as he knows his alphabet, that the picture of a chair or table, or anything else, drawn from *one point of sight*, or as seen by one eye placed in that point, is *necessarily dissimilar* to another drawing of the same object taken from another point of sight, or seen by the other eye placed in a point 2½ inches distant from the first? (1856, pp. 17–18).

Clearly, Brewster was confusing the knowledge of the existence of retinal disparity with the demonstration of the use to which it is put. Palpable though the truth of dissimilar projections may be, there is no discussion of it in Brewster's writing prior to Wheatstone's first memoir.

Not content with slighting Wheatstone in this regard, Brewster went further and introduced a contender for the invention of a stereoscope – James Elliot, a teacher of mathematics in Edinburgh. Four years earlier, Elliot had written to the Editors of the *Philosophical Magazine* stating

> I constructed a stereoscope, in everything but name, more than thirteen years ago, which, though since neglected by me, is still in existence, and can be produced, with evidence of its date. I do not state this with a view to detract at all from the merit or originality of Professor Wheatstone's invention, as mine was never made public. I mention the circumstance rather as a curious fact than anything else (1852, p. 397).

The letter was occasioned by the reprinting of Wheatstone's first memoir in the *Philosophical Magazine* of 1852. Wheatstone replied: "Had your correspondent, Mr. Elliot, attended to the original date of my first memoir . . . he would have seen that there was no ground for impugning the originality of my researches" (1852, p. 478). Following Wheatstone's letter is a retraction from Elliot via the editors, indicating "that had he been aware that Professor Wheatstone had produced his Stereoscope so early as 1838", he would not have sent the earlier letter. Brewster was less charitable. He must have contacted Elliot subsequently to learn more details of his ocular stereoscope, because no mention is made of him or his instrument in Brewster's anonymous article on binocular vision and the stereoscope, published in the *North British Review* of May, 1852. In *The Stereoscope* Brewster wrote of Elliot's endeavours thus:

> Previous to or during the year 1834, he had resolved to construct an instrument for uniting two dissimilar pictures, or of constructing a stereoscope – but he delayed doing so till the year 1839. . . . This simple stereoscope, without lenses or mirrors, consisted of a wooden box 18 inches long, 7 broad, and 4½ deep, and at the bottom of it, or rather at its farther end, was placed a slide containing two dissimilar pictures of a landscape as seen by each eye (Brewster, 1856, p. 19).

Because the aid of photography was not then available to him, Elliot drew two landscapes on a transparent surface, with three distances (or disparities), corresponding to the moon, a cross and a withered tree stump. These drawings are reproduced in Fig. 5, in the manner used by Elliot, namely with convergence at some point beyond the plane of the pictures.*

Having employed these means to denegrate Wheatstone's achievement in his own publication, it is not surprising to find Brewster repeating the claims through such an august public organ as *The Times*. In an initial, anonymous and mischievous letter Brewster compared Elliot's simple "stereoscope" with an even simpler device – a card with two holes in it – described by M. Faye in the French journals *Cosmos* and *Comptes Rendus*. Wheatstone was mentioned in passing, and only with respect to the optical tube method for separating the images to the eyes. This letter and the ensuing correspondence are reprinted in Article 2.12. Reading Brewster's second letter, one can feel, with Wheatstone, that "It is difficult to deal with Sir David Brewster's reasoning". However, the reply did elicit evidence that stereoscopes – both reflecting and refracting – were made in 1832 for Wheatstone. Brewster had earlier, in *The Stereoscope*, made great play regarding Wheatstone's statement in his second memoir (2.10, section 18) that he had for many years used prisms to refract two dissimilar pictures so that they appeared in the same position. Brewster's third letter admits of yet another contestant for priority – one "Theophilus" (George Maynard) – who wrote an article on binocular vision, in 1836, for a Toronto newspaper. Theophilus did state that the distance of objects could be determined by parallax, analogous to the manner in which the distances of heavenly bodies were calculated. However, parallax was referred to differences in visible directions rather than disparities, and so his views were more closely akin to Brewster's than Wheatstone's. Theophilus did present one of the most frequently cited examples of the advantages acruing to stereoscopic vision – the difficulty in threading a needle with only one eye open!

In his final reply to "so disputatious an antagonist as Sir D. Brewster" Wheatstone vented his spleen, and unleashed his considerable scholarship on Brewster. The latter had argued that Aguilonius had stated the principle of the stereoscope. A brief section, in which Aguilonius lapsed into Greek, was cited by Brewster. Even this was a cause for contention being differently translated and interpreted by each. Wheatstone did deliver a delightful *coup de grâce* in his statement "It is evident that Sir David has looked upon Aguilonius through a pseudoscope".

It is strange that the debate did not hinge more on pseudoscopic issues: no mention was made by either combatant of the seventeenth century binocular

---

* Mr. Elliot appears recently to have re-entered the controversy, but in a somewhat different guise. Dudley (1951) mentioned in his book *Stereoptics*, a simple stereoscope invented in 1834 by one Helioth. Because Dudley's book is devoid of a bibliography or any other means of tracing Helioth, it is possible that this is a confusion for Elliot. The stereoscopes attributed to Elliot and Helioth bear striking resemblance. Unfortunately, this chance, and possibly incorrect, reference has become enshrined in some text books of perception: Kaufman (1974) referred to the Helioth-Wheatstone stereoscope on the basis of Dudley's unsupported comment, and Schiff (1980) repeated this on Kaufman's authority!

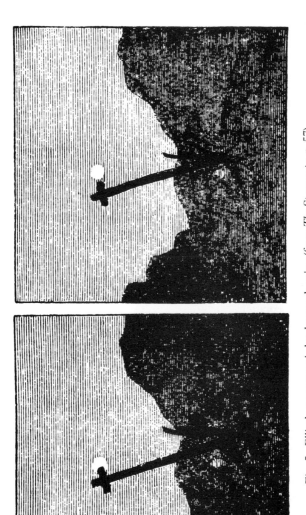

Fig. 5. Elliot's stereoscopic landscape drawing (from *The Stereoscope*, p. 57).

microscope. Because Wheatstone was well aware of it he cannot have considered it of any relevance to the debate. Had it have been deemed of any assistance to Brewster, assuming he knew of it, he would surely have introduced it.

Brewster was not one to allow a dispute to end without having the final word. This he did via another organ – *The Photographic Journal*. It is clear that his opinions regarding the history of stereoscopic vision did not change with *The Times*. He remained convinced that the principles of the stereoscope were understood by the ancients, but proof, in the form of an instrument or stereoscopic drawings, was still wanting. Fortuitously, he must have thought, this was provided indirectly by his friend James Forbes.* In a brief note (Article 2.13) Brewster cited the description by Alexander Crum Brown of two drawings (shown in Fig. 6) by Jacopo Chimenti, a sixteenth century Florentine artist, displayed in a museum in Lille. Brown found that by converging his eyes the two pictures could be combined binocularly to give the appearance of stereoscopic depth. To Brewster this circumstantial and second-hand evidence was conclusive: "we cannot for a moment doubt that they are binocular drawings intended by the artist to be united into relief either by the eye or by an instrument". Furthermore, an imaginary web was woven enmeshing Chimenti with Porta who was, Brewster assured his audience, aware of both the principle and the construction of the stereoscope.

Brewster had to rely on the observations and descriptions of Crum Brown because he was unable, initially, to obtain photographs or copies of the drawings. It is evident from the second article (2.14) that Wheatstone, much to Brewster's chagrin, had obtained a photographic copy of Chimenti's drawings in 1860. Moreover, Wheatstone was unable to see depth in the photographs when they were mounted in a stereoscope, nor could others who viewed them in London and in Paris. Not unexpectedly, when photographic copies did reach Brewster their stereoscopic nature was instantly evident. Reduced photographs were made for the stereoscope, and displayed by Brewster to a meeting of members of the Photographic Society of Scotland. The full stereoscopic relief was seen by all! One wonders whether anyone present would have had the temerity to question Sir David's conclusions. At the end of the meeting there was an astonishing

---

* James David Forbes (1809–1868) had been encouraged in his scientific pursuits early in his career by Brewster, following Forbes's anonymous correspondence (as a teenager) with the editor of the *Edinburgh Journal of Science* on certain aspects of optics. Brewster proposed Forbes for membership of the Royal Society of Edinburgh at the age of 21. However, their friendship soured later when they were in competition for the chair of natural philosophy at Edinburgh University, to which Forbes was appointed in 1833. That was the second unsuccessful attempt Brewster had made to secure this esteemed post. Forbes succeeded Brewster as Principal of the United College of St. Salvator and St. Leonard in St. Andrews, when Brewster was appointed Principal of the University at which he had been unable to obtain a chair. It was to the young Forbes that Brewster wrote, in 1830, "I cannot tolerate the idea of a Professorship being an object of your ambition, if you mean a Scotch one. There is no profession so incompatible with original enquiry as a Scotch Professorship, where one's income depends on the number of pupils" (Shairp, Tait and Adams-Reilly, 1873, p. 59).

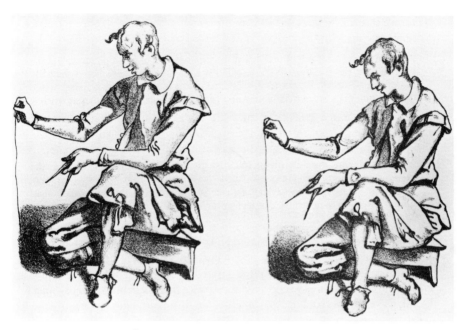

Fig. 6. Reproductions of the Chimenti drawings. These are copies of woodcuts which appeared in *The Photographic Journal* of 1862, and they were supplied to the journal by the Rev. J. B. Reade. The left and right figures are transposed relative to the originals (photographs of which can be seen in Gill, 1969). Brewster argued that the original drawings should be viewed with the eyes converged to a point in front of the pictures, so that they could be combined binocularly. The woodcuts were transposed in order to facilitate viewing with the aid of a book stereoscope.

remark by a Professor Archer that a box found in the Liverpool museum looked like a stereoscope and bore the date 1670! Could this have been the instrument that Brewster required to complete his argument? It would appear not. Archer's box was a binocular telescope, and its correct date was 1726 (see Emerson, 1864a).

The controversy over the Chimenti drawings did not end there, although Wheatstone did not pursue it further. The subsequent issues of *The Photographic Journal* are littered with claims and counter-claims for their stereoscopic authenticity. However, it should be noted that the arguments presented have been based on observations of reproductions, whether graphic or photographic, of the Chimenti drawings, and little account was made for any distortions that might have been introduced as a consequence of this.

The issue of accurate copying was considered of great importance by Professor E. Emerson, an American who had followed the controversy over the Chimenti pictures. Indeed, he entered it by publishing a note in the *American Journal of Science*:

> I have made a careful examination of the photographs of these pictures, and the truth is that the trifling stereoscopic and pseudoscopic qualities about them are evidently accidental. To prove this let anyone execute a pen-and-ink sketch, and then let him make as perfect a copy of it as he can without careful measurements. Now place these two drawings in a stereoscope, and you get the same kind of effect seen in the Chimenti drawings, and for the same reason; the drawings will vary more or less from each other. All that is necessary, then, to impose upon ordinary eyes, is to find which way the sum of the variations predominates, mount the drawings accordingly, and, mirabile dictu! you have produced a stereoscopic picture (the pseudoscopic portion being overlooked) drawn by hand; you have done the very thing that Sir David Brewster has repeatedly declared was quite beyond human skill! If Professor Wheatstone gets no heavier blow than this, his fame as a discoverer is secure (1862, p. 315).

Brewster's retort to this is reprinted in Article 2.15. He cast aspersions both on Emerson's logic and method. None the less, Brewster, together with P. G. Tait, performed the type of experiment suggested by Emerson: schoolchildren were given Chimenti pictures to copy and these were then examined stereoscopically. Depth was not perceived in their combination. Brewster reiterated his arguments regarding the stereoscopic nature of Chimenti's drawings, and asked what other interpretation an historian of science would place upon their existence.

Brewster so misinterpreted Emerson's earlier work that the latter addressed four scathing and scholarly replies to him in *The British Journal of Photography* (Emerson, 1864). In the first, he corrected errors of fact in Brewster's article, and gave more detail regarding the copies drawn from photographs of the Chimenti drawings. Emerson also determined the date and nature of Professor Archer's "seventeenth century stereoscope". The second retort listed the improbabilities of the drawings being stereoscopic, not the least of which was the size of the originals – about 30 × 21 cm. The conclusions of four independent "witnesses" were presented, none of whom experienced stereoscopic depth. The third notice contained illustrations of one of his own sketched copies, and one by the American authority on optics, Ogden Rood. The final reply contained the most convincing evidence – detailed measurements of the pictures made by himself and independently by a Professor Towler. The left and right pictures differed in overall size, there were many vertical and horizontal discrepancies, but the latter were not in a systematic direction. The conclusion was clear:

> As Sir David Brewster desires particulars, we enumerate: a stereoscopic left knee, a pseudoscopic dress hanging over it, a stereoscopic left arm, but a pseudoscopic back, a pseudoscopic stool, and a pseudoscopic left foot, and a right foot still more pseudoscopic relatively to the left foot and the stool – and so we might go over the whole picture and show a *melange* of pseudoscopic and stereoscopic lines, producing precisely the commingled and uncertain effect which a drawing and an ordinary copy of it would produce if adjusted for the stereoscope (Emerson, 1864, p. 204).

Helmholtz came to much the same conclusion, and gave the following, sober assessment of the pictures:

> The two pictures of the man were certainly made from different positions, but I must admit that it seems to me very unlikely that Chimenti intended them for a stereoscopic experiment, because the stool, the dividers, and the plumb line, which could easily have been drawn correctly, are treated as unessentials and all drawn so irregularly and so differently that they cannot be combined. Had the artist desired to test a theory, it is more than likely that he would have drawn the easy things correctly and the difficult parts, such as the man, more inaccurately. It seems more probable to me that the artist was not quite satisfied with the first figure and did it over again from another point of view, using the same sheet of paper quite by accident (1925, p. 363).

Brewster was either wise enough or old enough (he was then in his ninth decade) not to write further on this topic, although near-universal opprobrium was unlikely to have been the reason. In his final article (2.15) Brewster had made great play on the interpretation an historian of science would make on the existence of the Chimenti drawings. Perhaps in an historical sense, much more significance should be given to the controversy itself rather than to the stimulus that elicited it. The Chimenti pictures represented a highly charged reflection of a problem that was bound to occur: how can differences in stereoscopic experience when viewing the same figure be reconciled? If one individual reports depth in a pair of pictures and another does not, which report should be given credence?

The issue of the Chimenti drawings was resolved, essentially, by resort to physics – by measurements of the dimensions of the pictures. Those marvels of the machine age, the stereoscopes, had produced "hitherto unobserved phenomena", but visual science had not invested the same ingenuity into how the phenomena might be measured. Mechanical sophistication was not matched by behavioural precision. Ironically, while the Chimenti controversy was raging in Britain the potential solution to this problem was emerging in Germany – in the guise of Fechner's *Elemente der Psychophysik* (1860).

2.2. Brewster: "Observations on the vision of impressions on the retina, in reference to certain supposed discoveries respecting vision announced by Mr. Charles Bell". *Edinburgh Journal of Science*, 1825, **2**, 1–9.*

There is no branch of physical science which has made less progress than that which relates to the optical functions of the eye. Although the phenomena of vision are constantly presented to our consideration, and although experiments without number, and speculations without end, have been accumulated, yet

* Read before the Royal Society of Edinburgh, 6 December, 1824.

during the last century no prominent discovery has been made respecting the physiology of this most important organ.

It was, therefore, with no inconsiderable satisfaction, that I observed in the *Philosophical Transactions* for 1823, a paper by Mr. Charles Bell, containing an account of discoveries which promised to throw a new light not only upon the optical, but upon the metaphysical questions which have so long been agitated respecting vision. In studying that paper, however, these expectations have been disappointed. After a careful repetition of the experiments which it contains, and a minute investigation of the phenomena to which it relates, I have no hesitation in stating, that its facts and reasonings are to a great extent incorrect and inconclusive.

In submitting the results of this inquiry to the Royal Society, I trust it will not be supposed that I am engaging their attention to a subject of a controversial nature. I have no inclination to offer any criticisms, or make any comments upon those parts of Mr. Bell's paper, which are open to controversy. My only object is to establish certain scientific facts and laws of vision which have been misunderstood or perverted; and I shall but ill perform the task I have undertaken, if I leave the subject in any doubt, or fail to impress upon those who hear me, the same conviction of their certainty which I entertain myself.

In order that these facts and doctrines maintained by Mr. Bell may not be misinterpreted, I shall state them in his own words.

> When the eye is at rest, as in sleep, or even when the eyelids are shut, the sensation on the retina being then neglected, *the voluntary muscles resign their office, and the involuntary muscles draw the pupil under the upper eyelid.* This is the condition of the organ during perfect repose.
>
> On the other hand, there is an inseparable connexion between the exercise of the sense of vision, and the exercise of the voluntary muscles of the eye. When an object is seen we enjoy too senses; there is an impression upon the retina; but we receive also the idea of position or relation, which it is not the office of the retina to give. It is by *the consciousness of the degree of effort put upon the voluntary muscles that we know the relative position of an object to ourselves.* The relation existing between the office of the retina and of the voluntary muscles, may be illustrated in this manner.
>
> Let the eyes be fixed upon an illuminated object, until the retina be fatigued, and in some measure exhausted by the image, then closing the eyes the figure of the object will continue present to them: and it is quite clear that nothing can change the place of this impression on the retina. But notwithstanding that the impression on the retina cannot be changed, the idea thence arising may. For, by an exertion of the voluntary muscles of the eyeball the body seen will appear to change its place, and *it will, to our feeling, assume different positions according to the muscle which is exercised.* If we raise the pupil we shall see the body elevated, or if we depress the pupil, we shall see the body placed below us; and all this takes place while the eyelids are shut, and when no new impression is conveyed to the retina. The state of the retina is here associated with a consciousness of muscular exertion; and it shows that vision, in its extended sense, is a compound operation, the *idea of position of an object having relation to the activity of the muscles.*

If we move the eye by the voluntary muscles, while this impression continues upon the retina, we shall have the notion of place and relation raised in the mind; but if the motion of the eyeball be produced BY ANY OTHER CAUSE, *by the involuntary muscles or by pressure from without,* we shall have no corresponding change of sensation.

If we make the impression on the retina in the manner described, and shut the eyes, *the image will not be elevated, although the pupils be actually raised,* as it is their condition to be when the eyes are shut, because there is here no sense of voluntary exertion. If we sit at some distance from a lamp, which has a cover of ground glass, and fix the eye on the centre of it, and then shut the eye and contemplate the phantom in the eye; and if, while the image continues to be present of a fine blue colour, *we press the eye aside with the finger, we shall not move that phantom or image,* although the circle of light produced by the pressure of the finger against the eyeball moves with the motion of the finger.

May not this be accounted for in this manner: The motion produced in the eyeball not being performed by the appropriate organs, the voluntary muscles, *it conveys no sensation of change* to the sensorium, and is not associated with the impression on the retina, so as to affect the idea excited in the mind? It is owing to the same cause, that, when looking on the lamp, by pressing one eye, we can make two images, and we can make the one move over the other. But if we have received the impression on the retina so as to leave the phantom visible when the eyelids are shut, *we cannot, by pressing one eye, produce any such effect. We cannot, by any degree of pressure, make that image appear to move*; but the instant that the eye moves by its voluntary muscles, the image changes its place; that is, we produce the two sensations necessary to raise this idea in the mind; we have the sensation on the retina combined with the consciousness or sensation of muscular activity. – *Phil. Trans.* 1823, pp. 177–180.

The passage now quoted contains three important results:

1. That when an impression is made upon the retina by strong light, this impression, in the form of a coloured spectrum, remains absolutely fixed and immoveable, if the eyeball is moved by the pressure of the finger, or by any other external cause than that of the voluntary muscles of the eyeball.

2. That during sleep, or upon the closing of the eyelids, the voluntary muscles resign their office, and the involuntary muscles draw the pupil under the upper eyelid.

3. That during this involuntary motion or displacement of the globe of the eye, the spectral impression continues absolutely fixed and immoveable.

From these results, Mr. Bell draws the highly important conclusion, that "it is by the consciousness of the degree of effort put upon the voluntary muscles, that we know the relative position of an object to ourselves," or that "the notion of place or relation is raised in the mind;" and hence he explains the old paradox of an inverted picture upon the retina producing the appearance of an erect object.

In estimating the value of this singular conclusion, we shall first admit its truth, as well as the correctness of the facts from which it is deduced, in order to form some notion of the consequences in which it will involve us.

Since the notion of place or relation depends solely on the consciousness of exerting the voluntary muscles of the eyeball, let the observer, with a spectral impression on his retina, close his eye, and turn round his head either in a vertical or a horizontal plane, *by the muscles of his neck alone*. It will now be found, that the spectrum follows the motion of the head; and hence we must conclude, that the notion of place or relation depends on the exercise of the muscles of the neck, as those of the eyeball have been entirely at rest.

But as there may exist some undiscovered sympathy between the muscles of the neck and those of the eyeball, let the observer, with his eyes closed be now placed upon a stool, to which an assistant communicates a rotatory motion through the intermedium of a leathern belt. In this case also, it will be found that the spectrum revolves with the stool in the same manner as if the eyeball had performed the same angular motion by the action of its voluntary muscles. Hence we must conclude, that the notion of place or relation depends on the muscles of the assistant's arm, conveyed by some sympathetic action to the observer's eye along the leathern belt; a result so inadmissible, that, to use the sentence which Mr. Bell directs against the illustrious Kepler, "The mind might as well follow the ray out of the eye, and like the spider, feel along the line."

In order to view this subject under another aspect, let us suppose that, by cutting the voluntary muscles, the eyeball is left to float in its socket; or, what is the same thing, that these muscles have lost their power of giving motion to the eyeball. In such a case, will the eye retain its notions of place or relation? or will it lose them entirely? It is quite clear that the impression of external objects on the retina will not be affected by this condition of the voluntary muscles; and therefore it follows, that if the notion of place is lost, the eye must either see the object erect as usual, or inverted, or in some intermediate position, or what is more probable, in all these positions at once. For if it has *a determinate position*, the eye will only have exchanged its notion of true position for a notion of false position, a result too absurd to be for a moment entertained. Fortuntely for this argument, Mr. Bell has actually described a case under the care of Dr. Macmichael, which occurred after his paper was read. "In this case," says he, "which shows the consequences of the eye and eyelids being rendered immoveable, the surface of the eye is totally insensible, and the eye remains fixed and directed straight forward, *whilst the vision is entire*." If there ever was an *experimentum crucis*, which could settle at once a controverted question, we have one in the case now quoted. Dr. Macmichael's patient preserved his vision entire, when "the outward apparatus was without sensibility and motion," and when there was no consciousness of effort in the voluntary muscles to convey the notions of place and relation.

Although mathematicians have acknowledged the legitimacy of the *reductio ad absurdum*, which constitutes the principal feature of the preceding argument, yet we fear this will not be admitted in physical science, unless it is accompanied with an acknowledgment of our ignorance respecting the facts and principles which the paralogism involves. I shall therefore proceed to an examination of the facts themselves.

1. The leading fact which has misled Mr. Bell in this inquiry, is the alleged immobility of the spectral impression, when the eye is displaced by the pressure of the finger. This spectrum is by no means immoveable. It is quite true that it moves through a very small space; but this space, small as it is, is the precise quantity through which it ought to move according to the principles of optics; and the explanation of this fact leads us to investigate the difference between the vision of external objects, and that of impressions upon the retina.

In order to understand this difference, let A (Fig. 1) be the eye of the observer, and O an external object, whose image at P is seen along the axis of vision POM. Let the eye be pushed upwards, suppose $1/10$th of an inch, into the position B, the external object O remaining fixed. The image of O upon the retina will now be raised from P to Q in the elevated eye at B. Hence the object O will now be seen in the direction QON, having descended, by the elevation of the eye, from M to N.

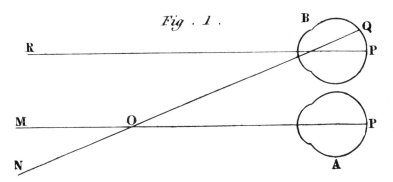

Fig . 1 .

Let the eye be now brought back to its original position A, and let the object O be the lamp with ground glass used by Mr. Bell. The spectral impression will therefore be made upon the retina at P, and will remain on that spot till it is effaced. If the eye A is now raised to B, the impression will still be at P in the elevated eye, and it will be seen in the direction PR parallel to PM, having risen only $1/10$th of an inch, or the height through which the eye has been raised by pressure. This small space is not very visible to an ordinary observer, when his head is at liberty to move; but if the head is carefully fixed, the motion of the spectrum becomes quite apparent. Hence it is obvious that Mr. Bell has been first misled by not observing the motion of the spectrum, and secondly, by supposing that the vision of an impression followed the same law as the vision of an external object. The difference between these two cases of vision which Mr. Bell has overlooked, consists in this, that in *ordinary vision* the object forms a new image upon a new part of the retina, after the eye is pushed up; whereas in *spectral vision*, the original object has nothing to do after the eye is displaced, the spectrum itself which retains its place on the retina being now the only object of perception.

2. The *second* fact announced by Mr. Bell is, that during sleep, or upon the closing of the eyelids, the eyeball is involuntarily turned up beneath the upper eyelid, and so far even as to withdraw the pupil from the faint light which that eyelid transmits.

This singular result stands in direct contradiction to the opinion of Soemmering and other anatomists, who consider the eyeball as perfectly stationary when the eyelids are shut; but as Mr. Bell has deduced his opinion from direct experiment, it requires to be strictly examined. I have frequently and carefully repeated the experiment which he describes, and I find that no such motion of the eyeball takes place upon shutting the eyelids; but that, on the contrary, they remain perfectly stationary. I am informed also by Dr. Knox, that he saw a case of a protrusion of the iris through the cornea, which could very readily be distinguished even when the eyelids were closed; and that the protuberance occupied the same position whether the eyelids were open or shut.

The impossibility of the existence of such a motion may be deduced also from other principles. When the observer, with a spectrum in his eye, closes his eyelids, Mr. Bell admits that the spectrum remains stationary, which is undoubtedly the case; but as we have already demonstrated that the spectrum actually follows the movements of the eye as it ought to do, upon the ordinary principles of optics, the absolute immobility of the impression, upon shutting the eyelids, becomes an incontrovertible proof, that when the eye is closed, the eyeball is not displaced by the action of any involuntary muscles.

In order to strengthen his arguments for the existence of this involuntary revolution of the eyeball, Mr. Bell has stated, in a very ingenious manner, the final cause of such an arrangement.

> The purpose of this rapid insensible motion of the eyeball will be understood on observing the form of the eyelids, and the place of the lachrymal gland. The margins of the eyelids are flat, and when they meet, they touch only at their outer edges, so that when closed, there is a gutter left between them and the cornea. If the eyeball were to remain without motion, the margins of the eyelids would meet in such a manner on the surface of the cornea, that a certain portion would be left untouched, and the eye would have no power of clearing off what obscured the vision, at that principal part of the lucid cornea, which is in the very axis of the eye; and if the tears flowed, they would be left accumulated on the centre of the cornea; and winking, instead of clearing the eye, would suffuse it. To avoid these effects, and to sweep and clear the surface of the cornea, at the same time that the eyelids are closed, the eyeball revolves, and the cornea is rapidly elevated under the eyelid. – *Phil. Trans.* 1823, p. 169.

Unfortunately for these views, the clearing away of the lubricating fluid which is left in the groove between the closed eyelids has not been accomplished by

Almighty wisdom. Those who are familiar with this case of experiments, will have no difficulty in observing the ridge of accumulated fluid remaining after the eye is opened, and gradually falling to its level by the united forces of gravity and capillary attraction. In order to perceive this effect, let the eye be directed to a small point of light, such as the image of a candle diminished by reflexion from a convex surface, and let this image be brought near the eye, so that the pencils of rays which diverge from it may have their foci a great way behind the retina. When the eye is open, the image of this luminous point will be a circular disc of light, or a section of the cone of rays formed by the refraction of the eye. If, when looking at this circular disc, shown in A in Fig. 2, we shut the eyelids, and then open them gradually, examining at the same time the appearance of the disc, we shall at first observe it to have the compressed form shown at B, occasioned by the ridge of fluid, and then gradually extending itself into its regular circular form, an effect which may be produced at once by the operation of winking; the only one which nature has combined with the ordinary motion of the eyeball for the purpose of smoothing the outer surface of the cornea.

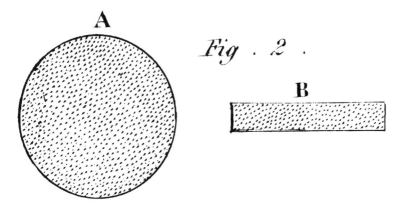

In concluding these remarks, I cannot avoid expressing a wish that Mr. Bell will re-examine his own observations, and repeat with care those to which I have had occasion to refer, before he proceeds to his ulterior object of establishing upon such a basis an arrangement of the nerves of the eye, and a distinction of them according to their uses. Such an arrangement must be affected by the facts upon which it is founded; and the present advanced state both of human and comparative anatomy, requires that all their classifications, and particularly their most difficult ones, should not rest on contested *data*, or be regulated by ambiguous principles.

Before quitting this subject, I am desirous of stating to the society some views connected with the preceding observations, and relating to a more recondite affection of the eye, which it seems to receive through the agency of the mind.

When the eye is not exposed to the impressions of external objects, or when it is insensible to these impressions, in consequence of the mind being engrossed with its own operations, any object of mental contemplation which has either been called up by the memory, or created by the imaginaton, will be seen as distinctly as if it had been formed from the vision of a real object. In examining these mental impressions, I have found that they follow the motions of the eyeball exactly like the spectral impressions of luminous objects, and that they resemble them also in their apparent immobility when the eyeball is displaced by an external force. If this result (which I state with much diffidence, from having only my own experience in its favour) shall be found generally true by others, it will follow that the objects of mental contemplation may be seen as distinctly as external objects, and will occupy the same local position in the axis of vision, as if they had been formed by the agency of light.*

Hence all the phenomena of apparitions may depend upon the relative intensities of these two classes of impressions, and upon their manner of accidental combination. In perfect health, when the mind possesses a control over its powers, the impressions of external objects alone occupy the attention, but in the unhealthy condition of the mind, the impressions of its own creation, either overpower, or combine themselves with the impressions of external objects; – the mental spectra in the one case appearing alone, while in the other they are seen projected among those external objects to which the eyeball is directed.

2.3. Brewster: "On the optical illusion of the conversion of cameos into intaglios, and of intaglios into cameos, with an account of other analogous phenomena". *Edinburgh Journal of Science*, 1826, **4**, 99–108. (Published anonymously)

The remarkable phenomena to which we propose at present to direct the attention of our readers, while they possess all the interest which belongs to them as physical facts, have attached to them another kind of interest, not less deserving of attention. To those who are in the practice of exercising a presumptuous confidence in their own judgments, and who trust in the indications of their senses as infallible guides, we would recommend the particular study of this class of deceptions. They will here find their judgments deluded, where every thing is favourable to the discovery of the truth; and even when they are aware of the source of the deception, they will find themselves again brought under its dominion, and again released from it, by the operation of the most trivial

---

* These results, and several others which I shall have occasion to explain in another paper, confirm, in a remarkable manner, the views of my friend Dr Hibbett, in his able work on the Philosophy of Apparitions.

circumstances which they are not able to discover, and the influence of which, if they do discover them, they are not able to appreciate. If all this takes place in matters of simple observation, where the senses of sight and of touch are allowed their undisturbed exercise, how much more liable must they be to error, where their passions, their prejudices, or their feelings, concur in promoting the delusion, or even in any remote degree prepare the mind for its reception.

The class of deceptions to which we allude, were, so far as we know, first noticed at one of the early meetings of the Royal Society of London, when a compound microscope, on a new construction, was exhibited. When the members were looking through it at a guinea, some of them saw the head upon the coin depressed, while others considered it to be raised, as it was in reality.

This deception was studied by Dr Philip Frederick Gmelin of Wurtemburg, who communicated the following observations upon it to the Royal Society of London in 1744.

Being informed by a friend, says he, that if a common seal was applied to the focus of a compound microscope, or optical tube, which has two or three convex or plano-convex lenses, that part which is cut the deepest in it would appear very convex, and so on the contrary; and that sometimes, but very seldom it would appear in the same state as to the naked eye. I was desirous to make the observation myself, and found it constantly to happen as my friend told me. I thought the experiment worthy of being farther prosecuted; and, accordingly, on the 16th of last April, the morning not being very clear, but in a pretty light chamber, I viewed a watch hanging against a plain wall, through the optical tube; the whole of it appeared concave, and fixed into the wall. I also observed some flies that were running about the wall, and they appeared in like manner. I also viewed a small globe of a thermometer filled with red spirit, and this also seemed hollow, and fixed within the frame. I found the same to happen with the round parts of garments of all colours, and with the brazen protuberances of a small cabinet; all which appeared concave, and deeply sunk into the cloth and wood. I also viewed a small stag's head, cut in wood, and hanging horizontally on the wall; this also appeared concave, and fixed into the wall.

After this, I observed a ball of one of Fahrenheit's thermometers, full of quicksilver: but it did not change its natural convexity; nor did the empty glass ball of the inverted thermometer hanging against the wall, though the lower ball of the same, filled with red spirit, and that also of Fahrenheit's, filled with spirit, lost their convexity. Hence, I presently concluded, that white or shining uncoloured bodies, appear under the focus of this tube in the same manner as they appear to the naked eye; *at the same time, I must fairly acknowledge, that an assisting friend has sometimes made observations directly opposite to mine in the same circumstances; nay, in a darker day, I myself have found my observations quite contrary to those I had made the day before.* Hence, though the observations with the seal held constantly the same, I imagined there must be some particular circumstances hitherto undiscovered, in which these objects appeared thus perverted. I therefore endeavoured to discover some certain laws, according to which these perverted objects appeared when exposed to these foci, and some others according to which they constantly appeared as when they were exposed to the naked eye. After various experiments, I partly obtained my end.

As often as I viewed any object, rising upon a plane, of what colour soever, provided it was neither white nor shining, with the eye and optical tube directly opposite to it, the elevated parts appeared depressed, and the depressed parts elevated, as it happened in the seal, as often as I held the tube perpendicularly, and brought it in such a manner, that its whole surface almost covered the last glass of the tube; and in like manner it happened under the compound microscope. But as often as I viewed any of the other objects depending perpendicularly from a perpendicular plane, in such a manner that the tube was supported in a horizontal situation directly opposite to it, the same always happened, and the appearance was not altered, when the object hung obliquely or even horizontally. I was mightily delighted with the observation of a tobacco-pipe, which had a porcelain bowl of a snowy whiteness, and a tube of horn almost black, and hung obliquely from a beam; the bowl preserved its natural convexity, and the tube was deeply sunk, and seemed to be almost immersed in the wall. I also observed, that when I placed the watch horizontally upon a horizontal plane, and then looked on it perpendicularly, near the window, it no longer appeared so depressed, and surrounded with a shady ring; whence I began to *suspect, that all those fallacies were owing to shade,* just as painters can elevate or depress a figure, by making the ground lighter or deeper. Thus, when the raised object was so placed between the windows, that it must *be illuminated on all sides*, it did not change its convexity. But at last I discovered a method of making objects always appear with their natural convexity. If any object hung against a wall, or was contiguous to it in any situation whatsoever, I viewed sideways, in such a manner as not to oppose the tube directly against it, but below the eminence near the plain at some distance. By those means, the protuberance of the instrument and other objects always appeared to me of their true natural convexity. With regard to the seal, I held it in such a manner, that the whole circumference was perpendicular, or rather a little inclined. Then I applied the lower side of the tube exactly to the upper margin of the disc of the seal, so that the tube formed an obtuse angle with the seal; then, carefully preserving the same situation, I very gently raised the tube from the rim of the seal upon its face; and then I always saw the seal with its true natural face. But why all these things happen exactly after the same manner, I do not pretend to determine; nor why white, or uncoloured transparent bodies, rising in any manner above any plain, afford an exception from that rule of vision, and do not appear depressed when viewed after the method above mentioned.

In the year 1780, this subject occupied the attention of David Rittenhouse, president of the American Philosophical Society, who gave a correct explanation of the illusion, by referring it to the inversion of the shadow by the eye-tube. He employed in his observations an eye-piece, having two lenses placed at a distance greater than the sum of their focal distances; and by throwing a reflected light on the cavities observed, in a direction opposite to that of the light, which came from his window, he was able to see them raised into elevations, by looking through a tube without any lenses. Mr Rittenhouse also observed, that, by putting his finger into the cavity, the illusion ceased to take place.

Having thus given a brief detail of the experiments of Gmelin and Rittenhouse, we shall proceed to explain more minutely the principles on which this illusion depends.

It will afterwards be seen, that inverting telescopes and microscopes are not necessary to the production of this illusion; but it may be best seen by viewing with the eye-piece of an achromatic telescope the engraving upon a seal, when

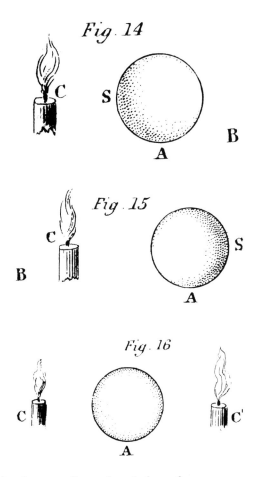

illuminated either by a candle or the window of an apartment. This eye-piece inverts the objects to which it is applied like the compound microscope, and the excavations or depressions of the seal are immediately raised up into elevations like a cameo, or a bas-relief. The cause of this illusion will be understood from Fig. 14, where A represents a spherical cavity illuminated by a candle C. The shadow of the cavity will of course be on the left side S, and, therefore, if we view it through an inverting eye-piece or microscope, the cavity will be seen as at A, Fig. 15, with its shadow on the right hand S of the cavity. As the candle C remains where it was, the observer instantly concludes, that what was formerly a cavity, must now be a spherical elevation or segment of a sphere, as nothing but a raised body could have its shadow on the right hand S. If a second candle is now placed on the right hand side of A, so that it is between two candles, and is equally illuminated by both, the elevation will again sink into a cavity, as in Fig. 16.

If the object A, in place of being a cavity, is actually the raised segment of a solid sphere, the same phenomena will be observed, the inverting eye-piece converting it into a cavity. These two experiments may be made most successfully with a seal, and an impression taken from it.

It cannot therefore be doubted, that the optical illusion of the conversion of a cameo into an intaglio, and of an intaglio into a cameo, by an inverting eye-piece, is the result of an operation of our own minds, whereby we judge of the forms of bodies by the knowledge we have acquired of light and shadow. The greater our knowledge is, of this subject, the more readily does the illusion seize upon us; while, if we are but imperfectly acquainted with the effects of light and shadow, the more difficult is it to be deceived. If the hollow is not polished, but ground, and the surface round and of uniform colour and smoothness, almost every person, whether young or old, will be subject to the illusion; but if the object is the raised impression of a seal upon wax, we have often found that, when viewed with the eye-piece, it still seemed raised to the three youngest of six persons, while the three eldest were subject to the deception. By such trifling, and often unappreciable circumstances, is our judgment affected, that the same person at one moment sees the convexity raised, and at another time depressed, though viewed as nearly as possible under the same circumstances. This remarkable effect no doubt arises from the introduction of some casual reflected lights, which the slightest change of position will produce.

Having thus seen how our judgment concerning elevations and depressions is affected by our degree of knowledge of the effects of light and shade, and by unappreciable causes, we shall proceed to consider how our judgment is again deceived by the introduction of new circumstances.

Let the depression A, illuminated by one candle, as in Fig. 14, be converted into an elevation as in Fig. 15, by the application of an inverting eye-piece; then, if another candle C', Fig. 16, is introduced so as to illuminate the depression A in the same manner, and with nearly the same intensity as C does, the elevation will fall down into a depression. The cause of this is obvious: the application of the inverting eye-piece produces no effect whatever, for both the sides of the cavity are symmetrically illuminated. In moving round the second candle C' from its position C', so as to stand beside C, it is curious to observe the progress of the deception by which the depression is again changed into an elevation.

If, when the depression A, Fig. 17, is converted into an elevation, we introduce a small unpolished opaque body M, and place it either beside the hollow or in it, so that the body M, and its shadow m, may be distinctly seen by the microscope, we shall have the appearance shown in Fig. 18, the elevation having sunk into a depression. This correction of the deception arises from the introduction of a new illusion, namely, that which arises from the shadow m; for it is evident, that, as the body M appears to project its shadow in the direction Mm, the luminous body must be supposed to be on the same side D; and the evidence that this is the

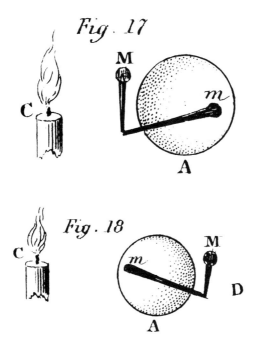

case, is more powerful than our knowledge that the candle is actually at C, because it co-exists along with our perception of the depression A, whereas our knowledge of the situation of the candle is an act of recollection.

This correction of the delusion may be effected in another manner, which is perhaps more complete. If, in place of the unpolished body, we use a pin with a highly polished head, as shown at M, Fig. 19, and then apply the inverting eye-piece, we shall have the effect shown in Fig. 20, the cavity A appearing depressed. The image *s* of the candle C being seen by reflection in the polished head of the pin M, is seen by the application of the eye-piece at *s*, on the right hand side of M in Fig. 20, so that we immediately conceive, in opposition to our previous knowledge, that the candle must be at D; and hence the elevation falls into a depression the moment the pin head is pushed up into the field of view. The shadow M*m* has also its influence in the present case.

The next case in which this illusion is dispelled, is, when the sense of touch corrects the deduction formed through the medium of sight. Let the cavity A be raised into an elevation by the inverting eye-piece, as in Fig. 15. Then, if the cavity is sufficiently deep, and if we place the point of our finger in the cavity, the evidence which this gives us of its being a depression, is superior to the evidence of its being a cavity arising from the inversion of the shadow; the apparent elevation will of course sink into a depression; but the moment the finger is

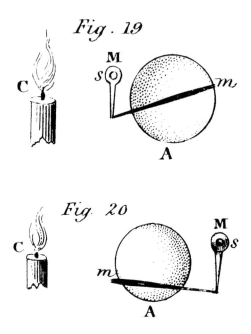

withdrawn, it will again rise into an elevation. If the cavity is a long groove, the part not touched by the finger will appear elevated, while the part touched by it will appear depressed!

Having thus considered some of the principal phenomena arising from the inversion of the object, we shall now proceed to explain some analogous facts which are owing to the semi-transparency of the body. If MN, Fig. 21, is a plate of mother-of-pearl, and A a cavity ground or turned in it; then if this cavity is illuminated by a candle C, or by a window at C, in place of there being a shadow at the side *s*, as there would have been had the body been opaque, there is a quantity of refracted light seen along the whole side *s*, next the candle. The consequence of this is, that the cavity appears as an elevation when seen only by the naked eye, as it is only an elevated surface that could have the side *s* illuminated. The fact which we have now stated, is, we think, a very important one, in so far as it may affect the labours of the sculptor. In some kinds of marble, the transparency is so great, that the depressions and elevations in the human face cannot be represented by it with any degree of accuracy; and, consequently, transparent marble ought never to be used for works of any importance.

Illusions arising from the same cause may be observed even when the surface of the object is perfectly plain and smooth. If MN, Fig. 22, is the surface of a mahogany table, MN *nm* a section of it, and *abc* a section of a knot in the wood, then it often happens, from the transparency of the thin edge at *a*, next the candle, that that side is illuminated while the opposite side at *c* is dark, the eye being

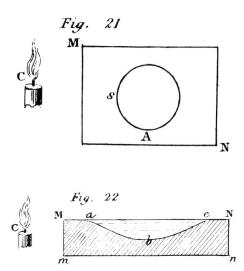

Fig. 21

Fig. 22

placed in the plane of the section *abc*. The consequence of this is, that the spot *abc* appears to be a hollow in the table.

Hence arises the appearance in certain plates of agate, which has obtained for it the name of *hammered agate*. The surface on which these cavities appears, is a section of small spherical aggregations of siliceous matter like *abc* in Fig. 22, which present exactly the same phenomenon, arising from the same cause as the knots in mahogany and other woods.

The very same phenomenon is often seen in mother-of-pearl. Indeed, it is so common in this substance, that it is almost impossible to find a mother-of-pearl counter which seems to have its surfaces flat, although they are perfectly so when examined by the touch. Owing to the refraction of the light by the different growths of the shell lying in different planes, the flattest surface seems to be inequal and undulating.

One of the finest deceptions which we have ever met with, arising from the disposition of light and shadow, presented itself on viewing through a telescope the surface of a growing field of corn, illuminated by the sun when near the horizon. This field, on Sir Walter Scott's estate at Abbotsford, was about two miles distant, and was divided into furrows, which were directed to the eye of the observer, as shown in Fig. 23, where AB, CD, EF, represent the furrows. These furrows are of course depressed, and the growing corn rises gradually from two adjacent ones towards the middle *mn*, *op*, so that the surfaces A*m*C, C*o*E were convex. The drills of corn on the highest summits *mn*, *op*, caught the rays of the setting sun, which shone upon them very obliquely in the direction S*s*,* and

* No letters S or s are shown in Fig. 3. (Ed.)

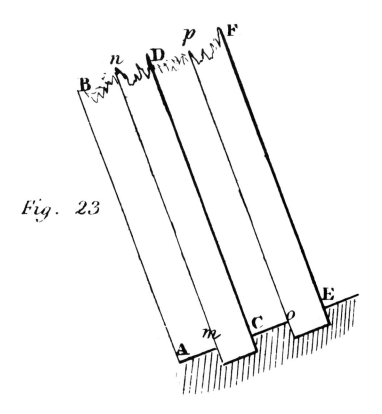

Fig. 23

illuminated their summits laterally, while the furrows AB, CD, EF, were in shadow. The consequence of this disposition of the light and shade was, that the whole field seemed to be trenched, and the corn to be growing in the trenches as well as upon the elevated beds between them. The half furrow AB *nm* being shaded on its edge AB, and illuminated on its edge *mn*, became the elevated part of the trenched ground, while the other half *mn* CD appeared the sunk part, in consequence of the side *mn* being illuminated, and its other side CD in shade. At a certain period of the day, this deception did not take place, and it was dispelled the moment the sun had set. This very singular illusion we have seen on several days in July. The telescope had no effect whatever in producing it, as it showed objects erect.

An illusion of an analogous nature we once observed when looking at the Abbey Church of Paisley, where the clustered columns of a Gothic pillar all sunk into hollow flutings. The cause of this deception was not discovered, but it must have arisen from some mistaken notion respecting the direction in which the object was illuminated.

The last species of illusion of this nature, and perhaps the most remarkable of all of them, may be produced by a continued effort of the mind to deceive itself. If we take one of the intaglio moulds used for making the bas-reliefs of that able artist Mr Henning, and direct the eye to it steadily without noticing surrounding objects, we may coax ourselves into the belief that the intaglio is actually a bas-relief. It is difficult at first to produce the deception, but a little practice never fails to accomplish it.

We have succeeded in carrying this deception so far, as to be able, by the eye alone, to raise a complete hollow mask of the human face into a projecting head. In order to do this, we must exclude the vision of other objects; and also the margin or thickness of the cast. This experiment cannot fail to produce a very great degree of surprise in those who succeed in it; and it will no doubt be regarded by the sculptor who can use it as a great auxiliary in his art.

D. B.

2.4. Wheatstone: "Contributions to the physiology of vision – Part the first. On some remarkable, and hitherto unobserved, phenomena of binocular vision". *Philosophical Transactions of the Royal Society*, 1838, **128**, 371–394.

---

§ 1.

When an object is viewed at so great a distance that the optic axes of both eyes are sensibly parallel when directed towards it, the perspective projections of it, seen by each eye separately, and the appearance to the two eyes is precisely the same as when the object is seen by one eye only. There is, in such case, no difference between the visual appearance of an object in relief and its perspective projection on a plane surface; and hence pictorial representations of distant objects, when those circumstances which would prevent or disturb the illusion are carefully excluded, may be rendered such perfect resemblances of the objects they are intended to represent as to be mistaken for them; the Diorama is an instance of this. But this similarity no longer exists when the object is placed so near the eyes that to view it the optic axes must converge; under these conditions a different perspective projection of it is seen by each eye, and these perspectives are more dissimilar as the convergence of the optic axes becomes greater. This fact may be easily verified by placing any figure of three dimensions, an outline cube for instance, at a moderate distance before the eyes, and while the head is kept perfectly steady, viewing it with each eye successively while the other is closed. Figure 13 represents the two perspective projections of a cube; *b* is that seen by the right eye, and *a* that presented to the left eye; the figure being supposed to be placed about seven inches immediately before the spectator.

The appearances, which are by this simple experiment rendered so obvious, may be easily inferred from the established laws of perspective; for the same object in relief is, when viewed by a different eye, seen from two points of sight at a distance from each other equal to the line joining the two eyes. Yet they seem to have escaped the attention of every philosopher and artist who has treated of the subjects of vision and perspective. I can ascribe this inattention to a phenomenon leading to the important and curious consequences, which will form the subject of the present communication, only to this circumstance; that the results being contrary to a principle which was very generally maintained by optical writers, viz. that objects can be seen single only when their images fall on corresponding points of the two retinæ, an hypothesis which will be hereafter discussed, if the consideration ever arose in their minds, it was hastily discarded under the conviction, that if the pictures presented to the two eyes are under certain circumstances dissimilar, their differences must be so small that they need not be taken into account.

It will now be obvious why it is impossible for the artist to give a faithful representation of any near solid object, that is, to produce a painting which shall not be distinguished in the mind from the object itself. When the painting and the object are seen with both eyes, in the case of the painting two *similar* pictures are projected on the retinæ, in the case of the solid object the pictures are *dissimilar*; there is therefore an essential difference between the impressions on the organs of sensation in the two cases, and consequently between the perceptions formed in the mind; the painting therefore cannot be confounded with the solid object.

After looking over the works of many authors who might be expected to have made some remarks relating to this subject, I have been able to find but one, which is in the Trattato della Pittura of Leonardo da Vinci.* This great artist and ingenious philosopher observes, "that a painting, though conducted with the greatest art and finished to the last perfection, both with regard to its contours, its lights, its shadows and its colours, can never show a relievo equal to that of the natural objects, unless these be viewed at a distance and with a single eye. For," says he,

> if an object C (Fig. 1) be viewed by a single eye at A, all objects in the space behind it, included as it were in a shadow ECF cast by a candle at A, are invisible to the eye at A; but when the other eye at B is opened, part of these objects become visible to it; those only being hid from both eyes that are included, as it were, in the double shadow CD, cast by two lights at A and B, and terminated in D, the angular space EDG beyond D being always visible to both eyes. And the hidden space CD is so much the shorter, as the object C is smaller and nearer to the eyes. Thus the object

---

* See also a Treatise of Painting, p. 178. London, 1721; and Dr. Smith's Complete System of Optics, vol. ii. r. 244, where the passage is quoted.

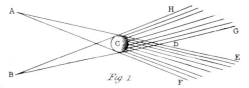

Fig. 1.

C seen with both eyes becomes, as it were, transparent, according to the usual definition of a transparent thing; namely, that which hides nothing beyond it. But this cannot happen when an object, whose breadth is bigger than that of the pupil, is viewed by a single eye. The truth of this observation is therefore evident, because a painted figure intercepts all the space behind its apparent place, so as to preclude the eyes from the sight of every part of the imaginary ground behind it.

Had Leonardo da Vinci taken, instead of a sphere, a less simple figure for the purpose of his illustration, a cube for instance, he would not only have observed that the object obscured from each eye a different part of the more distant field of view, but the fact would also perhaps have forced itself upon his attention, that the object itself presented a different appearance to each eye. He failed to do this, and no subsequent writer within my knowledge has supplied the omission; the projection of two obviously dissimilar pictures on the two retinæ when a single object is viewed, while the optic axes converge, must therefore be regarded as a new fact in the theory of vision.

§ 2.

It being thus established that the mind perceives an object of three dimensions by means of the two dissimilar pictures projected by it on the two retinæ, the following question occurs: What would be the visual effect of simultaneously presenting to each eye, instead of the object itself, its projection on a plane surface as it appears to that eye? To pursue this inquiry it is necessary that means should be contrived to make the two pictures, which must necessarily occupy different places, fall on similar parts of both retinæ. Under the ordinary circumstances of vision the object is seen at the concourse of the optic axes, and its images consequently are projected on similar parts of the two retinæ; but it is also evident that two exactly similar objects may be made to fall on similar parts of the two retinæ, if they are placed one in the direction of each optic axis, at equal distances before or beyond their intersection.

Figure 2 represents the usual situation of an object at the intersection of the optic axes. In Fig. 3 the similar objects are placed in the direction of the optic axes before their intersection, and in Fig. 4 beyond it. In all these three cases the mind perceives but a single object, and refers it to the place where the optic axes meet. It will be observed, that when the eyes converge beyond the objects, as in Fig. 3, the right hand object is seen by the right eye, and the left hand object by the left

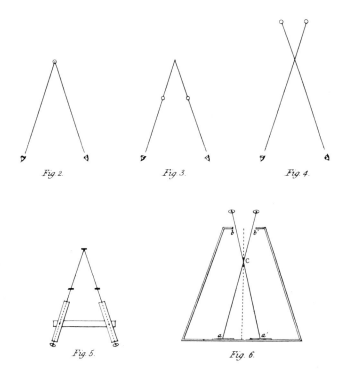

Fig 2.   Fig 3.   Fig 4.

Fig 5.   Fig 6.

eye; while when the axes converge nearer than the objects, the right hand object is seen by the left eye, and conversely. As both of these modes of vision are forced and unnatural, eyes unaccustomed to such experiments require some artificial assistance. If the eyes are to converge beyond the objects, this may be afforded by a pair of tubes (Fig. 5) capable of being inclined towards each other at various angles, so as to correspond with the different convergences of the optic axes. If the eyes are to converge at a nearer distance than that at which the objects are placed, a box (Fig. 6) may be conveniently employed; the objects *aa'* are placed distant from each other, on a stand capable of being moved nearer the eyes if required, and the optic axes being directed towards them will cross at *c*, the aperture *bb'* allowing the visual rays from the right hand object to reach the left eye, and those from the left hand object to fall on the right eye; the coincidence of the images may be facilitated by placing the point of a needle at the point of intersection of the optic axes *c*, and fixing the eyes upon it. In both these instruments (Figs. 5 and 6) the lateral images are hidden from view, and much less difficulty occurs in making the images unite than when the naked eyes are employed.

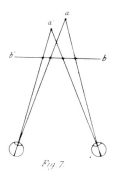

Fig. 7.

Now if, instead of placing two exactly similar objects to be viewed by the eyes in either of the modes above described, the two perspective projections of the same solid object be so disposed, the mind will still perceive the object to be single, but instead of a representation on a plane surface, as each drawing appears to be when separately viewed by that eye which is directed towards it, the observer will perceive a figure of three dimensions, the exact counterpart of the object from which the drawings were made. To make this matter clear I will mention one or two of the most simple cases.

If two vertical lines near each other, but at different distances from the spectator, be regarded first with one eye and then with the other, the distance between them when referred to the same plane will appear different; if the left hand line be nearer to the eyes, the distance as seen by the left eye will be less than the distance as seen by the right eye; Fig. 7 will render this evident; aa' are vertical sections of the two original lines, and bb' the plane to which their projections are referred. Now if the two lines be drawn on two pieces of card, at the respective distances at which they appear to each eye, and these cards be afterwards viewed by either of the means above directed, the observer will no longer see two lines on a plane surface, as each card separately shows; but two lines will appear, one nearer to him than the other, precisely as the original vertical lines themselves. Again, if a straight wire be held before the eyes in such a position that one of its ends shall be nearer to the observer than the other is, each eye separately referring it to a plane perpendicular to the common axis, will see a line differently inclined; and then if lines having the same apparent inclinations be drawn on two pieces of card, and be presented to the eyes as before directed, the real position of the original line will be correctly perceived by the mind.

In the same manner the most complex figures of three dimensions may be accurately represented to the mind, by presenting their two perspective projections to the two retinæ. But I shall defer these more perfect experiments until I describe an instrument which will enable any person to observe all the phenomena in question with the greatest ease and certainty.

In the instruments above described the optic axes converge to some point in a plane before or beyond that in which the objects to be seen are situated. The adaptation of the eye, which enables us to see distinctly at different distances, and which habitually accompanies every different degree of convergence of the optic axes, does not immediately adjust itself to the new and unusual condition; and to persons not accustomed to experiments of this kind, the pictures will either not readily unite, or will appear dim and confused. Besides this, no object can be viewed according to either mode when the drawings exceed in breadth the distance of the two points of the optic axes in which their centres are placed.

These inconveniences are removed by the instrument I am about to describe; the two pictures (or rather their reflected images) are placed in it at the true concourse of the optic axes, the focal adaptation of the eye preserves its usual adjustment, the appearance of lateral images is entirely avoided, and a large field of view for each eye is obtained. The frequent reference I shall have occasion to make to this instrument, will render it convenient to give it a specific name, I therefore propose that it be called a Stereoscope, to indicate its property of representing solid figures.

§ 3.

The stereoscope is represented by Figs. 8 and 9; the former being a front view, and the latter a plan of the instrument. AA′ are two plane mirrors, about four inches square, inserted in frames, and so adjusted that their backs form an angle of 90° with each other; these mirrors are fixed by their common edge against an upright B, or which was less easy to represent in the drawing, against the middle line of a vertical board, cut away in such manner as to allow the eyes to be placed before the two mirrors. CC′ are two sliding boards, to which are attached the upright boards DD′, which may thus be removed to different distances from the mirrors. In most of the experiments hereafter to be detailed, it is necessary that each upright board shall be at the same distance from the mirror which is opposite to it. To facilitate this double adjustment, I employ a right and a left-handed wooden screw, rl; the two ends of this compound screw pass through the nuts $ee′$, which are fixed to the lower parts of the upright boards DD′, so that by turning the screw pin p one way the two boards will approach, and by turning it the other they will recede from each other, one always preserving the same distance as the other from the middle line f. EE′ are pannels, to which the pictures are fixed in such manner that their corresponding horizontal lines shall be on the same level: these pannels are capable of sliding backwards and forwards in grooves on the upright boards DD′. The apparatus having been described, it now remains to explain the manner of using it. The observer must place his eyes as near as possible to the mirrors, the right eye before the right hand mirror, and the left eye before the left hand mirror, and he must move the sliding pannels EE′

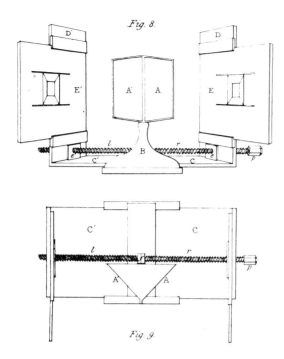

Fig. 8.

Fig. 9.

to or from him until the two reflected images coincide at the intersection of the optic axes, and form an image of the same apparent magnitude as each of the component pictures. The pictures will indeed coincide when the sliding pannels are in a variety of different positions, and consequently when viewed under different inclinations of the optic axes; but there is only one position in which the binocular image will be immediately seen single, of its proper magnitude, and without fatigue to the eyes, because in this position only the ordinary relations between the magnitude of the pictures on the retina, the inclination of the optic axes, and the adaptation of the eye to distinct vision at different distances are preserved. The alteration in the apparent magnitude of the binocular images, when these usual relations are disturbed, will be discussed in another paper of this series, with a variety of remarkable phenomena depending thereon. In all the experiments detailed in the present memoir I shall suppose these relations to remain undisturbed, and the optic axes to converge about six or eight inches before the eyes.

If the pictures are all drawn to be seen with the same inclination of the optic axes, the apparatus may be simplified by omitting the screw *rl* and fixing the upright boards DD′ at the proper distances. The sliding pannels may also be dispensed with, and the drawings themselves be made to slide in the grooves.

§ 4.

A few pairs of outline figures, calculated to give rise to the perception of objects of three dimensions when placed in the stereoscope in the manner described, are represented from Figs. 10 to 20. They are one half the linear size of the figures actually employed.* As the drawings are reversed by reflection in the mirrors, I will suppose these figures to be the reflected images to which the eyes are directed in the apparatus; those marked *b* being seen by the right eye, and those marked *a* by the left eye. The drawings, it has been already explained, are two different projections of the same object seen from two points of sight, the distance between which is equal to the interval between the eyes of the observer; this interval is generally about 2½ inches.

a and *b*, Fig. 10 will, when viewed in the stereoscope, present to the mind a line in the vertical plane, with its lower end inclined towards the observer. If the two component lines be caused to turn round their centres equally in opposite directions, the resultant line will, while it appears to assume every degree of inclination to the referent plane, still seem to remain in the same vertical plane.

Fig. 11. A series of points all in the same horizontal plane, but each towards the right hand successively nearer the observer.

Fig. 12. A curved line intersecting the referent plane, and having its convexity towards the observer.

Fig. 13. A cube.

Fig. 14. A cone, having its axis perpendicular to the referent plane, and its vertex towards the observer.

Fig. 15. The frustum of a square pyramid; its axis perpendicular to the referent plane, and its base furthest from the eye.

Fig. 16. Two circles at different distances from the eyes, their centres in the same perpendicular, forming the outline of the frustum of a cone.

The other figures require no observation.

For the purposes of illustration I have employed only outline figures, for had either shading or colouring been introduced it might be supposed that the effect was wholly or in part due to these circumstances, whereas by leaving them out of consideration no room is left to doubt that the entire effect of relief is owing to the simultaneous perception of the two monocular projections, one on each retina. But if it be required to obtain the most faithful resemblances of real objects, shadowing and colouring may properly be employed to heighten the effects. Careful attention would enable an artist to draw and paint the two component pictures, so as to present to the mind of the observer, in the resultant perception, perfect identity with the object represented. Flowers, crystals, busts, vases,

---

* The figures reproduced opposite are slightly smaller than those in the original Plate, being about 0.4 of the linear size of the figures actually employed. (Ed.)

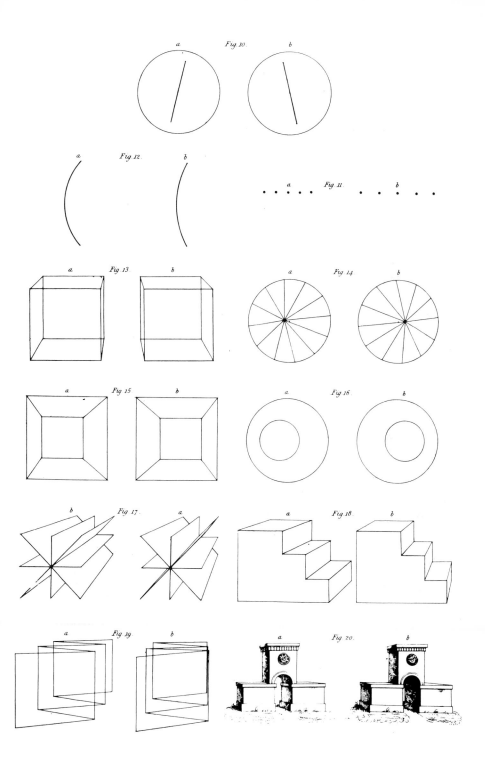

instruments of various kinds, &c., might thus be represented so as not to be distinguished by sight from the real objects themselves.

It is worthy of remark, that the process by which we thus become acquainted with the real forms of solid objects, is precisely that which is employed in descriptive geometry, an important science we owe to the genius of Monge, but which is little studied or known in this country. In this science, the position of a point, a right line or a curve, and consequently of any figure whatever, is completely determined by assigning its projections on two fixed planes, the situations of which are known, and which are not parallel to each other. In the problems of descriptive geometry the two referent planes are generally assumed to be at right angles to each other, but in binocular vision the inclination of these planes is less according as the angle made at the concourse of the optic axes is less; thus the same solid object is represented to the mind by different pairs of monocular pictures, according as they are placed at a different distance before the eyes, and the perception of these differences (though we seem to be unconscious of them) may assist in suggesting to the mind the distance of the object. The more inclined to each other the referent planes are, with the greater accuracy are the various points of the projections referred to their proper places; and it appears to be a useful provision that the real forms of those objects which are nearest to us are thus more determinately apprehended than those which are more distant.

§ 5.

A very singular effect is produced when the drawing originally intended to be seen by the right eye is placed at the left hand side of the stereoscope, and that designed to be seen by the left eye is placed on its right hand side. A figure of three dimensions, as bold in relief as before, is perceived, but it has a different form from that which is seen when the drawings are in their proper places. There is a certain relation between the proper figure and this, which I shall call its *converse* figure. Those points which are nearest the observer in the proper figure are the most remote from him in the converse figure, and *vice versâ*, so that the figure is, as it were, inverted; but it is not an exact inversion, for the near parts of the converse figure appear smaller, and the remote parts larger than the same parts before the inversion. Hence the drawings which, properly placed, occasion a cube to be perceived, when changed in the manner described, represent the frustum of a square pyramid with its base remote from the eye: the cause of this is easy to understand.

This conversion of relief may be shown by all the pairs of drawings from Figs. 10 to 19. In the case of simple figures like these the converse figure is as readily apprehended as the original one, because it is generally a figure of as frequent occurrence; but in the case of a more complicated figure, an architectural design, for instance, the mind, unaccustomed to perceive its converse, because it never occurs in nature, can find no meaning in it.

§ 6.

The same image is depicted on the retina by an object of three dimensions as by its projection on a plane surface, provided the point of sight remain in both cases the same. There should be, therefore, no difference in the binocular appearance of two drawings, one presented to each eye, and of two real objects so presented to the two eyes that their projections on the retina shall be the same as those arising from the drawings. The following experiments will prove the justness of this inference.

I procured several pairs of skeleton figures, i.e. outline figures of three dimensions, formed either of iron wire or of ebony beading about one tenth of an inch in thickness. The pair I most frequently employed consisted of two cubes, whose sides were three inches in length. When I placed these skeleton figures on stands before the two mirrors of the stereoscope, the following effects were produced, according as their relative positions were changed. 1st. When they were so placed that the pictures which their reflected images projected on the two retinæ were precisely the same as those which would have been projected by a cube placed at the concourse of the optic axes, a cube in relief appeared before the eyes. 2ndly. When they were so placed that their reflected images projected exactly similar pictures on the two retinæ, all effect of relief was destroyed, and the compound appearance was that of an outline representation on a plane surface. 3rdly. When the cubes were so placed that the reflected image of one projected on the left retina the same picture as in the first case was projected on the right retina, and conversely, the converse figure in relief appeared.

§ 7.

If a symmetrical object, that is one whose right and left sides are exactly similar to each other but inverted, be placed so that any point in the plane which divides it into these two halves is equally distant from the two eyes, its two monocular projections are, it is easy to see, inverted fac-similes of each other. Thus Fig. 15, *a* and *b* are symmetrical monocular projections of the frustum of a four-sided pyramid, and Figs. 13, 14, 16 are corresponding projections of other symmetrical objects. This being kept in view, I will describe an experiment which, had it been casually observed previous to the knowledge of the principles developed in this paper, would have appeared an inexplicable optical illusion.

M and M' (Fig. 21) are two mirrors, inclined so that their *faces* form an angle of 90° with each other. Between them in the bisecting plane is placed a plane outline figure, such as Fig. 15*a*, made of card all parts but the lines being cut away, or of

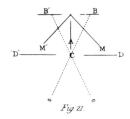

Fig 21

wire. A reflected image of this outline, placed at A, will appear behind each mirror at B and B', and one of these images will be the inversion of the other. If the eyes be made to converge at C, it is obvious that these two reflected images will fall on corresponding parts of the two retinæ, and a figure of three dimensions will be perceived; if the outline placed in the bisecting plane be reversed, the converse skeleton form will appear; in both these experiments we have the singular phenomenon of the conversion of a single plane outline into a figure of three dimensions. To render the binocular object more distinct, concave lenses may be applied to the eyes; and to prevent the two lateral images from being seen, screens may be placed at D and D'.

§ 8.

An effect of binocular perspective may be remarked in a plate of metal, the surface of which has been made smooth by turning it in a lathe. When a single candle is brought near such a plate, a line of light appears standing out from it, one half being above, and the other half below the surface; the position and inclination of this line changes with the situation of the light and of the observer, but it always passes through the centre of the plate. On closing the left eye the relief disappears, and the luminous line coincides with one of the diameters of the plate; on closing the right eye the line appears equally in the plane of the surface, but coincides with another diameter; on opening both eyes it instantly starts into relief.* The case here is exactly analogous to the vision of two inclined lines (Fig. 10) when each is presented to a different eye in the stereoscope. It is curious, that an effect like this, which must have been seen thousands of times, should never have attracted sufficient attention to have been made the subject of philosophic observation. It was one of the earliest facts which drew my attention to the subject I am now treating.

Dr. Smith† was very much puzzled by an effect of binocular perspective which

---

* The luminous line seen by a single eye arises from the reflection of the light from each of the concentric circles produced in the operation of turning; when the plate is not large the arrangement of these successive reflections does not differ from a straight line.
† System of Optics, vol. ii. p. 388. and r. 526.

he observed, but was unable to explain. He opened a pair of compasses, and while he held the joint in his hand, and the points outwards and equidistant from his eyes, and somewhat higher than the joint, he looked at a more distant point; the compasses appeared double. He then compressed the legs until the two inner points coincided; having done this the two inner legs also entirely coincided, and bisected the angle formed by the outward ones, appearing longer and thicker than they did, and reaching from the hand to the remotest object in view. The explanation offered by Dr. Smith accounts only for the coincidence of the points of the compasses, not for that of the entire leg. The effect in question is best seen by employing a pair of straight wires, about a foot in length. A similar observation, made with two flat rulers, and afterwards with silk threads, induced Dr. Wells to propose a new theory of visible direction in order to explain it, so inexplicable did it seem to him by any of the received theories.

§ 9.

The preceding experiments render it evident that there is an essential difference in the appearance of objects when seen with two eyes, and when only one eye is employed, and that the most vivid belief of the solidity of an object of three dimensions arises from two different perspective projections of it being simultaneously presented to the mind. How happens it then, it may be asked, that persons who see with only one eye form correct notions of solid objects, and never mistake them for pictures? and how happens it also, that a person having the perfect use of both eyes, perceives no difference in objects around him when he shuts one of them? To explain these apparent difficulties, it must be kept in mind, that although the simultaneous vision of two dissimilar pictures suggests the relief of objects in the most vivid manner, yet there are other signs which suggest the same ideas to the mind, which, though more ambiguous than the former, become less liable to lead the judgment astray in proportion to the extent of our previous experience. The vividness of relief arising from the projection of two dissimilar pictures, one on each retina, becomes less and less as the object is seen at a greater distance before the eyes, and entirely ceases when it is so distant that the optic axes are parallel while regarding it. We see with both eyes all objects beyond this distance precisely as we see near objects with a single eye; for the pictures on the two retinæ are then exactly similar, and the mind appreciates no difference whether two identical pictures fall on corresponding parts of the two retinæ, or whether one eye is impressed with only one of these pictures. A person deprived of the sight of one eye sees therefore all external objects, near and remote, as a person with both eyes sees remote objects only, but that vivid effect arising from the binocular vision of near objects is not perceived by the former; to supply this deficiency he has recourse unconsciously to other means of acquiring more accurate information. The motion of the head is the principal means he employs.

That the required knowledge may be thus obtained will be evident from the following considerations. The mind associates with the idea of a solid object every different projection of it which experience has hitherto afforded; a single projection may be ambiguous, from its being also one of the projections of a picture, or of a different solid object; but when different projections of the same object are successively presented, they cannot all belong to another object, and the form to which they belong is completely characterized. While the object remains fixed, at every movement of the head it is viewed from a different point of sight, and the picture on the retina consequently continually changes.

Every one must be aware how greatly the perspective effect of a picture is enhanced by looking at it with only one eye, especially when a tube is employed to exclude the vision of adjacent objects, whose presence might disturb the illusion. Seen under such circumstances from the proper point of sight, the picture projects the same lines, shades and colours on the retina, as the more distant scene which it represents would do were it substituted for it. The appearance which would make us certain that it is a picture is excluded from the sight, and the imagination has room to be active. Several of the older writers erroneously attributed this apparent superiority of monocular vision to the concentration of the visual power in a single eye.*

There is a well-known and very striking illusion of perspective which deserves a passing remark, because the reason of the effect does not appear to be generally understood. When a perspective of a building is projected on a horizontal plane, so that the point of sight is in a line greatly inclined towards the plane, the building appears to a single eye placed at the point of sight to be in bold relief, and the illusion is almost as perfect as in the binocular experiments described in §§ 2, 3, 4. This effect wholly arises from the unusual projection, which suggests to the mind more readily the object itself than the drawing of it; for we are accustomed to see real objects in almost every point of view, but perspective representations being generally made in a vertical plane with the point of sight in a line perpendicular to the plane of projection, we are less familiar with the appearance of other projections. Any other unusual projection will produce the same effect.

§ 10.

If we look with a single eye at the drawing of a solid geometrical figure, it may be imagined to be the representation of either of two dissimilar solid figures, the figure intended to be represented, or its converse figure (§ 5.). If the former is a very usual, and the latter a very unusual figure, the imagination will fix itself on the original without wandering to the converse figure; but if both are of ordinary

---

* "We see more exquisitely with one eye shut than with both, because the vital spirits thus unite themselves the more, and become the stronger: for we may find by looking in a glass whilst we shut one eye, that the pupil of the other dilates." – Lord Bacon's Works, Sylva Sylvarum, art. Vision.

occurrence, which is generally the case with regard to simple forms, a singular phenomenon takes place; it is perceived at one time distinctly as one of these figures, at another time as the other, and while one figure continues it is not in the power of the will to change it immediately.

The same phenomenon takes place, though less decidedly, when the drawing is seen with both eyes. Many of my readers will call to mind the puzzling effect of some of the diagrams annexed to the problems of the eleventh book of Euclid; which, when they were attentively looked at, changed in an arbitrary manner from one solid figure to another, and would obstinately continue to present the converse figures when the real figures alone were wanted. This perplexing illusion must be of common occurrence, but I have only found one recorded observation relating to the subject. It is by Professor Necker of Geneva, and I shall quote it in his own words from the Philosophical Magazine, Third Series, vol. i. p. 337.

> The object I have now to call your attention to is an observation which has often occurred to me while examining figures and engraved plates of crystalline forms; I mean a sudden and involuntary change in the apparent position of a crystal or solid represented in an engraved figure. What I mean will be more easily understood from the figure annexed (Fig. 22). The rhomboid AX is drawn so that the solid angle A should be seen the nearest to the spectator, and the solid angle X the farthest from him, and that the face ACDB should be the foremost, while the face XDC is behind. But in looking repeatedly at the same figure, you will perceive that at times the apparent position of the rhomboid is so changed that the solid angle X will appear the nearest, and the solid angle A the farthest; and that the face ACDB will recede behind the face XDC, which will come forward, which effect gives to the whole solid a quite contrary apparent inclination.

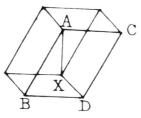

Fig 22.

Professor Necker attributes this alteration of appearance, not to a mental operation, but to an involuntary change in the adjustment of the eye for obtaining distinct vision. He supposed that whenever the point of distinct vision on the retina is directed on the angle A, for instance, this angle seen more distinctly than the others is naturally supposed to be nearer and foremost, while the other angles seen indistinctly are supposed to be farther and behind, and that the reverse takes place when the point of distinct vision is brought to bear on the angle X.

That this is not the true explanation, is evident from three circumstances: in the first place, the two points A and X being both at the same distance from the eyes, the same alteration of adjustment which would make one of them indistinct would make the other so; secondly, the figure will undergo the same changes whether the focal distance of the eye be adjusted to a point before or beyond the place in which the figure is drawn; and thirdly, the change of figure frequently occurs while the eye continues to look at the same angle. The effect seems entirely to depend on our mental contemplation of the figure intended to be represented, or of its converse. By following the lines with the eye with a clear idea of the solid figure we are describing, it may be fixed for any length of time; but it requires practice to do this or to change the figure at will. As I have before observed, these effects are far more obvious when the figures are regarded with one eye only.

No illusion of this kind can take place when an object of three dimensions is seen with both eyes while the optic axes make a sensible angle with each other, because the appearance of the two dissimilar images, one to each eye, prevents the possibility of mistake. But if we regard an object at such a distance that its two projections are sensibly identical, and if this projection be capable of a double interpretation, the illusion may occur. Thus a placard on a pole carried in the streets, with one of its sides inclined towards the observer, will, when he is distant from it, frequently appear inclined in a contrary direction. Many analogous instances might be adduced, but this will suffice to call others to mind; it must however be observed, that when shadows, or other means capable of determining the judgement are present, these fallacies do not arise.

§ 11.

The same indetermination of judgement which causes a drawing to be perceived by the mind at different times as two different figures, frequently gives rise to a false perception when objects in relief are regarded with a single eye. The apparent conversion of a cameo into an intaglio, and of an intaglio into a cameo, is a well-known instance of this fallacy in vision; but the fact does not appear to me to have been correctly explained, nor the conditions under which it occurs to have been properly stated.

This curious illusion, which has been the subject of much attention, was first observed at one of the early meetings of the Royal Society.* Several of the members looking through a compound microscope of a new construction at a guinea, some of them imagined the image to be depressed, while others thought it to be embossed, as it really was. Professor Gmelin, of Wurtemburg, published a paper on the same subject in the Philosophical Transactions for 1745; his

---

* Birch's History, vol. ii. p. 348.

experiments were made with telescopes and compound microscopes which inverted the images; and he observed that the conversion of relief appeared in some cases and not in others, at some times and not at others, and to some eyes also and not to others. He endeavoured to ascertain some of the conditions of the two appearances; "but why these things should so happen," says he, "I do not pretend to determine."

Sir David Brewster accounts for the fallacy in the following manner*:–

> A hollow seal being illuminated by a window or a candle, its shaded side is of course on the same side with the light. If we now invert the seal with one or more lenses, so that it may look in the opposite direction, it will appear to the eye with the shaded side furthest from the window. But as we know that the window is still on our left hand, and as every body with its shaded side furthest from the light must necessarily be convex or protuberant, we immediately believe that the hollow seal is now a cameo or bas-relief. The proof which the eye thus receives of the seal being raised, overcomes the evidence of its being hollow, derived from our actual knowledge and from the sense of touch. In this experiment the deception takes place from our knowing the real direction of the light which falls on the seal; for if the place of the window, with respect to the seal, had been inverted as well as the seal itself, the illusion could not have taken place. The illusion, therefore, under our consideration is the result of an operation of our own minds, whereby we judge of the forms of bodies by the knowledge we have acquired of light and shadow. Hence the illusion depends on the accuracy and extent of our knowledge on this subject; and while some persons are under its influence, others are entirely insensible to it.

These considerations do not fully explain the phenomenon, for they suppose that the image must be inverted, and that the light must fall in a particular direction; but the conversion of relief will still take place when the object is viewed through an open tube without any lenses to invert it, and also when it is equally illuminated in all parts. The true explanation I believe to be the following. If we suppose a cameo and an intaglio of the same object, the elevations of the one corresponding exactly to the depressions of the other, it is easy to show that the projection of either on the retina is sensibly the same. When the cameo or the intaglio is seen with both eyes, it is impossible to mistake an elevation for a depression, for reasons which have been already amply explained; but when either is seen with one eye only, the most certain guide of our judgement, viz. the presentation of a different picture to each eye, is wanting; the imagination therefore supplies the deficiency, and we conceive the object to be raised or depressed according to the dictates of this faculty. No doubt in such cases our judgement is in a great degree influenced by accessory circumstances, and the intaglio or the relief may sometimes present itself according to our previous knowledge of the direction in which the shadows ought to appear; but the real cause of the phenomenon is to be found in the indetermination of the judgement arising from our more perfect means of judging being absent.

* Natural Magic, p. 100.

Observers with the microscope must be particularly on their guard against illusions of this kind. Raspail observes* that the hollow pyramidal arrangement of the crystals of muriate of soda appears, when seen through a microscope, like a striated pyramid in relief. He recommends two modes of correcting the illusion. The first is to bring successively to the focus of the instrument the different parts of the crystal; if the pyramid be in relief, the point will arrive at the focus sooner than the base will; if the pyramid be hollow, the contrary will take place. The second mode is to project a strong light on the pyramid in the field of view of the microscope, and to observe which sides of the crystal are illuminated, taking however the inversion of the image into consideration if a compound microscope be employed.

The inversion of relief is very striking when a skeleton cube is looked at with one eye, and the following singular results may in this case be observed. So long as the mind perceives the cube, however the figure be turned about, its various appearances will be but different representations of the same object, and the same primitive form will be suggested to the mind by all of them: but it is not so if the converse figure fixes the attention; the series of successive projections cannot then be referred to any figure to which they are all common, and the skeleton figure will appear to be continually undergoing a change of shape.

§ 12.

I have given ample proof that objects whose pictures do not fall on corresponding points of the two retinæ may still appear single. I will now adduce an experiment which proves that similar pictures falling on corresponding points of the two retinæ may appear double and in different places.

Present, in the stereoscope, to the right eye a vertical line, and to the left eye a line inclined some degrees from the perpendicular (Fig. 23); the observer will then perceive, as formerly explained, a line, the extremities of which appear at different distances before the eyes. Draw on the left hand figure a faint vertical line exactly corresponding in position and length to that presented to the right eye, and let the two lines of this left hand figure intersect each other at their centres. Looking now at these two drawings in the stereoscope, the two strong lines, each seen by a different eye, will coincide, and the resultant perspective line will appear to occupy the same place as before; but the faint line which now falls on a line of the left retina, which corresponds with the line of the right retina on which one of the coinciding strong lines, viz. the vertical one, falls, appears in a different place. The place this faint line apparently occupies is the intersection of that plane of visual direction of the left eye in which it is situated, with the plane of visual direction of the right eye, which contains the strong vertical line.

* Nouveau Système de Chimie Organique, 2me edit. t. 1. p. 333.

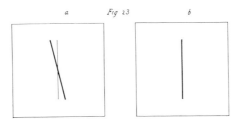

This experiment affords another proof that there is no necessary physiological connection between the corresponding points of the two retinæ, – a doctrine which has been maintained by so many authors.

§ 13. *Binocular vision of images of different magnitudes.*

We will now inquire what effect results from presenting similar images, differing only in magnitude, to analogous parts of the two retinæ. For this purpose two squares or circles, differing obviously but not extravagantly in size, may be drawn on two separate pieces of paper, and placed in the stereoscope so that the reflected image of each shall be equally distant from the eye by which it is regarded. It will then be seen that, notwithstanding this difference, they coalesce and occasion a single resultant perception. The limit of the difference of size within which the single appearance subsists may be ascertained by employing two images of equal magnitude, and causing one of them to recede from the eye while the other remains at a constant distance; this is effected merely by pulling out the sliding board C (Fig. 8) while the other C′ remains fixed, the screw having previously been removed.

Though the single appearance of two images of different size is by this experiment demonstrated, the observer is unable to perceive what difference exists between the apparent magnitude of the binocular image and that of the two monocular images; to determine this point the stereoscope must be dispensed with, and the experiment so arranged that all three shall be simultaneously seen; which may be done in the following manner:– The two drawings being placed side by side on a plane before the eyes, the optic axes must be made to converge to a nearer point as at Fig. 4, or to a more distant one as at Fig. 3, until the three images are seen at the same time, the binocular image in the middle, and the monocular images at each side. It will thus be seen that the binocular image is apparently intermediate in size between the two monocular ones.

If the pictures be too unequal in magnitude, the binocular coincidence does not take place. It appears that if the inequality of the pictures be greater than the difference which exists between the two projections of the same object when seen in the most oblique position of the eyes (*i.e.* both turned to the extreme right or to the extreme left), ordinarily employed, they do not coalesce. Were it not for the

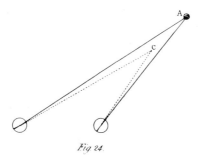

Fig 24.

binocular coincidence of two images of different magnitude, objects would appear single only when the optic axes converge immediately forwards; for it is only when the converging visual lines form equal angles with the visual base (the line joining the centres of the two eyes) as at Fig. 2, that the two pictures can be of equal magnitude; but when they form different angles with it, as at Fig. 24, the distance from the object to each eye is different, and consequently the picture projected on each retina has a different magnitude. If a piece of money be held in the position *a*, (Fig. 24) while the optic axes converge to a nearer point *c*, it will appear double, and that seen by the left eye will be evidently smaller than the other.

§ 14. *Phenomena which are observed when objects of different forms are simultaneously presented to corresponding parts of the two retinæ*

If we regard a picture with the right eye alone for a considerable length of time it will be constantly perceived; if we look at another and dissimilar picture with the left eye alone its effect will be equally permanent; it might therefore be expected, that if each of these pictures were presented to its corresponding eye at the same time the two would appear permanently superposed on each other. This, however, contrary to expectation, is not the case.

If *a* and *b* (Fig. 25) are each presented at the same time to a different eye, the common border will remain constant, while the letter within it will change alternately from that which would be perceived by the right eye alone to that which would be perceived by the left eye alone. At the moment of change the letter which has just been seen breaks into fragments, while fragments of the letter which is about to appear mingle with them, and are immediately after

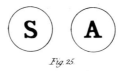

Fig. 25.

replaced by the entire letter. It does not appear to be in the power of the will to determine the appearance of either of the letters, but the duration of the appearance seems to depend on causes which are under our control: thus if the two pictures be equally illuminated, the alternations appear in general of equal duration; but if one picture be more illuminated than the other, that which is less so will be perceived during a shorter time. I have generally made this experiment with the apparatus, Fig. 6. When complex pictures are employed in the stereoscope, various parts of them alternate differently.

There are some facts intimately connected with the subject of the present article which have already been frequently observed. I allude to the experiments, first made by Du Tour, in which two different colours are presented to corresponding parts of the two retinæ. If a blue disc be presented to the right eye and a yellow disc to the corresponding part of the left eye, instead of a green disc which would appear if these two colours had mingled before their arrival at a single eye, the mind will perceive the two colours distinctly one or the other alternately predominating either partially or wholly over the disc. In the same manner the mind perceives no trace of violet when red is presented to one eye and blue to the other, nor any vestige of orange when red and yellow are separately presented in a similar manner. These experiments may be conveniently repeated by placing the coloured discs in the stereoscope, but they have been most usually made by looking at a white object through differently coloured glasses, one applied to each eye.

In some authors we find it stated, contrary to fact, that if similar objects of different colour be presented one to each eye, the appearance will be that compounded of the two colours. Dr. Reid* and Janin are among the writers who have fallen into this inconsiderate error, which arose no doubt from their deciding according to previous notions, instead of ascertaining by experiment what actually does happen.

§ 15.

No question relating to vision has been so much debated as the cause of the single appearance of objects seen by both eyes. I shall in the present section give a slight review of the various theories which have been advanced by philosophers to account for this phenomenon, in order that the remarks I have to make in the succeeding section may be properly understood.

The law of visible direction for monocular vision has been variously stated by different optical writers. Some have maintained with Drs. Reid and Porterfield, that every external point is seen in the direction of a line passing from its picture on the retina through the centre of the eye; while others have supposed with Dr.

* Enquiry, Sect. xiii.

Smith that the visible direction of an object coincides with the visual ray, or the principal ray of the pencil which flows from it to the eye. D'Alembert, furnished with imperfect data respecting the refractive densities of the humours of the eye, calculated that the apparent magnitudes of objects would differ widely on the two suppositions, and concluded that the visible point of an object was not seen in either of these directions, but sensibly in the direction of a line joining the point itself and its image on the retina; but he acknowledged that he could assign no reason for this law. Sir David Brewster, provided with more accurate data, has shown that these three lines so nearly coincide with each other, that "at an inclination of 30°, a line perpendicular to the point of impression on the retina passes through the common centre, and does not deviate from the real line of visible direction more than half a degree, a quantity too small to interfere with the purposes of vision." We may, therefore, assume in all our future reasonings the truth of the following definition given by this eminent philosopher: – "As the interior eye-ball is as nearly as possible a perfect sphere, lines perpendicular to the surface of the retina must all pass through one single point, namely the centre of its spherical surface. This one point may be called the centre of visible direction, because every point of a visible object will be seen in the direction of a line drawn from this centre to the visible point."

It is obvious, that the result of any attempt to explain the single appearance of objects to both eyes, or, in other words, the law of visible direction for binocular vision, ought to contain nothing inconsistent with the law of visible direction for monocular vision.

It was the opinion of Aguilonius, that all objects seen at the same glance with both eyes appear to be in the plane of the horopter. The horopter he defines to be a line drawn through the point of intersection of the optic axes, and parallel to the line joining the centres of the two eyes; the plane of the horopter to be a plane passing through this line at right angles to that of the optic axes. All objects which are in this plane, must, according to him, appear single because the lines of direction in which any point of an object is seen coincide only in this plane and nowhere else; and as these lines can meet each other only in one point, it follows from the hypothesis, that all objects not in the plane of the horopter must appear double, because their lines of direction intersect each other, either before or after they pass through it. This opinion was also maintained by Dechales and Porterfield. That it is erroneous, I have given, I think, sufficient proof, in showing that, when the optic axes converge to any point, objects before or beyond the plane of the horopter are under certain circumstances equally seen single as those in that plane.

Dr. Wells's "new theory of visible direction" was a modification of the preceding hypothesis. This acute writer held with Aguilonius, that objects are seen single only when they are in the plane of the horopter, and consequently that they appear double when they are either before or beyond it; but he attempted to make this single appearance of objects only in the plane of the horopter to depend on other principles, from which he deduced, contrary to Aguilonius, that the objects which are doubled do not appear in the plane of the horopter, but in other places which are determined by these principles. Dr. Wells was led to his new theory by a fact which he accidentally observed, and which he could not reconcile with any existing theory of visible direction; this fact had, though he was unaware of it, been previously noticed by Dr. Smith; it is already mentioned in § 8, and is the only instance of binocular vision of relief which I have found recorded previous to my own investigations. So little does Dr. Wells's theory appear to have been understood, that no subsequent writer has attempted either to confirm or disprove his opinions. It would be useless here to discuss the principles of this theory, which was framed to account for an anomalous individual fact, since it is inconsistent with the general rules on which that fact has been now shown to depend. Notwithstanding these erroneous views, the "essay upon single vision with two eyes" contains many valuable experiments and remarks, the truth of which are independent of the theory they were intended to illustrate.

The theory which has obtained greatest currency is that which assumes that an object is seen single because its pictures fall on corresponding points of the two retinæ, that is on points which are similarly situated with respect to the two centres both in distance and position. This theory supposes that the pictures projected on the retinæ are exactly similar to each other, corresponding points of the two pictures falling on corresponding points of the two retinæ. Authors who agree with regard to this property, differ widely in explaining why objects are seen in the same place, or single, according to this law. Dr. Smith makes it to depend entirely on custom, and explains why the eyes are habitually directed towards an object so that its pictures fall on corresponding parts in the following manner:–

> When we view an object steadily, we have acquired a habit of directing the optic axes to the point in view; because its pictures falling upon the middle points of the retinas, are then distincter than if they fell upon any other places; and since the pictures of the whole object are equal to one another, and are both inverted with respect to the optic axes, it follows that the pictures of any collateral point are painted upon corresponding points of the retinas.

Dr. Reid, after a long dissertation on the subject, concludes,

> that by an original property of human eyes, objects painted upon the centres of the two retinæ, or upon points similarly situated with regard to the centres, appear in the same visible place; that the most plausible attempts to account for this property of the eyes have been unsuccessful; and therefore, that it must be either a primary law of our constitution, or the consequence of some more general law which is not yet discovered.

Other writers who have admitted this principle have regarded it as arising from anatomical structure and dependent on connexion of nervous fibres; among these stand the names of Galen, Dr. Briggs, Sir Isaac Newton, Rohault, Dr. Hartley, Dr. Wollaston and Professor Müller.

Many of the supporters of the theory of corresponding points have thought, or rather have admitted, *without thinking*, that it was not inconsistent with the law of Aguilonius; but very little reflection will show that both cannot be maintained together; for corresponding lines of visible direction, that is, lines terminating in corresponding points of the two retinæ, cannot meet in the plane of the horopter unless the optic axes be parallel, and the plane be at an infinite distance before the eyes. Some of the modern German writers* have inquired what is the curve in which objects appear single while the optic axes are directed to a given point, on the hypothesis that objects are seen single only when they fall on corresponding points of the two retinæ. An elegant proposition has resulted from their investigations, which I shall need no apology for introducing in this place, since it has not yet been mentioned in any English work.

R and L (Fig. 26) are the two eyes; CA, C′A the optic axes converging to the point A; and CABC′ is a circle drawn through the point of convergence A and the centres of visible direction CC′. If any point be taken in the circumference of this circle, and lines be drawn from it through the centres of the two eyes CC′, these lines will fall on corresponding points of the two retinæ DD′; for the angles ACB, AC′B being equal, the angles DCE, D′C′E′ are also equal; therefore any point placed in the circumference of the circle CABC′ will, according to the hypothesis, appear single while the optic axes are directed to A, or any other part in it.

I will mention two other properties of this binocular circle: 1st. The arc subtended by two points on its circumference contains double the number of degrees of the arc subtended by the pictures of these points on either retina, so that objects which occupy 180° of the supposed circle of single vision are painted on a portion of the retina extended over 90° only; for the angle DCE or D′C′E′ being at the centre, and the angle BCA or BC′A at the circumference of a circle, this consequence follows. 2ndly. To whatever point of the circumference of the circle the optic axes be made to converge, they will form the same angle with each other; for the angles CAC′, CBC′ are equal.

In the eye itself, the centre of visible direction, or the point at which the principal rays cross each other, is, according to Dr. Young and other eminent optical writers, at the same time the centre of the spherical surface of the retina, and that of the lesser spherical surface of the cornea; in the diagram (Fig. 26), to simplify the consideration of the problem, R and L represent only the circle of curvature of the bottom of the retina, but the reasoning is equally true in both cases.

The same reasons, founded on the experiments in this memoir, which disprove the theory of Aguilonius, induce me to reject the law of corresponding points as

* *Tortual*, die Sinne des Menschen. Münster, 1827. *Bartels*, Beitrage zur Physiologie der Gesichtssinnes. Berlin, 1834.

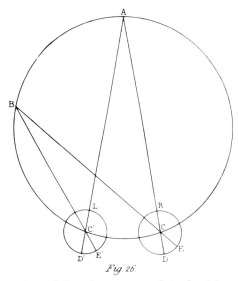

Fig. 26.

an accurate expression of the phenomena of single vision. According to the former, objects can appear single only in the plane of the horopter; according to the latter, only when they are in the circle of single vision; both positions are inconsistent with the binocular vision of objects in relief, the points of which they consist appearing single though they are at different distances before the eyes. I have already proved that the assumption made by all the maintainers of the theory of corresponding points, namely that the two pictures projected by any object in the retinæ are exactly similar, is quite contrary to fact in every case except that in which the optic axes are parallel.

Gassendus, Porta, Tacquet and Gall maintained, that we see with only one eye at a time though both remain open, one according to them being relaxed and inattentive to objects while the other is upon the stretch. It is a sufficient refutation of this hypothesis, that we see an object double when one of the optic axes is displaced either by squinting or by pressure on the eye-ball with the finger; if we saw with only one eye, one object only should under such circumstances be seen. Again, in many cases which I have already explained, the simultaneous affection of the two retinæ excites a different idea in the mind to that consequent on either of the single impressions, the latter giving rise to the idea of a representation on a plane surface, the former to that of an object in relief; these things could not occur did we see with only one eye at a time.

Du Tour* held that though we might occasionally see at the same time with both eyes, yet the mind cannot be affected simultaneously by two corresponding points of the two images. He was led to this opinion by the curious facts alluded to in § 14. It would be difficult to disprove this conjecture by experiment; but all that

* Act. Par. 1743. M. p. 334.

the experiments adduced in its favour, and others relating to the disappearance of objects to one eye really proves, is, that the mind is inattentive to impressions made on one retina when it cannot combine the impressions on the two retinæ together so as to resemble the perception of some external objects; but they afford no ground whatever for supposing that the mind cannot under any circumstances attend to impressions made simultaneously on points of the two retinæ, when they harmonize with each other in suggesting to the mind the same idea.

A perfectly original theory has been recently advanced by M. Lehot,[*] who has endeavoured to prove, that instead of pictures on the retinæ, images of three dimensions are formed in the vitreous humour which we perceive by means of nervous filaments extended thence from the retina. This theory would account for the single appearance to both eyes of objects in relief, but it would be quite insufficient to explain why we perceive an object of three dimensions when two pictures of it are presented to the eyes; according to it, also, no difference should be perceived in the relief of objects when seen by one or both eyes, which is contrary to what really happens. The proofs, besides, that we perceive external objects by means of pictures on the retinæ are so numerous and convincing, that a contrary conjecture cannot be entertained for a moment. On this account it will suffice merely to mention two other theories which place the seat of vision in the vitreous humour. Vallee,[†] without denying the existence of pictures on the retina, has advocated that we see the relief of objects by means of anterior foci on the hyaloid membrane; and Raspail[‡] has developed at considerable length the strange hypothesis, that images are neither formed in the vitreous humour nor painted on the retina, but are immediately perceived at the focus of the lenticular system of which the eye is formed.

§ 16.

It now remains to examine *why* two dissimilar pictures projected on the two retinæ give rise to the perception of an object in relief. I will not attempt at present to give the complete solution of this question, which is far from being so easy as at a first glance it may appear to be, and is indeed one of great complexity. I shall in this place merely consider the most obvious explanations which might be offered, and show their insufficiency to explain the whole of the phenomena.

It may be supposed, that we see but one point of a field of view distinctly at the same instant, the one namely to which the optic axes are directed, while all other points are seen so indistinctly, that the mind does not recognize them to be either

[*] Nouvelle Théorie de la Vision, Par. 1823.
[†] Traité de la Science du Dessein, Par. 1821, p. 270.
[‡] Nouveau Système de Chimie Organique, t. 2. p. 329.

single or double, and that the figure is appreciated by successively directing the point of convergence of the optic axes successively to a sufficient number of its points to enable us to judge accurately of its form.

That there is a degree of indistinctness in those parts of the field of view to which the eyes are not immediately directed, and which increases with the distance from that point, cannot be doubted, and it is also true that the objects thus obscurely seen are frequently doubled. In ordinary vision, it may be said, this indistinctness and duplicity is not attended to, because the eyes shifting continually from point to point, every part of the object is successively rendered distinct; and the perception of the object is not the consequence of a single glance, during which only a small part of it is seen distinctly; but is formed from a comparison of all the pictures successively seen while the eyes were changing from one point of the object to another.

All this is in some degree true; but were it entirely so, no appearance of relief should present itself when the eyes remain intently fixed on one point of a binocular image in the stereoscope. But on performing the experiment carefully, it will be found, provided the pictures do not extend too far beyond the centres of distinct vision, that the image is still seen single and in relief when this condition is fulfilled. Were the theory of corresponding points true, the appearance should be that of the superposition of the two drawings, to which however it has not the slightest similitude. The following experiments are equally decisive against this theory.

Exp. 1. Draw two lines about two inches long and inclined towards each other, as in Fig. 10, on a sheet of paper, and having caused them to coincide by converging the optic axes to a point nearer than the paper, look intently on the upper end of the resultant line, without allowing the eyes to wander from it for a moment. The entire line will appear single and in its proper relief, and a pin or a piece of straight wire may without the least difficulty be made to coincide exactly in position with it; or, if while the optic axes continue to be directed to the upper and nearer end, the point of a pin be made to coincide with the lower and further end or with any intermediate point of the resultant line, the coincidence will remain exactly the same when the optic axes are moved and meet there. The eyes sometimes become fatigued, which causes the line to appear double at those parts to which the optic axes are not fixed, but in such cases all appearance of relief vanishes. The same experiment may be tried with more complex figures, but the pictures should not extend too far beyond the centres of the retinæ.

Another and a beautiful proof that the appearance of relief in binocular vision is an effect independent of the motions of the eyes, may be obtained by impressing on the retinæ ocular spectra of the component figures. For this purpose the drawings should be formed of broad coloured lines on a ground of the complementary colour, for instance red lines on a green ground, and be viewed either in the stereoscope or in the apparatus, Fig. 6, as the ordinary figures are, taking care however to fix the eyes only to a single point of the compound figure; the drawings must be strongly illuminated, and after a sufficient time has elapsed to impress the spectra on the retinæ, the eyes must be carefully covered to exclude all external light. A spectrum of the object in relief will then appear before the closed eyes. It is well known, that a spectrum impressed on a single eye and seen in the dark, frequently alternately appears and disappears: these alternations do not correspond in the spectra impressed on the two retinæ, and hence a curious effect arises; sometimes the right eye spectrum will be seen alone, sometimes that of the left eye, and at those moments when the two appear together, the binocular spectrum will present itself in bold relief. As in this case the pictures cannot shift their places on the retinæ in whatever manner the eyes be moved about, the optic axes can during the experiment only correspond with a single point of each.

When an object, or a part of an object, thus appears in relief while the optic axes are directed to a single binocular point, it is easy to see that each point of the figure that appears single is seen at the intersection of the two lines of visible direction in which it is seen by each eye separately, whether these lines of visible direction terminate at corresponding points of the two retinæ or not.

But if we were to infer the converse of this, viz. that every point of an object in relief is seen by a single glance at the intersection of the lines of visible direction in which it is seen by each eye singly, we should be in error. On this supposition, objects before or beyond the intersection of the optic axes should never appear double, and we have abundant evidence that they do. The determination of the points which shall appear single seems to depend in no small degree on previous knowledge of the form we are regarding. No doubt, some law or rule of vision may be discovered which shall include all the circumstances under which single vision by means of non-corresponding points occurs and is limited. I have made numerous experiments for the purpose of attaining this end, and have ascertained some of the conditions on which single and double vision depend, the consideration of which however must at present be deferred.

Sufficient, however, has been shown to prove that the laws of binocular visible direction hitherto laid down are too restricted to be true. The law of Aguilonius assumes that objects in the plane of the horopter are alone seen single; and the law of corresponding points carried to its necessary consequences, though these consequences were unforeseen by its first advocates, many of whom thought that it was consistent with the law of Aguilonius, leads to the conclusion, that no object appears single unless it is seen in a circle passing through the centres of visible direction in each eye and the point of convergence of the optic axes. Both of these are inconsistent with the single vision of objects whose points lie out of the plane in one case and the circle in the other; and that objects do appear single under circumstances that cannot be explained by these laws, has, I think, been placed beyond doubt by the experiments I have brought forward. Should it be hereafter proved, that all points in the plane or in the circle above mentioned are seen single, and from the great indistinctness of lateral images it will be difficult to give this proof, the law must be qualified by the admission, that points out of them do not always appear double.

2.5. Brewster: "On the law of visible position in single and binocular vision, and on the representation of solid figures by the union of dissimilar plane pictures on the retina". *Transactions of the Royal Society of Edinburgh*, 1844, **15**, 349–368.

In the course of an examination of Bishop Berkeley's "New Theory of Vision," the foundation of the Ideal Philosophy, I have found it necessary to repeat many old experiments, and to make many new ones, in reference to the functions of the eye as an optical instrument. I had imagined that many points in the physiology of vision were irrevocably fixed, and placed beyond the reach of controversy; but though this supposition may still be true in the estimation of that very limited class of philosophers who have really studied the subject, yet it is mortifying to find that the laws of vision, as established by experiment and observation, are as little understood as they were in the days of Locke and Berkeley. Metaphysicians and physiologists have combined their efforts in substituting unfounded speculation for physical truth; and even substantial discoveries have been prematurely placed in opposition to opinions of which they are the necessary result.

In prosecuting this subject, my attention has been particularly fixed upon the interesting paper of my distinguished friend Professor Wheatstone, *"On some remarkable and hitherto unobserved phenomena of binocular vision."** It is impossible to over-estimate the importance of this paper, or to admire too highly the value and beauty of the leading discovery which it describes, namely, the perception of an object of three dimensions by the union of the two dissimilar pictures formed on the retinæ:– but, in seeking an explanation of this curious phenomenon, and in applying it to explain phenomena previously known, Mr Wheatstone has adduced experimental results, and drawn conclusions which stand in direct opposition to what was best established in our previous knowledge. Before entering, however, upon this branch of the subject, I must first explain the law of visible direction, and the phenomena of ocular parallaxes.

1. *On the Law of Visible Direction in Monocular Vision.*

Several philosophers had hazarded the opinion, that every external visible point is seen in the direction of a line passing from its picture on the retina through the centre of the eye considered as a sphere; while others maintained that every such

* Phil. Trans. 1838, p. 371.

point was seen in the direction of the refracted ray by which its image was formed.

The celebrated D'Alembert, in his *Doutes sur differents questions d'Optique*, maintains that the action of light upon the retina is conformable to the laws of mechanics; and he adds, that it is difficult to conceive how an object could be seen in any other direction than that of a line perpendicular to the curvature of the retina at the point where it is really excited. He then investigates, mathematically, how the apparent magnitudes of objects would be affected, on the two suppositions that the line of visible direction coincides either with the refracted ray, or with a line perpendicular to the retina at the point of excitement. On the *first* of these suppositions, he finds that the apparent magnitude of small objects would be increased about $1/13$th, and on the *second* supposition, a little more than $1/3$, or $\frac{6823}{18267}$. This last result is, as D'Alembert justly remarks, so contrary to experience, that we cannot suppose vision to be thus performed, however natural the supposition may appear. "In the direction of what line, then," he adds, "do we perceive objects, or visible points, which are not placed in the optical axis? This is a point which it appears very difficult to determine exactly and rigorously. As experience, however, proves that objects of small extent, which are within the range of our eyes, do not appear sensibly greater than they are in reality, it follows, that the visible point which sends a ray to the cornea, is seen sensibly in its place, and consequently in the direction of a line joining the point itself and its image on the retina. But why," D'Alembert adds, "is this the case? It is a fact which I will not undertake to explain."*

When we consider the data from which D'Alembert has deduced the preceding results, it is not easy to account for his having abandoned the inquiry as a hopeless one. He employs the dimensions of the eye as given by Petit and Jurin, and he assumes Jurin's index of refraction for the human crystalline lens, though it is almost exactly the same as that of an ox, as given by Hawksbee. These, indeed, were the best data he could procure; but he should have inquired if the most probable law of visible direction was compatible with any other dimensions of the eye, and any other refractive powers of the humours which were within the limits of probability; and above all, he ought to have examined experimentally the truth of his fundamental assumption, *that visible points are really seen in their true places when they are not in the axis of vision.*

Now it is quite certain that these points are not seen in their true direction, and that there is an *ocular parallax*, which is the measure of the deviation of the *visible* from the *true direction* of objects. This parallax is nothing in the axis of the eye, and it increases as the visible point is more and more distant from that axis; and hence it follows, that, during the motion of the eyeball, when the head is immoveable, visible objects not only change their place, but also their form.

Had the eye consisted of only *two* concentric coats, a *cornea* and a *retina*, filled with a homogeneous fluid, vision would have been performed by centrical

* *Opuscules Mathematiques*, Tom. I. Mem. ix. p. 266.

pencils; – the visible and the true direction of points would have coincided, and objects would have changed neither their form nor their position during the motion of this hypothetical eyeball round the common centre of the two coats. But as such an eye could not have afforded sufficiently distinct vision, the introduction of the crystalline lens became necessary; and it is owing to the secondary refractions at its surfaces and within its mass of variable density, that the parallax of visible direction is produced.

Fig. 1.

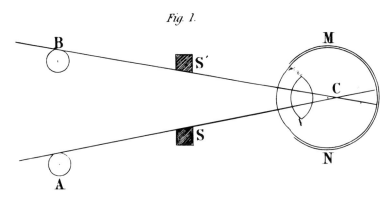

The following experiment will establish the existence, and explain the nature of this parallax. Let MN, Fig. 1, be the eyeball, C the centre of curvature of the retina, and also the centre of motion of the eyeball. Having placed an opaque screen S several inches from the eye, till its inner edge just eclipses a luminous object A, look away from the screen, and the object A will appear. Keeping the head steady, place another screen S'* so that, when viewed directly, it does not eclipse another luminous object B, the line CS'B just grazing the outer edge of B. When the screens and luminous objects, therefore, are so arranged that A is *invisible* when the axis of the eye is directed to S or to A, and B visible when the axis of the eye is directed to S' or B, – then by turning the eye from A to B, A will *appear*, and B will disappear, exhibiting the curious effect *of an invisible body appearing by looking away from it, and of a visible body disappearing by looking at it!*

Had the eyeball MN been our hypothetical one, these effects would not have been produced. All objects, near and remote, would have retained their relative positions and magnitudes during its rotation.

Hence it follows, that we are not entitled to reject any law of visible direction, because it gives a position to visible objects different from their real position.

Having removed this difficulty, I proceeded to examine the other data of D'Alembert. Making the eyeball and the retina spherical, he assumes that the centre of the latter is equidistant from the *foramen centrale* of the retina, and the

* The two screens S, S' may be the opposite edges of a triangular notch in a card held in the hand.

centre of the crystalline lens. This, however, is far from being the case. M. Du Tour, and Dr Thomas Young, have made the centre of curvature of the retina coincident with the centre of curvature of the spherical surface of the cornea, as in our hypothetical eye; and this centre, in place of being almost half-way between the apex of the posterior surface of the lens and the *foramen centrale*, is actually almost in contact with the latter! The dissections of Dr Knox and Mr Clay Wallace, of New York, give similar results. When we add to these considerations the fact that the refractive power of the crystalline lens assumed by D'Alembert is nearly *triple* of what it really is, we are entitled to reject the results of his calculations.

Assuming, then, the most correct anatomy of the eye, namely, that according to which the cornea and the retina are concentric, it is obvious that if there was no crystalline lens, pencils, incident perpendicularly on the cornea, would pass through the common centre, and fall perpendicularly upon the retina. Hence, in this case, the line of *visible* direction would coincide with the line of *real* direction, and also with the incident and intromitted ray. Now, the refractions at the crystalline are exceedingly small, and, at moderate inclinations to the axis, the deviations from the preceding law are very minute. At an inclination of 25° or 30°, a line perpendicular to the point of impression on the retina passes through the common centre already referred to, and does not deviate from the line of real visible direction more than half a degree, a quantity too small to interfere with the purposes of vision. The deviation, of course, increases with the inclination; but as there is no such thing as distinct vision out of the axis, and as the indistinctness increases with the inclination, it is impossible to ascertain, by ordinary observation, that any deviation exists. Hence the mechanical principle of D'Alembert, which he himself has rejected, and the law of visible direction, which I have established, are substantially true. As the Almighty has not made the eye achromatic, because it was unnecessary, so He has, in the same wise economy of His power, not given it the property of seeing visible points in their real direction.

Had it been necessary to make the visible ray coincident in direction with the incident ray, it might have been effected by giving such a form and variable density to the crystalline lens as to make the ray which it refracted across the axis of vision at the centre of curvature of the retina; and if the crystalline lens were such that this crossing point was variable, this variation might have been compensated by making the retina spheroidal, with a variable centre of curvature.

That a visible point is seen in the direction of a line perpendicular to the surface of the retina at which the image of the point is formed, may be established experimentally in the following manner. Having expanded the pupil by belladonna, look directly at a point in the axis of the eye. Its image will be formed by a cone of rays variously inclined from 85° to 90° to the surface of the retina. While the point is distinctly seen, intercept all these different rays in succession, and it will be found that each ray gives vision in the same direction, the visible point retaining its position. Hence it follows, that on the part of the retina in the axis of vision, all rays, however obliquely incident, give the same visible direction perpendicular to the surface of the membrane. That the same property is possessed by every other part of the retina cannot be doubted, and may be proved by direct experiment.

Although D'Alembert states it as unquestionable, that when the visual ray is in the axis of vision, or the optic axis, and passes to the retina without refraction, the point which emits it will be seen in the direction of a line passing from its image to the visible point; yet, after he has found that his mechanical principle is not correct, he gives loose reins to his scepticism, and maintains the extraordinary paradox, that objects even which are placed in the optical axis are not always seen in this axis. The following is the argument he employs, which I shall give in his own words.

If we direct the two optic axes AE, BE, Fig. 2, towards a star E, it is certain that this star appears much nearer to us than it really is: It is true that we estimate its distance only in a very imperfect and vague manner; but it is not less certain that this distance perceived, whether apparent or presumed, is greatly *below* the real distance. If, then, we see the star in each of the optical axes AE, BE, we should see it in each of these axes in the points *e, e,* which are incomparably nearer A and B than E. Thus we should see two stars *e, e,* and their apparent distance *ee* would be nearly equal to AB.

Fig. 2.

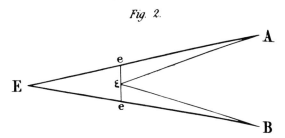

Observation, however, proves that we see only *one* star, and this star is seen nearly at the middle point *ε* of the line *ee* in the direction of lines A*ε*, B*ε*, different from the optic axes. It is true that these lines, though really different from the optic axes, deviate from them but very little, but still they do differ from them; and this experiment is sufficient to prove *that objects which are at a considerable distance from the eye are not seen exactly in the optical axis, even when we look at them directly.*

Whence, in general, nothing is less certain than this common principle in optics, that *objects are seen in the direction of the ray which they send to the eye.**

It is almost impossible to believe that D'Alembert is serious in maintaining these doctrines. The major proposition of his syllogism is absolutely incorrect. It is not true that we see the star E nearer than it is. The eye does not see distances directly: the mind only estimates them, and, according to its means of judging, it forms a right or a wrong opinion. The second proposition is equally incorrect. We

* *Opuscules Mathematiques*, Tom. I. Mem. ix. § iv. p. 273–4.

do not see the star along the lines Aε, Bε. We see it along the lines AE, BE, at the very place where it is, and whether we consider it nearer or more remote than it is, – whether we think that it touches our eye, or exists at the remotest verge of space, – the position of the optical axis of each eye remains as before, and our vision of the star is not affected by the truth or falsehood of our judgment.

2. *On the Law of Visible Direction in Binocular Vision.*

In admitting the correctness of the law of visible direction in monocular vision, which I have endeavoured to establish in the preceding section, Professor Wheatstone justly remarks, "that the result of any attempt to explain the single appearance of objects to both eyes, or, in other words, *the law of visible direction for binocular vision,* ought to contain nothing inconsistent with the law of visible direction for monocular vision."* Properly speaking, however, there is no such thing as a law of visible direction in binocular vision, because there is no such thing as *a centre* of visible direction, or *a line* of visible direction in binocular vision. When we see an object distinctly with both eyes, it is actually seen in *two* directions, and the point where these directions intersect each other determines the visible place of the object. But if we follow Mr Wheatstone in considering such a law as equivalent to the law which regulates "the single appearance of objects to both eyes," we can readily deduce it as a corollary from the law in monocular vision. A visible point is seen single with two eyes only when it is at the intersection of its lines of visible direction as given by each eye separately. It is obvious that this law does not harmonize with the doctrine of corresponding points, or with the binocular circle of the German physiologists. It is, however, rigorously true; for no philosopher can adopt the monstrous opinion that the functions and laws of vision which belong to each eye, acting separately, are subverted when they act in concert. Hence it is obvious that the single vision of points with *two* eyes, or with *two hundred* eyes, is the necessary consequence of the convergency of the *two*, or the *two hundred*, lines of visible direction to the same point in absolute space; and although we think that objects appear single with both eyes, yet it is only the points to which the optic axes and the lines of visible direction converge that are actually seen single, and the unity of the perception is obtained by the rapid survey which they eye takes of every part of the object.

The phenomenon of an erect object from an inverted picture on the retina, which has so unnecessarily perplexed metaphysicians and physiologists, is a demonstrable corollary from the law of visible direction for points. The only difficulty which I have ever experienced in studying this subject, has been to discover where any difficulty lay. An able writer, however, in a recent number of *Blackwood's Magazine,*† in discussing the Berkleyan theory of vision, has started a difficulty of a very novel kind, and has called upon me personally to solve it. Were

* Phil. Trans. 1838, p. 388.   † June 1842, vol. li. p. 830.

this the proper place for such a discussion, I should willingly enter upon it; but I must content myself with stating, that the doctrine which the very ingenious author calls the *ordinary optical doctrine*, was never maintained by any optical writer whatever, and that the doctrine which he substitutes in its place is that which all optical writers implicitly adopt, though they have thought it too elementary to require illustration. A visible point which throws out *two* separate particles of light, an *upper* and an *under*, will be inverted on the retina, but a *smaller* visible point, which throws out only *one* particle of light, cannot be *inverted*, because *inversion* implies a change in the relative position of *two* visible points.

3. *On the Vision of Objects of Three Dimensions.*

(1.) *By Monocular Vision.* – If we look with one eye at a solid body, for example a six-sided pyramid with its apex directed to the eye, and uniformly illuminated, we recognise at a single glance that it is not a drawing of the pyramid. When the eye adjusts itself to distinct vision of its apex, all the more distant parts are seen indistinctly, but the eye quickly surveys the whole, adjusting itself to distinct vision of its base and of its edges, and by these successive efforts, at one time contracting the pupil and the eyebrows to see the near parts, and expanding them to see the more remote ones, it obtains a knowledge of the relative distance of its different parts. The vision of the pyramid thus obtained is nearly perfect. There is no inequality of illumination produced by the act of single vision; and there is no flickering in the outlines of the figure. The only apparent imperfection is, that when we see one point very distinctly we do not see the other parts with equal distinctness; but this imperfection is unavoidable in vision, whether with one or two eyes; and, in place of being a defect, is the very means by which we judge of the relative distance of its parts. If we saw all its lines and parts with equal distinctness, without moving the eyeball, or without altering the mechanism for its adjustment, we should not have been able to distinguish the pyramid from its projection upon a plane surface.

Hence we draw the conclusion that the vision of bodies of three dimensions with one eye is perfect.

(2.) *By Binocular Vision.* – If we now place the pyramid before both eyes, so that the pictures of it on each retina are nearly similar, the one being the reflected image of the other, we shall see the pyramid with great distinctness. It will appear more luminous with the two eyes, and if the observer wished to estimate the distance of its apex, or any other point of it, from himself, the convergency of *both* eyes to that point would enable him to form a more correct judgment than with a single eye. These, doubtless, are advantages, but they do not in the least degree improve our vision of the pyramid, which is independent of them. More light may injure vision as well as improve it; and if we could project a foot-rule from each eye, and read upon it the distance of every part of the pyramid, the vision of it would not in the slightest degree be affected. May we not add also, that the intromission of scattered light through *two* eyes in place of one, and the possible dissimilarity, however small, between the curvatures and densities of their humours, which would give rise to two pictures of different magnitudes, would entitle us to give the preference to single vision, in reference to its power of giving us a distinct view of objects of three dimensions.

Hence, we conclude, that when the pyramid is placed in a position of symmetry between the two eyes, *binocular* is not superior to *monocular vision*.

But if the pyramid is so placed that the left eye sees only *four* faces of it, while the right eye sees all the *six*, then the *monocular* vision of the pyramid is more distinct that the *binocular* one. The vision of faces 1, 2, 3, and 4 is sufficiently distinct with two eyes; but the faces 5, 6, being seen only with one eye, are less luminous than the other faces, and as the optic axes do not perform their functions with the same accuracy when the object to which they are directed is visible only to one eye, the part of the object seen by single vision will not unite with that seen by double vision; and, in the case of the pyramid, we shall observe its apex actually projecting upon the faces 5, 6, of the pyramid, and destroying the symmetry of the picture. When all the faces but No. 6 are seen by the left eye, vision is still unsatisfactory with both eyes, and yet more so when only *three* of the faces are seen by the left eye.

Hence we conclude that, in these cases, *binocular* is *inferior* to *monocular* vision.

Let us next suppose that the object viewed is a table knife, so placed that, when the back of it is towards the observer, the *left* side of the blade is seen by the *left* eye, and the *right* side of the blade by the *right* eye. As the back is seen by both eyes, the picture presented to the mind is a compound of one double and two single sensations, and, consequently, a very unsatisfactory representation of the object.

Hence we conclude that, in this case, *binocular* is still more inferior to *monocular* vision.

These results stand in direct opposition to those given by Professor Wheatstone, who considers it an established fact, "*that the most vivid belief of the solidity of an object of three dimensions arises from two different perspective projections of it being simultaneously presented to the mind.*" Before entering, however, upon this branch of the subject, I must examine Mr Wheatstone's views respecting the *binocular* vision of figures of different magnitudes.

4. *On the Binocular Vision of Figures of Different Magnitudes.*

Mr Wheatstone seems to have been the first person who made experiments on the binocular vision of unequal figures. Having drawn on separate pieces of paper "two squares or circles, differing obviously, but not extravagantly, in size;" he

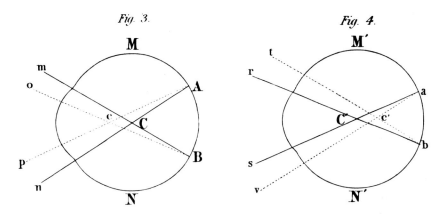

Fig. 3.   *Fig. 4.*

placed them in the stereoscope, and concluded from his observations that the *two unequal pictures* "coalesced, and occasioned a single resultant perception;" and that the binocular image thus perceived was apparently intermediate in size between the two unequal monocular ones. This perfect coalescence of the two images he considers as demonstrated, and he deduces from it the important conclusion, that, if it were otherwise, "objects would appear single only when the optic axes converge immediately forwards." That is, we see objects single when the optic axes converge laterally in virtue of the coincidence of two unequal images.

These extraordinary results are obviously subversive of the established laws of vision, but especially of the law of visible direction; and if they are true, they must arise from a sudden change in the properties of the humours, or in the functions of the retina. The lesser image may become greater, or the greater less, by a variation in the refractive density or the form of the cornea and the crystalline lens, or, what would be more probable, the retina may become subject to a new law of visible direction. Assuming this to be the case, we must suppose the change of law to take place in each eye, so that the *larger* image must be seen *less*, and the *smaller* image seen *greater*, than they really are. Now, this change must take place instantaneously at the moment of coalescence, for the two images retain their proper magnitude till their apparent union takes place; and the eye must recover its ordinary functions as instantaneously, for the moment we intercept one of the images the other resumes its proper size.

In order to understand what the nature of this supposed change actually is, let MN, M'N' (Figs 3, 4) be the two eyes, AB the larger image, and *ab* the smaller one; then if C be the centre of curvature of the retina, the points A, B will be seen in the directions, A*n*, B*m* intersecting at C, and the points *a*, *b* in the directions *as*, *br* intersecting at C'. But when these separate images coalesce, in consequence of AB becoming less and *ab* greater, the points A, B, *a*, *b* must be seen in the directions A*p*, B*o*, *av*, *bt*, intersecting at new centres of visible direction *c*, *c'*, the one farther from, and the other nearer to, the retina. If we now shift the *larger* picture to the *right* eye, and the smaller to the *left* eye, the function of the retina will be again changed: the *left* eye MN will have its lines of visible direction as in Fig. 4, and the *right* eye as in Fig. 3. Such an oscillation of the *binocular centre* of visible direction on each side of the *monocular centre*, produced solely during the attempt to unite unequal images, would indicate a function of the retina so extraordinary, that the most incontrovertible experiments, and the universal experience of accurate observers, could alone give it credibility.

There is no doubt that the two unequal images appear to coalesce; but if we make the outlines of the squares and circles luminous, by pricking small holes in their outlines, and exposing them to very strong light, we shall find it impossible to produce a coincidence. The best way to make this experiment is to take two lines, AB, *ab*, Fig. 5, of unequal lengths, and with a large pin to perforate the lines at A, B, *a*, *b*, so that when we attempt to unite them, as at Fig. 6, we shall see with

Fig. 5.

A   B   a   b

Fig. 6.

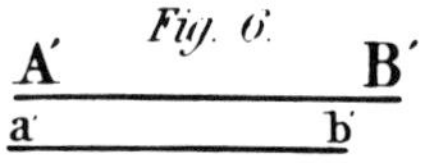

A'   B'

a'   b'

perfect distinctness their four luminous extremities. When the point *a* is made to pass into A, I have never succeeded in making *b* pass into B. Whenever there is an appearance of this, either turn round the paper, or the head, so as to separate the lines as in Fig. 6, and it will be invariably seen that if *a* springs out of A, *b* will spring out of a point between A and B. The apparent coincidence, therefore, of AB with *ab*, Fig. 6, when it is seen, arises from the disappearance of one or other of the extremities of the two lines.

But Mr Wheatstone has described another very interesting experiment, of the same character as that which we have been examining, and he regards it as "proving that similar pictures, falling on corresponding points of the two retinæ, may appear double and in different places." Draw a strong vertical line, AB, Fig. 7, and another CD inclined some degrees to it, and also a faint line *mn* parallel to AB, and cutting CD at its centre S', then, according to Mr Wheatstone, the two strong lines AB, CD, when seen with different eyes in the stereoscope, or brought together by looking at a nearer object, "will coincide, and the resultant perspective line (CD) will appear to occupy the same place as before; but the faint line (*mn*) which now falls on a line of the left retina, which corresponds with the line of the right retina, on which one of the coinciding strong lines, viz., the vertical one (AB) falls, appears in a different place." In repeating this experiment, I have occasionally observed an apparent coincidence similar to that which is described in the preceding passage; but after numerous and varied observations, made with lines *coloured* and *uncoloured, opaque* and *transparent, similar* and *dissimilar* both in strength and form, I have no hesitation in affirming that the phenomenon described by Mr Wheatstone is an illusion, arising from the actual disappearance of one or more parts, or even of the whole of one of the lines, and from the difficulty of observing the separation or superposition of images in the circumstances under which the experiment is made.

The following are a few of the variations of the experiment which I have found the best calculated to exhibit the real place of the combined images.

1. In Mr Wheatstone's form of the lines shewn in Fig. 7, the *strong* line AB assumes more readily the appearance of uniting with the *similarly strong line* CD; but if *mn* is a *strong* line and CD a *weak* one (Fig. 11), or an *interrupted* one, AB will unite with *mn*, and not even apparently with CD. In like manner, if AB be a *weak* line, it will unite with the *weak* line *mn* rather than with CD. (See Fig. 12.)

Now, the apparent coalescence of similar lines arises from the fact, that when corresponding, or nearly corresponding, parts of the retinæ are impressed with similar images, one of the two more readily vanishes, independent of its liability to vanish from its being out of the axis of vision. Whenever two images interfere with one another so as to impede vision, one of them disappears – or rather, is not taken cognisance of by the eye. Hence it is, that many sportsmen shoot with both eyes open; and hence it is that, in very oblique vision, one of the eyes resigns its office, and leaves the other to view the object distinctly and singly.*

But, in point of fact, AB, Fig. 7, does not coalesce with CD. If the eye strives to see distinctly any object at the point S', then AB coalesces with *mn*. If the eye looks fixedly at C when A is united with C, AS will unite with CS' and SB with S'*n*; and if the eye is fixed intently on D when B and D are united, SB will coalesce with S'D and AS with *m*S'. In these two last cases, the coalescence arises from the same cause as the coalescence of dissimilar forms in Mr Wheatstone's fundamental experiment, as I shall now shew.

2. If we join C*m*, D*n*, Fig. 7 (as is done in Fig. 8), we may regard AB and C*m*S' *n*D as dissimilar images of a solid, consisting of two triangles C*m*S', D*n*S', united at their apex. In this case, AS, Fig. 8, will coincide with CS' and SB with S'*n*. If the two dissimilar images are, as in Figs 9, 10, 11, and 12, AB will not appear to coalesce with CD. In Fig. 13, the coalescence is not complete; but it becomes so by removing the portion *ab* of the line AB the part A*a* coalescing with C, and *b*B with D. In Fig. 14, the line AB will not coalesce with CD; but each separate portion of AB will, when the other two portions are concealed or removed, coalesce with the corresponding portion of CD.

* The fact of objects seen obliquely not being double, is ascribed by Mr Wheatstone to the coalescence of the images of different magnitudes given by each eye.

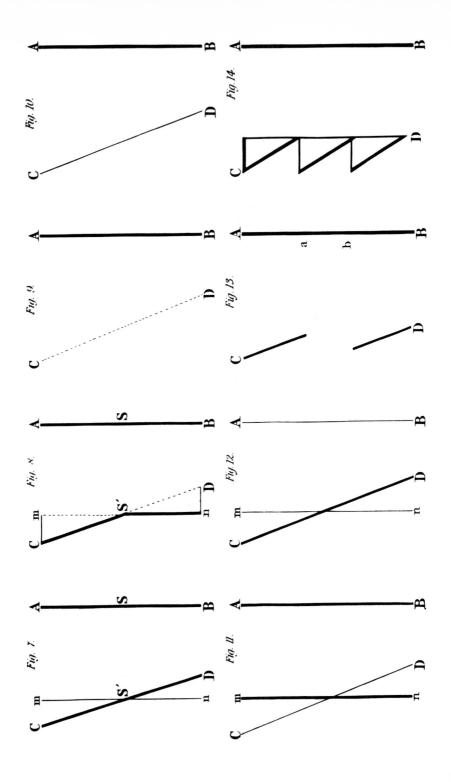

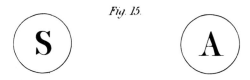

Fig. 15.

The *ocular equivocation*, as it may be called, which is produced by the capricious disappearance and reappearance of images formed on nearly corresponding parts of the retina of each eye, is placed beyond a doubt by Mr Wheatstone's own experiments.* Having inscribed the letters A, S, Fig. 15, in two equal circles, he unites the circles, and finds, that, while the common border remains constant, "the letter within it will change alternately" from A to S. At the instant of change, the letter "breaks into fragments; while fragments of the letter which is about to appear, mingle with them, and are immediately replaced by the entire letter." I have long ago† described an affection of the retina, of an analogous kind, which illustrates the subject under consideration.

> If we look very steadily and continuously with both eyes at a double pattern – such as one of those on a carpet – composed of two single patterns of different colours, supppose *red* and *green*; and if we direct the mind particularly to the contemplation of the *red* one, the *green* pattern will sometimes vanish entirely, leaving the *red* one alone visible; and, by the same process, the *red* one may be made to disappear.

When we join to these various facts the remarkable phenomena of the disappearance of objects seen out of the axis of vision by one or by both eyes,‡ we shall find it difficult to believe that two similar unequal figures can coalesce; or that "similar pictures, falling upon corresponding points of the two retinæ, may appear double, and in different places."

5. *On the Cause of the Perception of Objects in Relief by the Coalescence of Dissimilar Pictures.*

Mr Wheatstone concludes his interesting paper with an inquiry into the cause "*why* two dissimilar pictures, projected on the two retinæ, give rise to the perception of an object in relief." "I will not attempt," he adds, "at present, to give the complete solution of this question, which is far from being so easy as at a first glance it may appear to be, and is, indeed, one of great complexity. I shall, in this place, merely consider the most obvious explanations which might be offered, and shew their insufficiency to explain the whole of the phenomena."

Mr Wheatstone then proceeds to describe the process of vision in the same

---

* *Phil. Trans.* 1838, p. 386, § 14.
† *Letters on Natural Magic*, p. 54.
‡ See *Letters on Natural Magic.* Lett. III., p. 54.

manner as we have done in § 3; but impressed with the conviction that his previous results are correct, he adds, "All this is *in some degree true*; but were it *entirely so*, no appearance of relief should present itself when the eyes remain intently fixed on one point of a binocular image in the stereoscope." He then gives the following experiment as decisive on the subject: – "Draw two lines, about two inches long, and inclined towards each other as in Fig. 7, on a sheet of paper; and having caused them to coincide by converging the optic axes to a point nearer than the paper, look intently on the upper end of the resultant line, without allowing the eyes to wander from it for a moment. The *entire line will appear* single, and in its proper relief," &c. After making this experiment with the greatest care, we admit that it may *appear* single, without being single. To us it does not appear single, but exactly the same as a line having the same length and the same position appears in ordinary vision. Now, though this latter line appears single to most eyes, yet it is certain that every point of it is double and indistinct, excepting the point on which the attention is fixed, and to which the optic axes converge. The vision of objects in relief from the union of dissimilar pictures, is performed by the very same process as the vision of real objects in relief by the ordinary agency of our two eyes; and in establishing this principle, the true cause of the phenomenon discovered by Mr Wheatstone will be readily obtained.

Mr Wheatstone considers it as experimentally established, "that the most vivid belief of the solidity of an object of three dimensions arises from two different perspective projections of it being simultaneously presented to the mind;" and that "the simultaneous vision of two dissimilar pictures suggests the relief of objects in the most vivid manner." Having already explained in, § 3, the true process by which solid bodies are seen in relief, I shall now endeavour to shew, that, in the vivid relief produced by the union of two dissimilar plane pictures, this union is merely a necessary accessory, and not the cause of the phenomenon in question.

When two of the images of two perfectly similar objects are united either by looking at a nearer or a remote object, the compound image, thus formed, is seen at the place where the two optic axes converge, and is larger and more remote than the single image if we look at a more distant object, and smaller and nearer if we look at a nearer object.* The best mode of conducting this class of experiments is to suspend two equal rings by invisible fibres, or to cement them upon a large plate of glass, whose surface and figure are not visible to the observer. The object of this arrangement is to prevent the observer from having any knowledge of their distance from the eye. When the rings, thus placed, are doubled, interpose an aperture, so as to permit only the united rings to be seen; and it will be found that they appear at the place to which the optic axes converge, appearing smaller and nearer, or larger and more remote, according as the optic axes are

---

* Several curious facts establishing this result have been given by Dr Smith in his *Compleat System of Optics*, vol. ii. 387–389; and *Remarks*, § 526–527.

converged to a point nearer or more distant than the actual rings. In both these cases, the similar rings are seen in identically the same manner, having the same apparent magnitude and position as if a similar real ring were placed as an object at the spot to which the optic axes converge. Let us now apply these facts to the vision of the apparent solid produced *in consequence* of the union of two dissimilar plane pictures of it. For this purpose, I shall take the case of the frustum of a cone, after having considered the process by which we see a real frustum of a cone by both eyes – the nature of the compound picture which we do see – and the cause of the apparent single picture of which the mind takes cognizance.

When we look at the real frustum of a cone (ABCD, placed as in Fig. 16), the right eye R sees a solid, whose projection is *a'b'*CD, or *abcd*, Fig. 17; and the left eye to a solid, whose projection is A'B'CD, or ABCD, Fig. 17. The smaller circle CD appears nearer to the observer than the base AB, because the eye cannot see it distinctly without adjusting itself to the distance RC, LD, and converging its optic axes to that distance. Each eye, acting alone, sees the cone single, and the various points of its outline are seen more or less distinct, according as they are more or less remote from the point to which the eye is for the instant adjusted. But so rapid is the motion of the eye, and so quickly does it survey the whole of the solid, that it obtains a most distinct perception of its form, its surface, and its solidity. When we view the cone with *both eyes*, we have the same indistinctness of outline when the optic axes are converged to a single point: but in addition to this, we have the greater indistinctness arising from every point of the figure being seen *double*, except the single point to which the axes are converged. But this imperfection, too, is scarcely visible, from the rapid view which the eyes take of the whole solid, converging their axes upon every point of it, and thus seeing each point in succession single and distinct. Hence, we must draw a marked distinction between the vision of the solid (as an optical fact) when the eyes are fixed upon one point of it, and the resultant perception of its figure arising from the union of all the separate sensations received by the two eyes.

Let ABCD, Fig. 16, be the solid frustum of a cone, having its axis MN produced, bisecting at O the distance LR between the two eyes L, R. Draw AL, AR, BL, BR; and also CL, CR, and DL, DR. Then, if we look at this solid with the left eye L only, the projection of it will be as shewn in Fig. 17 at ABCD, and in Fig. 16 at A'B'CD; AC being much greater than DB, and the summit-plane CD appearing on the right-hand side of the centre of the base AB. The reason of this is obvious from Fig. 16, where the left eye L sees the sides AC under the angle ALC, while it sees the other side DB under the much smaller angle BLD; the apparent magnitude being in the one case A'C, and in the other DB'. In like manner, the right eye R sees DB under the large angle BRD, and with an apparent magnitude D*b'*; while it sees AC under the smaller angle ARC, and with an apparent magnitude C*a'*. Hence it follows, that, with both eyes, we shall see the solid in perfect symmetry, with its summit CD concentric with AB; and hence

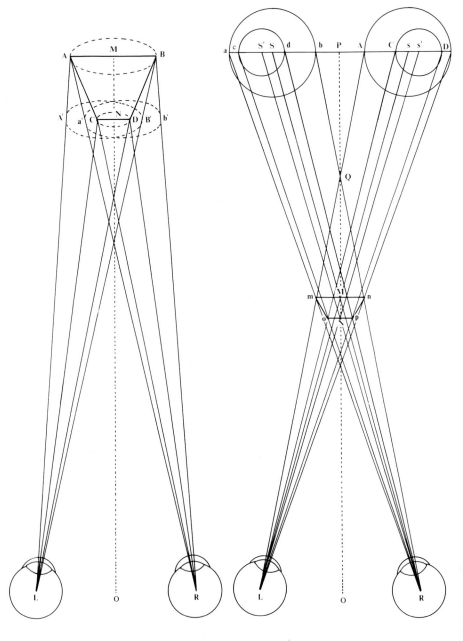

Fig 16   *Fig 17*

the reason is obvious why the two dissimilar pictures in the retina give a resultant picture corresponding with the solid itself.

Quitting our solid frustum of a cone, let us now suppose that its two dissimilar projections ABCD, *abcd*, Fig. 17, are united by the two eyes L, R, converging their axes to a point nearer the observer. By drawing lines from A, B, C, D, *a, b, c, d*, to L and R, the centres of visible direction, it will be seen that the circles AB, *ab* at the base, can be united only by converging the optical axes to M, and the summit circles CD, *cd* only by convering the axes to N. Hence, *mnop* will represent the solid frustum of a cone, whose axis is MN. Now, all the rays which flow from any point of the two projections AB, *ab*, cross each other at the figure *mnop*; and, consequently, this figure is seen by both eyes in identically the same manner as if the rays which really emanate from the plane figures had emanated from their points of intersection, that is, from the outlines of the solid figure *mnop*.

In order to see the base *mn*, the optic axes must be converged to M, or any other point of the base; and in order to see the summit *op* distinctly, the axes must be converged to N. But the distance MN is so very small, that the whole outline *mnop* will be seen with great distinctness; though it is certain that every point of it, but one, is seen double.

The height MN of the cone, Fig. 17, is equal to:

$$cot = \tfrac{1}{2}A - \tfrac{1}{2}A'$$

A, A' being the angles of the optic axes LMR, LNR, and OL or OR radius. But as these angles are not known, we may find MN thus: – Let D = distance OP; *d* = S*s*, the distance of the two points united at M; *d'* = S's', the distance of the two points united at N; C = LR = 2½ inches. Then

$$MP = \frac{Dd}{C+d}; NP = \frac{Dd'}{C+d'}; \text{ and } MN = \frac{Dd'}{C+d'} - \frac{Dd}{C+d}$$

When the two figures are united by converging the axes beyond P, the base *mn* of the line will be nearest the eye; and, consequently, the cone will appear *hollow*. In this case,

$$M'N' = \frac{Dd}{C-d} - \frac{Dd'}{C-d'}$$

and the cone will be much larger than in the other case. If we make

D   = 9.24 inches,
C   = 2.50; then
d   = 2.42;
d'   = 2.14; and
MN = 0.283, the height of the cone. Whereas, in the second case,
       M'N' = 18.9 feet!

Considering that the summit-plane *op* rises above the base *mn*, in consequence of the convergency of the optic axes at N, it may be asked, how it happens that the frustum still appears a solid, and the plane *op*, where it is, when the optic axes are converged to another point M, so as to see the base *mn* distinctly? Should not the relief disappear, when the condition on which it depends is not fulfilled? But, instead of the relief disappearing, the summit-plane *op* maintains its position there as fixedly as if it belonged to the real solid; and it ought to do so, for the rays emanate from it in exactly the same manner, and from identically the same image on the retina as if it were a real solid. Now, by the mere advance of the intersection of the optic axes from M to N, the rays from the circles AB, CD, &c. still produce the same picture on the retina of each eye, and the only effect of the advance of the point of convergence from N to M, is to throw that picture a little to the *right* side of the optic axes of the *left* eye, and a little to the *left* of the optic axes of the *right* eye; so that the summit *op* still retains its place, and is merely seen double.

6. *On the Doctrine of Corresponding Points.*

Our celebrated countryman, Dr Reid, calls those *points* in the retina of each eye *corresponding*, which are similarly situated with respect to the *foramen centrale*, or centre of each retina; and he maintains that objects painted on those points have the same visible position. He observes "that the most plausible attempts to account for this property of the eyes have been unsuccessful, and that it must be either a primary law of our constitution, or the consequence of some more general law which is not yet discovered." This doctrine has been very generally admitted; and if great names could have given it currency, those of Newton and Wollaston, supported by a number of anatomists and metaphysicians, might have placed it, both optically and metaphysically, beyond the reach of challenge. The doctrine of the semidecussation of the fibres of the optic nerve, as explained by Newton, gave great support to the theory of corresponding points. The idea that each fibre of the nerve divided itself into two, one of which went to a given point in the retina of one eye, while the other went to the corresponding point in the retina of the other eye, seemed to be at once an explanation and a proof of the doctrine.

Whether the anatomical supposition be true or false is a matter of little consequence at present, as the doctrine which it supports is not true excepting in the single case where the optic axes are parallel, and in this case it is true only because it is a necessary consequence of the general law of visible direction.

Along with the theory of corresponding points, we must rank the *binocular circle* of the Germans in which it is embodied. Let R, L, Fig. 18, be the right and left eyes whose centres of visible direction are C, C′, and whose optic axes CA, C′A, converge to any point A. Through the three points A, C, C′, describe the circle ABCC′. This circle is called the *Binocular Circle*, because if we take any point B in its circumference, and draw BCE, BC′E′, the points E, E′ on the retinæ will be

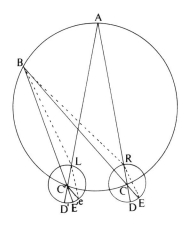

Fig 18.

corresponding points, that is, points equidistant from D (because the angles ACB, AC'B being equal, DC'E' and DCE are also equal), and consequently when the optic axes are directed to A, an object at B will have its image formed upon the corresponding points E, E', and will be seen single.

Now, when the optic axes are directed to A, a ray from B will fall upon the left eye at L with a greater angle of incidence than on the right eye at R; and consequently it will strike the retina at a point farther from D in the left eye than in the right eye; that is, if the ray BR is refracted to E, the ray BL will be refracted to some point *e*, and consequently the lines of visible direction EC, *e* C' will meet in a point without the circle ABC. The real *binocular curve*, therefore, is everywhere without the circle. Hence the doctrine of corresponding points is not true; and if it had been true, it would have been so because it was a necessary consequence of a law of visible direction.

7. *On the Vision of Cameos and Intaglios.*

The beautiful experiment of converting a *cameo* into an *intaglio*, and an *intaglio* into a *cameo*, by *monocular* vision, is well known. In 1825 I had occasion to investigate this subject, and in January 1826 I published an account of my observations, with an ample notice of the previous labours of other authors.*

Mr Wheatstone has ingeniously connected this optical fallacy with the union of dissimilar images on the retina, though he does not refer it to this union as its cause. After quoting my previous explanation of the illusion, he makes the

---

* This account was published anonymously in the *Edinburgh Journal of Science* for January 1826, No. VII. vol. iv. p. 97; and a popular abstract of it afterwards appeared in my *Letters on Natural Magic*, Letter V. p. 98.

following observations upon it. "These considerations do not *fully* explain the phenomenon, for they suppose that the image must be inverted, and that the light must fall in a particular direction; but the conversion of relief will still take place when the object is viewed through an open tube without any lenses to invert it, and also when it is equally illuminated in all parts."* In thus objecting to the *fulness* of my explanation, Mr Wheatstone has overlooked the great number of experiments by which I have supported it; and especially those facts in which I observed the fallacy when the object is viewed *without even an open tube, – without inversion; – with both eyes open*, and when it is *placed in broad daylight*. Mr Wheatstone then gives his own opinion as follows.

> If we suppose a cameo and an intaglio of the same object, the elevations of the one corresponding exactly to the depressions of the other, it is easy to shew that the projection of either on the retina is sensibly the same.† When the cameo or the intaglio is seen with both eyes, it is impossible to mistake an elevation for a depression; but when either is seen by one eye only, the most certain guide of our judgment, viz., the presentation of a different picture to each eye, is wanting; the imagination therefore supplies the deficiency, and we conceive the object to be raised or depressed according to the dictates of this faculty. No doubt, in such cases our judgment is in a great degree influenced by accessory circumstances, and the intaglio or the relief may sometimes present itself according to our previous knowledge of the direction in which the shadows ought to appear; but the *real cause* of the phenomenon is to be found in the *indetermination of the judgment*, arising from our more perfect means of judging being absent.‡

Now, what Mr Wheatstone calls the *real cause* of the illusion is no *cause* at all, – it is merely a previous state of the mind which is favourable to the operation of the real cause. Two eyes, like two witnesses, must always bear a better testimony to truth than one; and, in the present case, the want of the convergency of the optic axes to estimate the distance of the highest and lowest points of the cameo and the intaglio, undoubtedly favours the illusion, and allows the real cause to influence the judgment; but even here this admission has its limits, for in very shallow cameos and intaglios the illusion takes place with both eyes.§

Without repeating in this place the various facts respecting mother-of-pearl and other phenomena in which I observed the illusion when both eyes were used. I shall content myself with quoting the following observation, made in Egypt by Lady Georgiana Wolff. "Lady Georgiana," says the Rev. Mr Wolff, "observed a

---

* *Phil. Trans.* 1838, p. 383.
† This is true only when they are not seen obliquely. – D. B.
‡ *Phil. Trans.* 1838, p. 384.
§ When the cameo and intaglio are viewed very obliquely, one of the causes of deception disappears. In the case of a cameo appearing depressed, the depression disappears the instant that the shadow of the cameo encroaches distinctly upon the plane surface from which it is raised, because an intaglio never can, however obliquely viewed, throw a shadow upon the plane surface out of which it is excavated. For the same reason, an intaglio seen very obliquely will not rise into a cameo, because the shadow on the plane surface is wanting.

curious optical deception in the sand about the middle of the day, when the sun was strong; all the *foot-prints*, and *other marks that are indented in the sand, had the appearance of being raised out of it*; and at those times there was such a glare that it was unpleasant for the eye."*

8. *On the Change in the Apparent Position of the Drawings of Solid Bodies.*

Although this illusion may have been previously observed, yet I believe Professor Necker of Geneva is the first person who has described and explained it. He mentioned it to me in conversation in 1832; and afterwards sent me a notice of it, which I published in the London and Edinburgh Philosophical Journal.† Mr Necker describes the illusion in the following manner.

> The rhomboid AX, Fig. 19, is drawn so that the solid angle A should be seen the nearest to the spectator, and the solid angle X the farthest from him, and that the face ACBD should be the foremost while the face XDC is behind. But in looking repeatedly at the same figure, you will perceive that at times the apparent position of the rhomboid is so changed that the solid angle X will appear the nearest, and the solid angle A the farthest, and that the face ACDB will recede behind the face XDC, which will come forward; which effect gives to the whole solid a quite contrary apparent inclination.

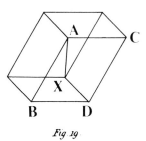

Fig 19

Professor Necker observed this change "as well with one as with both eyes," and he considered it as owing

> to an involuntary change in the adjustment of the eye for obtaining distinct vision. And that whenever the point of distinct vision on the retina was directed on the angle A, for instance, this angle seen more distinctly than the others, was naturally supposed to be nearer and foremost; while the other angles seen indistinctly were supposed to be farther away and behind. The reverse took place when the point of distinct vision was brought to bear upon the angle X.

Upon this explanation Mr Wheatstone makes the following observations:

> That this is not the true explanation is evident from *three* circumstances: in the *first* place, the two points A and X being both at the same distance from the eyes, the

---

* Journal of the Rev. Joseph Wolff, 1839, p. 189.
† Vol. i. p. 334.

same alteration of adjustment which would make one of them indistinct would make the other so; *secondly*, the figure will undergo the same changes whether the eye be adjusted to a point before or behind the plane in which the figure is drawn; and, *thirdly*, the change of figure frequently occurs while the eye continues to look at the same angle. The effect seems entirely to depend on our mental contemplation of the figure, or of its converse. By following the lines with the eye, with a clear idea of the solid figure we are describing, it may be fixed for any length of time; but it requires practice to do this, or to change the figure at will. As I have observed before, these effects are far more obvious when the figures are regarded with one eye only.

In a case of this kind, where one eminent individual assures us that he has proved his explanation to be true in *three* different ways, and another maintains that this explanation is evidently not the true one from *three* different circumstances, there must be a misapprehension to be removed, as well as a difficulty to be solved. It is impossible to read Mr Necker's paper without discovering that Mr Wheatstone has entirely mistaken his meaning, though the mistake is partly owing to Mr Necker's use of the phrase, "adjustment of the eye for obtaining distinct vision." Mr Wheatstone understands this to mean the adjustment of the eye to A or X, as if they were at different distances from the observer; whereas Mr Necker clearly refers to that indistinctness of vision which arises from distance on the retina from the *foramen centrale*, or point of distinct vision. When the eyes are converged upon A, X is seen indistinctly, and *vice versa*; and that this is Mr Necker's meaning is obvious from the following conclusion of his letter: "What I have said of the solid angles is equally true of the edges, – those edges upon which *the axis of the eye, or the central hole of the retina, are* directed, will always appear forward; so that now it appears to me certain that this little, at first so puzzling, phenomenon, depends upon the law of distinct vision." That this is the true cause of the phenomenon I have no hesitation in affirming. By hiding A with the finger, or making it indistinct with a piece of dimmed glass, or throwing a slight shadow over it, X appears forward, and continues so when these obscurations are removed and the same effect is produced by hiding X, A becoming then nearest to the eye. This experiment may be still more satisfactorily made by holding above the rhomboid a piece of ground glass (the ground side being farthest from the eye), and bringing one edge of it gradually down till it touches the point A, the other edge being kept at a distance from the paper. In this way AX, and all the lines diverging from A, become dimmer as they recede from A, and consequently A becomes the most forward point. A deep plano-convex lens, with its convex side ground, will answer the purpose still better, the apex of the lens being laid upon A or X; or the effect may be still farther improved by making the roughness increase either from the apex of a convex surface, or any fixed point of a plane one.

Following out his general opinion of the superiority of binocular vision, Mr Wheatstone remarks, that the illusion which we have been examining is most obvious with one eye. It is not so with my eyes; and I conceive it should not be so, as the convergency of the optic axes can have no efficacy in preventing illusion when the figure occupies a plane surface.

In the course of the investigation which I have now brought to a close, I have had occasion to observe many very interesting phenomena, which it would be out of place to describe at present. They relate partly to the effects produced by uniting unequal and dissimilar pictures which have a tendency to represent incompatible solids; – to the union of dissimilar pictures, when the parts of the solid which they tend to produce lie wholly or principally in a plane perpendicular to the line joining the eyes and to the plane of the optic axes;* – to the union of pictures, one of which is more or less turned round in its own plane; – to the phenomena exhibited by uniting the images of two similar real solids, the one elevated and the other depressed; – to the union of dissimilar plane figures, which should at the same time give a solid in relief, and in the converse of relief;† – and to the union of portions of dissimilar figures, those which are wanting in the one figure existing in the other. Among the singular effects produced under these various conditions, nothing is more remarkable than the tendency or desire, as it were, of the eyes, to unite and fix the two pictures hovering before them, to convert them into some figure of three dimensions (sometimes in relief, sometimes in the converse, and sometimes in both at the same time); and the suddenness with which the two images start into union, give birth to a solid figure on which the optic axes are converged, and release the eyes from that unnatural condition in which they had previously been placed.

St Leonards College, St Andrews,
January 1843.

2.6. Brewster: "On the conversion of relief by inverted vision". *Transactions of the Royal Society of Edinburgh*, 1844, **15**, 657–662.

Under the name *Conversion of Relief*, an expression first used by Mr Wheatstone, I include all those optical illusions which take place in the vision of cameos and intaglios, of elevations and depressions, whether they are produced with opaque or transparent bodies, – on surfaces with or without shadows, – in reflected or transmitted light, – while using one or both eyes, – or by erect or inverted vision. In these various forms of the phenomenon, the illusion is modified by certain

---

* Such as the magnified teeth of a saw, as in Fig. 14, or a thin section of a hexagonal prism whose axis is parallel to a line joining the eyes.
† In order to produce simultaneously this double effect, the lines of the pyramid, for example, which are to give the converse of relief, should be fainter than the other lines, or in different and feebler colours.

secondary causes, which were regarded both by Mr Wheatstone* and myself† as primary causes; so that we were led away, each in a different direction from the right path of inquiry.

The phenomenon occurs in its most general and simple form, when it is produced by viewing a shadowless depression, or elevation, made in an extended surface, through an inverting microscope, or the inverting eye-piece of a telescope, and at an angle intermediate between 0° and 90°. In so far as I know, the phenomenon has never been thus limited, and, consequently, no explanation of it has ever been given. That which I shall now submit to the Society is capable of the most rigorous demonstration; and when it is once in our possession, we can have no difficulty in recognising the secondary causes which increase or diminish the influence of the primary one, and which, in its absence, are sometimes the immediate cause of the illusion.

Let A, Fig. 1, be a deep spherical concavity, and A′, Fig. 2, a high spherical convexity in an extended horizontal table MN, M′N′, and let them be shadowless or illuminated by a *quaquaversus* light, like that of the sky. If the observer, placed at a moderate distance, view these objects in the directions EA, E′A′, either with one or with both eyes, his accurate appreciation of the distances EA, E′A′, will prove to him that A is a *concavity*, and A′ a *convexity*; but if EA, E′A′ approach to equality, either from the distance of the observer, or from the shallowness of A, or

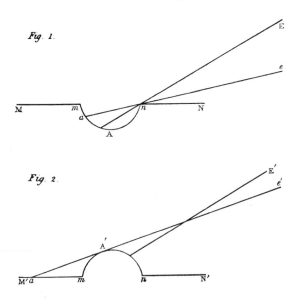

Fig. 1.

Fig. 2.

* *Phil. Trans.*, 1838, pp. 383, 384.
† *Edin. Trans.*, Vol. xv. p. 365; *Edin. Journal of Science*, Vol. iv. p. 97; and *Letters on Natural Magic*, p. 98.

the slight elevation of A', he will cease to recognise any difference in the distances EA, E'A', and will be unable to tell which is the convexity, and which the concavity. So great, indeed, is this uncertainty, that, from causes which he cannot discover, they will sometimes appear convex and sometimes concave. In this indetermination of the judgment, a touch of A, A' by the finger, or the introduction of a shadow, will remove or confirm the illusion, whatever it may be. The same result will be obtained, if we view A and A' vertically, with an erect or inverting eye-piece. In all these cases, we suppose that the circular, or rather the elliptical, base of the convexity or concavity is distinctly seen.

Let us now look at A, A', at obliquities varying from 0° to 90°. In Fig. 1 the *concavity* A will have an elliptical section at all obliquities, till, at 90°, it appears a straight line; but in the *convexity* the effect is very different. In passing from 0° to the position E', Fig. 2, the circular section of A' will appear an ellipse; but in passing from E' to 90°, the appearance of A' will lose all resemblance to A. When the eye is at *e'*, for example, the summit A' of the convexity will cover the point *a* of the table, and *am* will be invisible; and near 90°, the convexity A' will eclipse the whole surface of the table *m*M', however extended it may be, and will rise above it.

Let us now suppose that the eye at E, Fig. 3, views the concavity A through the inverting eye-piece EGH, the horizontal table MN must obviously be inverted as

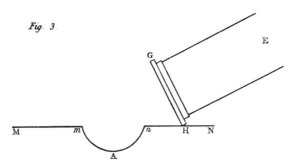

Fig. 3.

well as the hollow A; but the *apparent* change, produced by inversion, is very different from the real change. The surface MN, out of which A is excavated, and upon which the observer leans, and rests the lower end H of his inverting eye-piece, appears to remain where it was, and still to look upwards, in place of appearing inverted, and looking downwards. When he strikes the table with the end H of the eye-piece through which he looks, he believes that it is the lower end of the field of view that strikes the table, and rests upon it. With these convictions, he sees what is represented in Fig. 4. The concavity *m*A*n*, Fig. 3, appears inverted; and as the visible part of the concavity A*m*, Fig. 3, is nearest the eye in Fig. 4, and the invisible part A*n*, Fig. 3, farthest from the eye in Fig. 4, *m*A*n* must appear a concavity in Fig. 4, solely because it seems to rise out of the surface MN, which looks upward, as if it had not been inverted by the eye-piece.

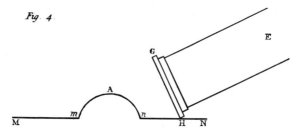

Fig. 4.

Now, in this experiment, the conversion of the concavity into a convexity depends on two separate illusions, one of which springs from the other. The *first* illusion is the belief that the surface MN is looking upwards, whereas it is really inverted, as shewn in Fig. 5; and the *second* illusion, which arises from the first, is, that the point *n* appears *farthest* from the eye, whereas it is *nearest* to it, as shewn in Fig. 5. All these observations are equally applicable *mutatis mutandis* to the vision of convexities; and hence it follows, that the conversion of relief, occasioned by the use of an inverting eye-piece, is not produced directly by the inversion, but by an illusion, in virtue of which we conceive the remotest side of the convexity or concavity to be nearest our eye when it is not.

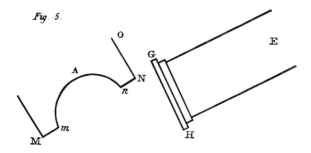

Fig. 5.

In order to demonstrate the correctness of this explanation, let the concavity *mAn* be made in a *narrow stripe* of wood, as in Fig. 5, and let it be viewed, as formerly, through the inverting eye-piece. It will now appear, as in Fig. 5, really inverted, and free from both the illusions which formerly took place. The narrow surface MN being now wholly included in the field of view, and the thickness NO of the stripe of wood distinctly seen, the inversion of the surface MN, which now looks downward, will be at once recognised. The edge *n* of the concavity will appear *nearest* the eye,* as it really is, and *the concavity, though inverted, will still appear a concavity*. The very same reasoning is applicable to a convexity on a narrow stripe of wood.

* The inversion of an object never makes the *nearer* part of an object *more remote*, nor the *remote* part *nearer*.

When, as in Fig. 4, the concavity is seen as a convexity, let it be viewed more and more obliquely. The *elliptical margin of the convexity will always be visible*, which is impossible in a real convexity; and the elevated apex will gradually sink till the elliptical margin becomes a straight line, and *the imaginary convexity completely levelled*. The struggle between truth and error is here so singular, that while one part of the Figure *m*A*n* has become concave, the other part retains its convexity!

In like manner, when a convexity is seen as a concavity, the concavity loses its true shape, as it is viewed more and more obliquely, till its remote elliptical margin is encroached upon by the apex of the convexity; and, towards an inclination of 90°, the concavity disappears altogether, under circumstances analogous to those already described.

If, in place of using an inverting eye-piece, we invert the concavity *m*A*n*, by looking at its image in the focus of a convex lens, it will sometimes appear a convexity, and sometimes not. In this form of the experiment the image of the concavity, and consequently its apparent depth, is greatly diminished. Hence any trivial cause, such as a preconception of the mind, or an approximation to a shadow, or a touch of the hollow by the point of the finger, will either produce a conversion, or prevent it.

In the preceding experiments we have supposed the convexity to be high and the concavity deep and circular, and we have supposed them also to be shadowless, or illuminated by a quaquaversus light, such as that of the sky in the open fields. This was done to get rid of all secondary causes, which interfere with and modify the normal cause when the concavities and convexities are shallow, and have distinct shadows, or when the concavity has the shape of an animal, or any body which we are accustomed to see convex.

Let us now suppose that a strong shadow is thrown upon the concavity. In this case the normal experiment, already explained and shewn in Fig. 5, is much more perfect and satisfactory. The illusion is complete, and invariable when the concavity is in an extended surface; and it as invariably disappears when it is in a narrow stripe.

In the secondary forms of the experiment, the inversion of the shadow becomes the principal cause of the illusion; but, in order that the result may be invariable, or nearly so, the concavities must be shallow, and the convexities a little raised. At great obliquities, however, this cause of the conversion of Form ceases to produce the illusion, and in varying the inclination from 0° to 90°, the cessation takes place sooner with deep than with shallow cavities. The reason of this is, that the shadow of a concavity is very different at great obliquities from the shadow of a similar convexity. The shadow never can emerge out of a cavity so as to darken the surface in which the cavity is made; whereas the shadow of a convexity soon extends beyond the outline of its base, and, finally, throws a long stripe of darkness over the surface on which it rests. Hence it is impossible to mistake a convexity for a concavity, whenever its shadow extends beyond its base.

When the concavity is a horse or a dog upon a seal, it will often rise into a convexity when seen through a single lens, which does not invert it; but the illusion disappears at great obliquities. In this case the illusion is favoured, or produced, by two causes: the first is, that the convex form of the horse or dog is the one which the mind is most disposed to seize; and the second is, that we use only one eye, with which we cannot measure depths as well as with two. The illusion, however, still takes place when we employ a lens *three* or more inches wide, so as to admit the use of both eyes, but it is less certain, as the binocular vision enables us to keep in check, to a certain degree, the other causes of illusion.

The influence of these secondary causes is strikingly displayed in the following experiment. In the armorial bearings upon a seal, the shield is often more deeply cut than the surrounding parts. With binocular vision the shallow parts rise into a convexity sooner than the shield, or continue so while the shield remains concave; but if we shut one eye, the shield then becomes convex like the rest. In these experiments with a single lens, a slight variation in the position of the seal, or a slight change in the direction or intensity of the illumination, or particular reflections from the interior of the stone, will favour or oppose the illusion. In viewing the shield, or the deepest portion, with a single lens, a slight rotation of the seal round the wrist, backwards and forwards, will remove the illusion, in consequence of the eye perceiving that the change in the perspective is different from what it should be.

In a paper in the *Edinburgh Journal of Science*, already referred to, I have described several other examples of the conversion of form, in which inverted vision is not employed. As seen by the naked eye, hollows in *mother of pearl*, and other semi-transparent bodies, rise into relief; and the same thing happens on surfaces of agate and woods of various kinds, when transparent circular portions are illuminated by refraction, at those parts of their circumference where they would have been illuminated had they been convexities.* But the most interesting cases of conversion of form are those in which *the mind alone* operates, and receives no aid either from inversion, shadow, or monocular vision.

If we take, as I have elsewhere remarked, one of the Intaglio moulds, used in making the bas-reliefs of that able artist Mr Henning, and direct the eyes to it steadily, without noticing surrounding objects, we may coax ourselves into the belief that the Intaglio is actually a bas-relief. It is difficult at first to produce the deception, but a little practice never fails to accomplish it. We have succeeded in carrying this deception so far as to be able, by the eye alone, to raise a complete hollow mask of the human face into a projecting head. In order to do this we must exclude the vision of other objects; and also the margin or thickness of the cast. This experiment cannot

---

* In examining, under the microscope, the shallow fluid cavities *within* the substance of a film of sulphate of lime, described in the *Edinburgh Transactions*, vol. x. p. 35, they frequently appeared as *elevations* on the surface of the plate next the eye.

fail to produce a very great degree of surprise in those who succeed in it; and it will, no doubt, be regarded by the sculptor (who can use it) as a great auxilliary in his art.*

From these observations it will be seen that the conversion of Form, excepting in the normal case, depends upon various causes which are effective only under particular conditions; such as the depth of the hollow or the elevation of the relief – the distance of the object – the sharpness of vision – the use of one or both eyes – the inversion of the shadow – the nature of the object – and the means used by the mind itself to produce the illusion. In the normal case, however, where the cavity or convexity is shadowless, and upon an extended surface, and where inverted vision is used, the conversion of Form depends solely on the illusion, which it is impossible to resist, that the side of the cavity or elevation next the eye is actually farthest from it – an illusion not produced by inversion, but by a false judgment respecting the position of the surface on which the form is placed.

St Leonard's College, St Andrews,
May 4. 1844.

2.7. Brewster: "On the knowledge of distance given by binocular vision". *Transactions of the Royal Society of Edinburgh*, 1844, **15**, 663–674.

In analysing Mr Wheatstone's beautiful discovery, that in binocular vision we see all objects of three dimensions by means of two dissimilar pictures on the retina, I trust I have satisfied the Society that the dissimilarity of these two pictures is in no respect the cause of our vivid perception of such objects, but, on the contrary, an unavoidable accompaniment of binocular vision, which renders it less perfect than vision with one eye. On the other hand, it is quite true that, in Mr Wheatstone's experiment of producing the perception of objects of three dimensions by the apparent coalescence of two dissimilar representations of such objects *in plano,* the dissimilarity of the pictures is necessary in the exhibition of that beautiful phenomenon.

In performing, with the eye alone, the various experiments detailed in a former paper, I was very much struck with the fact, that the apparent solid figure, produced by the union of its dissimilar pictures, never took its right position in absolute space: that is, in place of appearing suspended between the eye and the plane upon which the dissimilar figures were drawn, the base of the solid seemed to rest on that plane, whether its apex was nearer the eye or more remote than its component plane figures.

With the view of finding the cause of this, I placed the component figures on a

* *Edinburgh Journal of Science*, No. VIII. p. 109, Jan. 1826.

plate of glass suspended in the air, so as to have no vision of the surface on which they rested, and after uniting these figures by binocular vision, and concealing the two outstanding single figures, I obtained results which, though not entirely satisfactory, proved that there existed some disturbing cause which prevented the united image from placing itself in the *binocular centre,* or the intersection of the optical axes. This disturbing cause was simply the influence of other objects in the same field of view, whose distance was known to the observer.

In order to avoid all such influences, and to study the subject under a more general aspect, it occurred to me that these objects would be gained by using a numerous series of plane figures, such as those of flowers or geometrical patterns upon carpets or paper-hangings. These figures being always at equal distances from each other, and almost perfectly equal and similar, the coalescence of any pair of them, by directing the optic axes to a point between the paper-hangings and the eye, is accompanied with the coalescence of every other pair. When the observer, therefore, places himself in front of that side of a papered room in which there are neither doors nor windows, and conceals from his eye the floor, the roof, and the right and left hand sides of the room, the whole of the retina will be covered with the images of the united plane figures, and there will be no interposing objects to prevent him from judging of the distance of the picture that may be presented to him.

Let the observer, therefore, now place himself *three* feet in front of the papered wall, and unite two of the figures, suppose two flowers, at the distance of *twelve* inches. The whole wall will now be presented to his view, consisting of flowers as before, but each flower will be composed of two flowers superimposed at the binocular centre, or the point of convergence of the optical axes. If we call D the distance of the eyes from the wall or *three* feet, C the distance between the eyes or two-and-half inches, and *d* the distance between the similar parts of the two flowers, we shall have *x* the distance of the binocular centre from the wall,

$$x = \frac{D\,d}{C + d} = 30 \text{ inches nearly, and } D - x = 6 \text{ inches, the distance of the}$$

binocular centre from the middle point between the two eyes.

Hence the whole papered wall, with all its flowers, in place of being seen, as in ordinary vision, at the distance of *three* feet, *is now suspended in the air, at the distance of six inches from the observer.* In maintaining this view of the wall, the eye will, at first, experience a disagreeable sensation; but after a few experiments the sensation will disappear, and the observer will contemplate the new picture with the same satisfaction and absence of all strain as if he were looking directly at the wall itself: for there is a natural tendency in the eyes to unite two similar pictures, and to keep them united, provided they are not too distant.

When this picture is at first seized by the observer, he does not, for a while, decide upon its distance from himself. It sometimes appears to advance from the wall to its true position in the binocular centre, and, when it has taken its place, it has a very extraordinary character: – the surface seems slightly convex towards the eye; it has a sort of silvery transparent aspect, and looks more beautiful than the real paper; it moves, with the slightest motion of the head, either laterally or to or from the wall. If the observer, who is now *three* feet from the wall, retires from it, the suspended wall of flowers will follow him, moving father and father from the real wall, and also, but very slightly, farther and farther from the observer: that is, the distance of the observer from the real wall increases faster than the distance of the suspended wall from it, according to the law expressed by the preceding formula. The binocular centre, therefore, recedes from the eye as the observer retires, and the strain consequently diminishes.

In order to observe these phenomena in the most perfect manner, the paper should be pasted upon a large screen, previously unseen by the observer, unconnected with the roof or the floor, and placed in a large apartment. The deception will then be complete; and when the picture stands suspended before the observer, and within a few inches of himself, he may stretch out his hand and place it on the other side of the picture, and even hold a candle on the other side of it, so as to satisfy himself that in both cases the picture is between his hand and himself.

When we survey this picture with attention, several very curious phenomena present themselves. Some of the flowers, when narrowly examined, appear somewhat like real flowers. In some the stalk gradually retires from the general plane of the picture; in others, it rises above it: one leaf will come farther out than another, or the flower will appear thicker and more solid, deviating considerably from the plane representation of it seen by each eye separately. All this arises from slight and accidental irregularities in the two figures which are united, thus producing an approximation to three dimensions in the picture. If the distance, for example, of the ends of two stalks in two coalescing flowers is greater than the distance of corresponding points in other parts of the stalk, the end of the stalk will rise from the general surface of the figure, and *vice versa*. In like manner, if the distance between two corresponding leaves is greater than the distance between other two corresponding leaves, then the two first, when united, will appear nearer the eye than the other two, and hence the appearance of a solid flower is partially given to the combination. These effects are better seen in old and imperfectly made paper-hangings than in those which are more carefully executed.

In continuing our survey of the suspended image, another curious pheno-menon presents itself: a part of one of the pieces of paper, and sometimes a whole stripe from the roof to the floor, will retire behind the general plane of the image, or rise above it; thus displaying, on a large scale, an imperfection in the workman-ship which it would have required a very narrow inspection to discover. This defect arises from the paper-hanger having cut off too much of the white margin of one or more of the adjoining pieces, so that when the two halves of a flower are united, part of the middle of the flower is left out; and hence when this defective flower is united with the one on the right hand of it, and the one on the left hand united with the defective one, the united or corresponding portion, being at a less distance, will appear farther from the eye than those parts of the suspended image composed of complete flowers. In like manner, if the two portions of the flowers are not brought together, but separated by a small space, the opposite effect will be produced. This will be understood from Fig. 1, where MN, OP represent portions of two separate pieces of paper, each twenty-one inches wide. In this specimen, there are only two flowers in each piece, namely one white flower, A or B, and two halves. If the two halves C, D, are united as in the figure, it is obvious that the flower is incomplete, a part of the central circle of the corolla having been cut off from each half. If we now, by straining the eye, unite CD with B, and also with A, then, at the same time, E will be united with the second or left hand image of A, and G with the second or right hand image of B. But since a piece has been cut out of CD, the half $\alpha\alpha$ of A is nearer the half DD than the other half aa is to the other half CC; and, in like manner, the half bb of B is nearer the half CC than the other half $\beta\beta$ is to the other half DD. Hence, when the strained eyes unite $\alpha\alpha$ to DD, the binocular centre is more remote than when aa is united to C, and the same is true of the other halves; consequently, the halves DD and bb must appear, as it were, sunk in the wall, or as farther removed from the observer; and if the defective cutting exists along the line RS from the floor to the ceiling, the whole stripe of paper between RS and OP, from the floor to the ceiling, will appear sunk in the papered wall. But if the defect is confined to a portion only of the flowers, then a rectangular space of the breadth RO, and of a height equal to the defective portion, will appear sunk in the paper. If every junction has the same defect as that at RS, then the whole will appear to consist of equal stripes, every alternate one being raised and the other depressed.

In the preceding example, there are only *two* flowers in a breadth, and their distance is 10½ inches, which is also the breadth of the sunk stripes. But if the flowers are three or four in number, and their distance $\frac{21}{3}$, $\frac{21}{4}$ inches, the sunk stripes will vary according as we unite two flowers whose distances are in the one

Fig 1

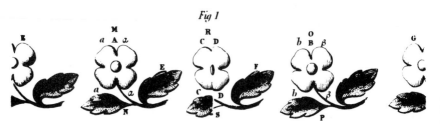

case 7 or 14 inches, and 5¼ or 10½ or 16¾ or 21 in the other. Calling B the breadth of the paper, n the number of flowers or figures in that breadth, and W the width of the sunk stripe, then we have $W = \dfrac{B}{n}$ or $\dfrac{2\,B}{n}$ or $\dfrac{3\,B}{n}$ according as we unite the two nearest, or the first and second flower, the first and third, or the first and fourth. When W = B, the sunk stripes will cover the whole paper, and all the flowers will lie in the same plane.

These results afford an accurate method of examining and discovering defects in the workmanship of paper-hangers, carpet-makers, painters, and other artists whose profession it is to combine a series of similar patterns in order to form an uniform and ornamental surface. The smallest defect in the similarity and equality in the figures or lines which compose a pattern, and any difference in the distance of the single figures, is instantly detected; and, what is remarkable, a small inequality of distance in a line perpendicular to the axis of vision, or in one dimension of space, is exhibited in a magnified form as a distance coincident with the axis of vision, and in an opposite dimension of space!

At the commencement of this class of experiments, it is difficult to realize, and very easy to dissolve, the singular binocular picture which we have been describing; but after the eyes have been drilled for a while to this species of exercise, the pictures become very persistent. Although the air-suspended image might be expected to disappear after closing one eye, and still more after having closed and re-opened both, yet I have found it in its original position in this latter case, and even after rubbing my eyes and shaking my head; and I have sometimes experienced a difficulty in ascertaining, after these operations, whether it was the real or the air-suspended wall that was before me. On some occasions a singular effect was produced. When the flowers on the paper are distant six inches, we may either unite two six inches distant, or two twelve inches distant. In the latter case, when the eyes have been accustomed to survey the suspended picture, I have found that, after shutting and opening them, I neither saw the picture formed by the two flowers twelve inches distant, nor the papered wall itself, but a picture formed by uniting the flowers six inches distant! The binocular centre had shifted its place, and instead of advancing to the wall, as is generally the case, and giving us ordinary vision of it, it advanced exactly as much as to unite the nearest flowers, just as on a ratchet wheel the detent slips over one tooth at a time; or, to speak more correctly, the binocular centre advanced in order to relieve the eyes from their strain, and when the eyes were opened, it had just reached that point which corresponded with the union of the flowers six inches distant.

In the construction of complex geometrical diagrams consisting only of fine lines, and in which similar figures are repeated at equal distances, it is very difficult to attain minute accuracy. The points of the compasses sink to different depths in the paper, and the lines which join such points seldom pass through their centres. Hence arises a general inaccuracy which the eye cannot detect; but if we examine such diagrams by strained binocular vision, their imperfections will be instantly displayed. Some parts will rise higher than others above the general level, and the whole will appear like several cobwebs placed at the distance of a tenth or a twelfth of an inch behind each other.*

In all the experiments made by Mr Wheatstone by the stereoscope, and in those described in my former paper, the dissimilar figures are viewed in a direction perpendicular to the plane on which they are drawn. A series of very interesting results, however, are obtained by uniting the images of lines meeting at an angular point, when the eye is placed at different heights above the plane of the paper, and at different distances from the angular point.

Let AC, BC (Fig. 2) be two lines meeting at C, the plane passing through them being the plane of the paper, and let them be viewed by the eys at E''', E'', E', E at different heights in a plane GMN perpendicular to the plane of the paper. Let R be the right eye and L the left eye, and when at E''' let them be strained so as to unite the points A, B. The united image of these points will be seen at the binocular centre D''', and the united lines AC BC will have the position D'''C.

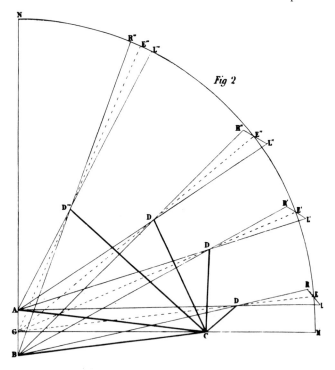

Fig 2

* This effect is finely seen in the diagram of the Homogeneous Curve, which forms Plate IX. of Mr Hay's work "On the Harmony of Form."

In like manner, when the eye descends to E'', E', E, the united image D'''C will rise and diminish, taking the positions D''C, D'C, DC till it disappears on the line CM, when the eyes reach M. If the eye deviates from the vertical plane GMN the united image will also deviate from it, and is always in a plane passing through the eye and the line GM.

If at any altitude EM the eye advances towards ACB in the line EG, the binocular centre D will also advance towards ACB in the line EG, and the image DC will rise and become shorter as its extremity D moves along DG, and after passing the perpendicular to GE it will increase in length. If the eye, on the other hand, recedes from ACB in the line GE, the binocular centre D will also recede, and the image DC will descend to the plane CM and increase in length.

The preceding diagram is, for the purpose of illustration, drawn in a sort of perspective, and therefore does not give the true positions and lengths of the united images. This defect, however, is remedied in Fig. 3, where E, E', E'', E''' is the middle point between the two eyes, the plane GMN being, as before, perpendicular to the plane passing through ACB. Now, as the distance of the eye from G is supposed to be the same, and as AB is invariable as well as the

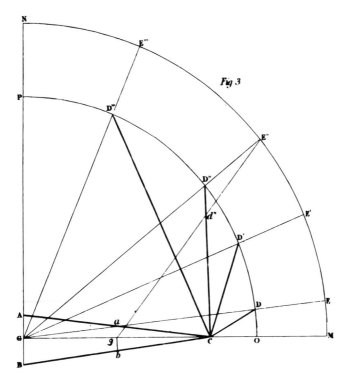

Fig. 3

distance between the eyes, the distance of the binocular centres O, D, D', D'', D''', P, from G will also be invariable, and lie in a circle ODP whose centre is G, and whose radius is GO, the point O being determined by the formula

$$GO = GD = \frac{GM \times AB}{AB + RL}.$$ Hence, in order to find the binocular centres D, D',

D'', D''', &c., at any altitude E, E' &c., we have only to join EG, E'G, &c., and the points of intersection D, D', &c., will be the binocular centres, and the lines DC, D'C, &c., drawn to C, will be the real lengths and inclinations of the united images of the lines AC, BC.

When GO is greater than GC there is obviously some angle A, or E''GM at

which D''C is perpendicular to GC. This takes place when cos. $A = \frac{GC}{GO}$ When

O coincides with C, the images CD, CD', &c., will have the same positions and magnitudes as the chords of the altitudes A of the eyes above the plane GC. In this case, the raised or united images will just reach the perpendicular when the eye is in the plane GCM, for since GC = GO, cos. A = 1, and A = 0°.

When the eye at any position, E'' for example, sees the points A and B united at D'', it sees also the whole lines AC, BC forming the image D''C. The binocular centre must, therefore, run rapidly along the line D''C: that is, the inclination of the optic axis must gradually diminish till the binocular centre reaches C, when all strain is removed. The vision of the image D''C, however, is carried on so rapidly, that the binocular centre returns to D'' without the eye being sensible of the removal and resumption of the strain which is required in maintaining a view of the united image D''C.

If we now suppose AB to diminish, the binocular centre will advance towards G, and the length and inclination of the united images DC, D'C, &c., will diminish also, and *vice versa*. If the distance RL (Fig. 2) between the eyes diminishes, the binocular centre will retire towards E, and the length and inclination of the images will increase. Hence persons with eyes more or less distant will see the united images in different places and of different sizes, though the quantities A and AB be invariable.

While the eyes at E'' are running along the lines AC, BC, let us suppose them to rest upon the points *a*, *b* equidistant from C. Join *ab*, and from the point *g*, where *ab* intersects GC, draw the line *g*E'', and find the point *d''* from the

formula $gd'' = \frac{gE'' \times ab}{ab + RL}.$ Hence the two points *a*, *b* will be united at *d''*, and

when the angle E''GC is such that the line joining D and C is perpendicular to GC, the line joining *d''*C will also be perpendicular to GC, the loci of the points D'' *d''* *d'* *d* will be in that perpendicular, and the image DC, seen by successive movements of the binocular centre from D'' to C, will be a straight line.

In the preceding observations we have supposed that the binocular centre D'', &c., is between the eye and the lines AC, BC; but the points A, C, and all the other points of these lines, may be united by fixing the binocular centre beyond AB. Let the eyes, for example, be at E''; then if we unite AB when the eyes converge to a point, $\varDelta''$ (not seen in the figure), beyond G, we shall have

$$G\varDelta'' = \frac{GE \times AB}{RL - AB}$$ and if we join the point $\varDelta''$ thus found and C, the line $\varDelta'$ C will

be the united image of AC and BC, the binocular centre ranging from $\varDelta''$ to C, in order to see it as one line. In like manner, we may find the position and length of the image $\varDelta'''$C, $\varDelta'$C, and $\varDelta$C corresponding to the position of the eyes at E''', E' and E. Hence all the united images of AC, BC: viz. C$\varDelta'''$, C $\varDelta''$, &c., will lie below the plane of ABC, and extend beyond a vertical line NB continued; and they will grow larger and larger, and approximate in direction to CG as the eyes descend from E''' to M. When the eyes are near to M, and a little above the plane of ABC, the line, when not carefully observed, will have the appearance of coinciding with CG, but stretching a great way beyond G. This extreme case represents the celebrated experiment with the compasses described by Dr Smith, and referred to by Professor Wheatstone. He took a pair of compasses, which may be represented by ACB, AB being their points, ACBC their legs, and C their joint; and having placed his eyes about E above their plane, he made the following experiment:–

> Having opened the points of a pair of compasses somewhat wider than the interval of your eyes, with your arm extended, hold the head or joint in the ball of your hand with the points outwards, and equidistant from your eyes, and somewhat higher than the joint. Then, *fixing your eyes upon any remote object* lying in the plane that bisects the interval of the points, you will first perceive two pair of compasses (each by being doubled with their inner legs crossing each other, not unlike the old shape of the letter W.) But by compressing the legs with your hand, the two inner points will come nearer to each other; and when they unite (having stopt the compression), the two inner legs will also entirely coincide and bisect the angle under the outward ones, and will appear more vivid, thicker and larger, than they do, so as to reach from your hand to the remotest object in view even in the horizon itself, if the points be exactly coincident.*

Owing to his imperfect apprehension of the nature of this phenomenon, Dr Smith has omitted to notice that the united legs of the compasses lie below the plane of ABC, and that they never can extend farther than the binocular centre at which their points A and B are united.

There is another variation of these experiments which possesses some interest, in consequence of its extreme case having been made the basis of a new theory of

* Smith's Optics, vol. ii. p. 388, § 977.

visible direction by the late Dr Wells.* Let us suppose the eyes of the observer to advance from E to N, and to descend along the opposite quadrant on the left hand of NG, but not drawn in Fig. 3, then the united image of AC, BC, will gradually descend towards CG, and become larger and larger. When the eyes are a very little above the plane of ABC, and so far to the left hand of AB, that CA points nearly to the left eye, and CB to the right eye, then we have the circumstances under which Dr Wells made the following experiment: – "If we hold two thin rules in such a manner that their sharp edges (AC, BC in Fig. 3) shall be in the optic axes, one of each, or rather a little below them, *the two edges will be seen united in the common axis* (GC in Fig. 3); and this apparent edge will seem of the same length with that of either of the real edges, when seen alone by the eye in the axis of which it is placed." This experiment, it will be seen, is the same with that of Dr Smith, with this difference only, that the points of the compasses are directed towards the eyes. Like Dr Smith, he has omitted to notice that the united image rises above GM, and he commits the opposite error of Dr Smith, in making the length of the united image too short.

If in this form of the experiment we fix the binocular centre beyond C, then the united images of AC, BC descend below GC, and vary in their length, and in their inclination to GC, according to the height of the eye above the plane of ABC, and its distance from AB.

It is a remarkable circumstance, that no examples have been recorded of false estimates of the distance of near objects, in consequence of the *accidental* binocular union of similar images. This has, no doubt, arisen from the rare occurrence of these circumstances or conditions, under which alone such illusions can be produced. In a room where the paper hangings have a small pattern, or similar figures recurring at the distance of 1, 1½, or 2 inches, a short-sighted person might very readily turn his eyes on the wall, when their axes converged to some point between him and the wall, which would unite one pair of the similar images; and, in this case, he would see the wall nearer him than the real wall, and moving with the motion of his head like something aerial. In like manner, a long-sighted person, with his optical axes converged to a point beyond the wall, might see an image of the wall more distant, and of an aerial character; – or a person who has taken too much wine, which often fixes the optical axes in opposition to the will, might, according to the nature of his sight, witness either of the illusions above mentioned.

In the preceding observations, we have confined ourselves to the binocular union of figures upon an opaque ground. This limitation almost necessarily precluded us from observing the results when the binocular centre is beyond the plane where these figures are situated, because it is not easy to adjust the eyes to a distant object, unless we look through the surfaces containing the figures. Now,

* Essay on Single Vision, &c., p. 44.

this is by far the most interesting form of the experiment, and it has the advantage of putting scarcely any strain upon the eyes, not only because the binocular centre is more distant, but because we cannot, in this way, unite figures whose distance exceeds 2½ inches, the interval between the eyes. Transparent patterns for these experiments may be cut out of stiff card paper, or thin plates of metal, or they may be made of paper pasted upon large panes of glass. Experiments may be made with trellis work, or with windows composed of small squares or lozenges; but the readiest pattern is the cane bottom of a chair, and I have performed my experiments by simply placing such a chair upon a high table, with its cane bottom in a vertical position. The distance of the centres of the eight-sided open figures in the direction of the width or depth of the chair, varies in different patterns from 0·54 to 0·76 of an inch. In order to simplify the calculations, we shall take the distance at 0·5, or half an inch. Then let

> D = 12 inches be the distance of the pattern from the eyes.
> d = 0·5 the distance of the centres of the similar figures.
> + $\varDelta$ = distance of suspended image from, and in front of, the pattern.
> − $\varDelta'$ = distance of suspended image from, and behind, the pattern.
> C = 2·5 the distance between the eyes.

Then we shall have

$$+\varDelta = \frac{Dd}{C + d} \text{and} - \varDelta' = \frac{Dd}{C - d}$$

Hence

> D − $\varDelta$ = distance of suspended image from the eye, and in front of the pattern, and
> D + $\varDelta'$ = its distance from the eye, and behind the pattern.

From these formulæ we have computed the following table, adapted to similar figures, whose centres are distant ½ an inch, 1, 1½, 2, and 2½ inches; but in reference to the positive values of $\varDelta$ and D, we may consider them as feet, 0·5 being in that case = 6 inches.

D Inches.	$d = 0·5$		$d = 1·0$		$d = 1·5$		$d = 2·0$		$d = 2·4$		$d = 2·5$	
	$+\varDelta$	$-\varDelta$	$+\varDelta$	$-\varDelta$	$+\varDelta$	$-\varDelta$	$+\varDelta$	$-\varDelta$	$+\varDelta$	$-\varDelta$	$+\varDelta$	$-\varDelta$
6	1	1·5	1·72	4	2·25	9	2·66	24	2·94	144	3	Infin.
12	2	3	3·43		4·50	18	5·33	48	5·88	288	6	Infin.
24	4	6	6·86	16	9	36	10·66	96	11·76	576	12	Infin.
48	8	12	13·7	32	18	72	21·33	192	23·52	1152	24	Infin.

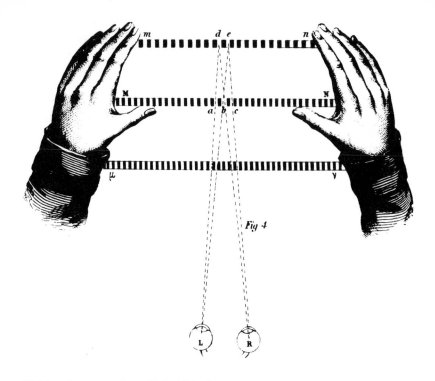

Fig 4

Taking the case where D is 12 inches, and uniting the two nearest openings where *d* is 0·5, let MN (Fig. 4) be a section of the transparent pattern, L, R the left and right eyes, L*ad*, L*be* lines drawn through the centres of two of the open figures *ab*, and R*bd*, R*ce* lines drawn through the centre of *b* and *c*, and meeting L*ad*, L*be* at *d* and *e*, *d* being the binocular centre when we look at it through *a* and *b*, and *e* the binocular centre when we look at it through *b* and *c*. Now, the right eye R sees the opening *b* at *d*, and the left eye L sees the opening *a* at *d*, hence the image at *d* consists of the similar images of *a* and *b* united. In like manner *e* consists of *b* and *c* united, and so on with all the rest, so that the observer at LR no longer sees the real pattern MN, but a suspended image of it at *mn*, *three* inches behind MN. If the observer now approaches MN, the image *mn* will approach to him, and if he recedes, *mn* will recede, being 1½ inches distant from MN when the observer is 6 inches from MN, and 12 inches from MN when he is 48 inches from MN, the image *mn* moving from MN with a velocity ¼th of that with which

the observer recedes. These two velocities are in the ratio of D to $\dfrac{Dd}{C-d}$.

Resuming the position in the figure where the observer is 12 inches distant from MN, let us consider the important results to which this experiment cannot fail to lead us. If the observer, with his eyes at LR, grasp the cane bottom or pattern at MN, as shewn in Fig. 4, his thumbs pressing upon MN, and his fingers trying to grasp *mn*, he will then *feel what he does not see*, and *see what he does not feel!* The real pattern is absolutely invisible at MN, and stands fixed at *mn*. The fingers may be passed through and through – now seen on this side of it – now in the middle of it, and now on the other side of it. If we next place the palms of each hand upon MN, feeling it all over, the result will be the same. No knowledge derived from touch – no measurement of real distances – no actual demonstration from previous or subsequent vision, that there is a real solid body at MN, and nothing at all at *mn*, will remove or shake the infallible conviction of the sense of sight that the object is at *mn*, and that dL or dR is its real distance from the observer. If the binocular centre be now drawn back to MN, the image *seen* will disappear, and the real object be seen at MN. If it be brought still farther back to *f*, the object MN will again disappear, and will be seen at $\mu\nu$, as described in a former part of this paper.

In making these experiments, the observer cannot fail to be struck with the remarkable fact, that though the openings at MN, *mn*, and $\mu\nu$, have all the same angular magnitude, that is, subtend the same angle at the eye, viz., dL*e*, dR*e*, yet those at *mn* appear larger than those at MN, and those at $\mu\nu$ smaller. If we cause the image *mn* to recede, and $\mu\nu$ to approach, the figures in *mn* will invariably *increase* as they *recede*, and those in $\mu\nu$ will *diminish* as they *approach* the eye, and their *visual magnitudes*, as we shall call them, will depend on the respective distances at which the observer, whether right or wrong in his estimate, conceives them to be placed.

Now, this is an universal fact, which the preceding experiments demonstrate; and though the estimate of magnitude thus formed is an erroneous one, yet it is one which neither reason nor experience is able to correct.

When we look at two equal lines, whose difference of distance is distinctly appreciable by the eye, either directly, or by inference, but whose difference of angular magnitude is not appreciable, the most remote must necessarily appear the smallest. For the same reason, if the remoter of two lines is really smaller than the nearer, and, therefore, its angular magnitude also smaller from both these causes, yet, even in this case, if the eye does not perceive distinctly the difference, the smaller and more remote line will appear the larger.*

---

* Malebranche seems to have been the first who introduced the *apparent* distance of objects as an element in our estimate of *apparent* magnitude. *De la Recherche de la Verité*, tom. i. liv. i.; tom. iii. p. 354. See also Bouguer, *Mem. Acad. Par.* 1755, p. 99. These views, however, have been abandoned by several subsequent writers, and the *real distance* of objects has been substituted for their *apparent* distance. Varignon, *Mem. Acad. Par.* 1717, p. 88. M. Lehot, for example, says, "L'expression de la grandeur visuelle d'un corps est egale à la grandeur reelle, multipliée par le logarithme de la *distance reelle* divisée par cette distance." *Nouvelle Théorie de la Vision*, 1er *Mem.* Suppl. p. 7, 8. Paris, 1823. This estimate of distance is incompatible with experiment and observation.

The law of visual magnitude, which regulates this class of phenomena, may be thus expressed.

If we call A the angular magnitude of the *nearest* of two lines or magnitudes whose apparent distance is d, a the angular magnitude of the remoter lines, whose apparent distance is D, and V, v the visual magnitudes of the two lines, then

$$V:v = A \times d:a \times D.$$

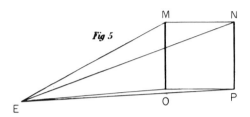

Now, let the two lines MO, NP. (Fig. 5) be the two sides of a quadrilateral figure seen obliquely by an eye at E, then, if the apparent distances of MO, NP, are such, that

$$A \times d > a \times D, \text{ then } V > v,$$

and the lines MN, OP, will converge to a vanishing point beyond N P. But if

$$A \times d = a \times D, \text{ then } V = v,$$

and the line MN, OP, will appear to be parallel. And if

$$A \times d < a \times D, \text{ then } V < v,$$

and the lines MN, OP, will converge to a vanishing point between MO and the observer.

These results may be considered as laying the foundation of a new art, to which we may give the name of *Visual Perspective*, in contradistinction to *Geometrical Perspective*. This art furnishes us with an immediate explanation of a great variety of optical illusions which have never yet been explained; and there is reason to believe that some of its principles were known to ancient architects, and even employed in modifying the nature and position of the lines and forms which enter into the construction of their finest edifices.

St Leonard's College, St Andrews,
April 10. 1844.

Appendix

When I wrote the paragraph in page 647,* I had no expectation of learning that any example of such an illusion had ever occurred. A friend, however, to whom I had occasion to shew the experiments, and who is short-sighted, mentioned to me that he had been on two occasions greatly perplexed by the vision of these suspended images. Having taken too much wine, and being in a papered room, he saw the wall suspended near him in the air; and on another occasion, when kneeling and resting his arms on a cane-bottomed chair, he had fixed his eyes on the carpet, which accidentally united the two images of the open-work, and threw the suspended image of the chair bottom to a distance, and beyond the plane on which his arms rested.

The following case, communicated to me by Professor Christison, is still more interesting.

> Some years ago, when I resided in a house where several rooms are papered with rather formally recurring patterns, and one, in particular, with stars only, I used occasionally to be much plagued with the wall suddenly standing out upon me, and waving, as you describe, with the movements of the head. I was sensible that the cause was an error as to the point of union of the visual axes of the two eyes; but I remember it sometimes cost me a considerable effort to rectify the error; and I found that the best way was to increase still more the deviation in the first instance. As this accident occurred most frequently while I was recovering from a severe attack of fever, I thought my near-sighted eyes were threatened with some new mischief; and this opinion was justified in finding that, after removal to my present house – where, however, the papers have no very formal pattern – no such occurrence has ever taken place. The reason is now easily understood from your researches.

2.8. Brewster: "Account of a new stereoscope". *Report of the British Association. Transactions of the Sections*, 1849, 6–7.

The ingenious stereoscope, invented by Professor Wheatstone for representing solid figures by the union of dissimilar plane pictures, is described in his very interesting paper "On some remarkable and hitherto unobserved Phænomena of Binocular Vision;" and in a paper published in a recent volume of the Edinburgh Transactions, Sir David Brewster has investigated the cause of the perception of objects in relief, by the coalescence of dissimilar pictures. Having had occasion to make numerous experiments on this subject, he was led to construct the stereoscope in several new forms, which, while they possess new and important properties, have the additional advantages of cheapness and portability. The first

* This is a misprint in the original. It probably refers to the second paragraph of this article. (Ed.)

and the most generally useful of these forms is the Lenticular Stereoscope. This instrument consists of two semilenses placed at such a distance that each eye views the picture or drawing opposite to it through the margin of the semilens, or through parts of it equidistant from the margin. The distance of the portions of the lens through which we look, must be equal to the distance of the centres of the pupils, which is, at an average, 2½ inches. The semilenses should be placed in a frame, so that their distance may be adjusted to different eyes. When we thus view two dissimilar drawings of a solid object, as it is seen by each eye separately, we are actually looking through two prisms, which produce a second or refracted image of each drawing, and when these second images unite, or coalesce, we see the solid object which they represent. But in order that the two images may coalesce without any effort or strain on the part of the eyes, it is necessary that the distance of similar parts of the two drawings be equal to *twice* the refraction produced by each lens. For this purpose, measure the distance at which the semilenses give the most distinct view of the drawings, and having ascertained, by using one eye, the amount of the refraction produced at the distance, or the quantity by which the image of one of the drawings is displaced, place the drawings at a distance equal to twice that quantity, that is, place the drawings so that the average distance of similar parts in each is equal to twice that quantity. If this is not correctly done, the eye of the observer will correct the error, by making the images coalesce, without being sensible that it is making any such effort. When the dissimilar drawings are thus united, the solid will appear standing, as it were, in relief, between the two plane representations of it. In looking through this stereoscope, the observer may probably be perplexed by the vision of *only the two dissimilar drawings.* This effect is produced by the strong tendency of the eyes to unite two similar, or even dissimilar drawings. No sooner do the refracted images emerge from their respective drawings, than the eyes, in virtue of this tendency, force them back into union; and though this is done by the convergency of the optic axes to a point nearer the eye than the drawings, yet the observer is scarcely conscious of the muscular exertion by which this is effected. This effect, when it does occur, may be counteracted by drawing back the eyes from the lenses, and shutting them before they again view the drawings. While the semilenses thus double the drawings and enable us to unite two of the images, they at the same time magnify them, – an advantage of a very peculiar kind, when we wish to give a great apparent magnitude to drawings on a small scale, taken photographically with the camera. The lenticular stereoscope may be made of any size. Sir David Brewster then described how we may see at the same time a *raised* and a *hollow* cone, the *former* being produced by the union of the *first* with the *second*, and the latter by the union of the *second* with the *third* figures. This method of exhibiting at the same time the raised and the hollow solid, enables us, he said, to give an ocular and experimental proof of the usual explanation of the cause of the large size of the horizontal moon, of her small size when in the meridian at a considerable altitude, and her intermediate apparent magnitude at an intermediate altitude. As the summit of the raised cone *appears* to be nearest the eye of the observer, the summit of the hollow cone furthest off, and that of the flat drawing on each side at an intermediate distance, these distances will represent the apparent distance of the moon in the zenith of the elliptical celestial vault, in the horizon, and at an altitude of 45°. The circular summits thus seen are in reality exactly of the same size, and at the same distance from the eye, and are therefore precisely in the same circumstances as the moon in the three positions already mentioned. If we now contemplate them in the stereoscope, we shall see the circular summit of the hollow cone the *largest,* like the *horizontal* moon, because it seems at the *greatest* distance from the eye; the circular summit of the *raised* cone the *smallest,* because it appears at the *least* distance, like the *zenith* moon; and the circular summit of the cones on each of an *intermediate* size, like the moon at an altitude of 45°, because their distance from the eye is intermediate. No change is produced in the apparent magnitude of these circles by making one or more of them less bright than the rest, and hence we see the incorrectness of the explanation of the size of the horizontal moon, as given by Dr. Berkeley. When the observer fails to see the object in relief from the cause already mentioned, but sees only the *two* drawings, if there are *two,* or the *three* drawings, if there are *three,* the plane of the drawings appears *deeply hollow*; and, what is very remarkable, if we look with the eccentric lenses at a flat table from above, it also appears deeply hollow, and if we touch it with the palm of our hand, *it is felt as hollow,* while we are looking at it, but the sensation of hollowness disappears on shutting our eyes. Sir David Brewster described a variety of forms in which he had constructed the stereoscope, by means of lenses, mirrors and prisms. The sense of sight, therefore, instead of being the pupil of the sense of touch, as Berkeley and others have believed, is, in this as in other cases, its teacher and its guide. Sir D. Brewster's simplified stereoscopes may not only be rendered portable, but may be constructed out of materials which every person possesses, and without the aid of an optician. A fuller account of these instruments will be found in the forthcoming volume of the Transactions of the Royal Scottish Society of Arts.

2.9. Brewster: "Description of several new and simple stereoscopes for exhibiting, as solids, one or more representations of them on a plane". *Transactions of the Royal Scottish Society of Arts*, 1851, 3, 247–259*

The ingenious stereoscope, invented by Professor Wheatstone, for representing solid figures by the union of dissimilar plane pictures, is described in his very interesting paper *On some remarkable and hitherto unobserved Phenomena of*

* Read before the Royal Scottish Society of Arts, 26th March 1849.

*Binocular Vision;** and in a paper published in a recent volume of the *Edinburgh Transactions*,† I have investigated the cause of the perception of objects in relief, by the coalescence of dissimilar pictures.

Having had occasion to make numerous experiments on this subject, I was led to construct the stereoscope in several new forms, which, while they possess new and important properties, have the additional advantages of cheapness and portability. The first and the most generally useful of these forms is,

1. *The Lenticular Stereoscope.*

This instrument consists of two semilenses placed at such a distance that each eye views the picture or drawing opposite to it, through the margin of the semilens, or through parts of it equidistant from the margin. The distance of the portions of the lens through which we look, must be equal to the distance of the centres of the pupils, which is, at an average, 2½ inches. The semilenses should be placed in a frame, so that their distance may be adjusted to different eyes, as shewn in Fig. 1.

When we thus view two dissimilar drawings of a solid object, as it is seen by each eye separately, we are actually looking through two prisms, which produce a second image of each drawing, and when these second images unite, or coalesce, we see the solid object which they represent. But in order that the two images may coalesce, without any effort or strain on the part of the eye, it is necessary that the distance of similar parts of the two drawings be equal to *twice* the separation produced by the prism. For this purpose, measure the distance at which the semilenses give the most distinct view of the drawings, and having ascertained, by using one eye, the amount of the refraction produced at that distance, or the quantity by which the image of one of the drawings is displaced, place the drawings at a distance equal to twice that quantity, that is, place the drawings so that the average distance of similar parts in each is equal to twice that quantity. If this is not correctly done, the eye of the observer will correct the error, by making the images coalesce, without being sensible that it is making any such effort. When the dissimilar drawings are thus united, the solid will appear standing, as it were, in relief, between the two plane representations of it.

In looking through this stereoscope, the observer may probably be perplexed by the vision of *only the two dissimilar drawings*. This effect is produced by the strong tendency of the eyes to unite two similar, or even dissimilar, drawings. No sooner do the refracted images emerge from their respective drawings, than the eye, in virtue of this tendency, force them back into union; and though this is done by the convergency of the optic axes to a point nearer the eye than the drawings, yet the observer is scarcely conscious of the muscular exertion by which this is

---

* Phil. Trans., 1838, p. 371.   † Vol. xv., part 3, p. 360.

effected. This effect, when it does occur, may be counteracted by drawing back the eyes from the lenses, and shutting them before they again view the drawings. It exists chiefly with shortsighted persons, for whom the stereoscope may be constructed with concave semilenses or quarters of lenses, placed as in Fig. 16, and when there are only *two* drawings, it may be prevented by a partition, which hides the right-hand drawing from the left eye, and the left-hand drawing from the right eye.

The instrument, as fitted up for use, is shewn in Fig. 2, where ABCD is a frame of tin or wood, consisting of an upper and a lower plate, and two ends, AB and CD: The semilenses are placed in CD, with an opening for the nose at NN, a part of the lower plate being cut away for this purpose. The *three* dissimilar drawings, as shewn at C, Fig. 4, are placed in the end AB, and are illuminated by the light which enters by the two open sides, AC, BD.* If the drawings are upon thin or transparent paper, or are executed as transparencies like the diagrams used in the magic lantern, the box ABCD may be closed, and the light admitted only through the end AB. In the form shewn in Fig. 2, where the drawings slide into an open frame, either opaque or transparent figures may be used. It is often convenient to have the drawings separate, so that, like the semilenses, they may be made to approach to or recede from one another; and when the drawings are thus separate, we can obtain the arrangement at B, Fig. 4, from the drawings at A, or all of them from the three drawings at C.

While the semilenses thus double the drawings and enable us to unite two of the images, they at the same time magnify them, – an advantage of a very peculiar kind, when we wish to give a great apparent magnitude to drawings on a small scale, taken photographically with the camera. But while the magnifying power of any lens is the same through whatever portion of it we look, its prismatic angle varies with the distance of that portion from the margin. In the semilens LL, for example, Fig. 3, the prismatic angle is a maximum at the margin A, less at A', and still less at A'', so that, when the drawing is very small, we can double it, and refract it sufficiently by looking through A'', when larger through A', and when larger still through A. By using a thicker lens, without changing the curvature of its surface, or its focal length, we can increase the prismatic angle at its margin, so as to produce any degree of refraction that may be required for the purposes of experiment, or for the duplication of large drawings.

It is obvious, from the very nature of the lenticular stereoscope, that it may be made of any size. The one from which Fig. 2 is copied is 8 inches long, and 5 inches at its widest end; but I have made them only *three* inches long, and have now before me a *microscopic stereoscope*, which can be carried in the pocket, and

---

* It is sometimes more convenient to close the sides, and leave the upper and under sides open, or we may cut off a circular segment from its upper and lower plate, as shewn in Fig. 2. The use of this opening in the lower plate is to illuminate the drawings when we turn the stereoscope and figures upside down, which increases the relief in a surprising degree.

which exhibits all the properties of the instrument to the greatest advantage.*

If we suppose the two figures at A, Fig. 4, to represent a cone, as seen by the right and left eye, the stereoscope will unite them into a *raised* cone, with the circular apex *nearest* the eye. If they are placed as at B, they will appear as a *hollow* cone, the apex being farthest from the eye. In Mr Wheatstone's stereoscope, the drawings must be turned upside down, in order that the *raised* and *hollow* cone may be seen in succession; but with the lenticular stereoscope, we have only to place *three* figures as at C, Fig. 4, and between A, B, Fig. 2, in order to see, at the same time, the *raised* and the *hollow* cone, the *former* being produced by the union of the *first* with the *second*, and the latter by the union of the *second* with the *third* figures.

This method of exhibiting at the same time the raised and the hollow solid, enables us to give an ocular and experimental proof of the usual explanation of the cause of the large size of the horizontal moon, of her small size when in the meridian at a considerable altitude, and her intermediate apparent magnitude at an intermediate altitude. As the summit of the raised cone *appears* to be nearest the eye of the observer, the summit of the hollow cone farthest off, and and that of the flat drawing on each side at an intermediate distance, these distances will represent the apparent distance of the moon in the zenith of the elliptical celestial vault, in the horizon, and at an altitude of 45°. The circular summits thus seen are in reality exactly of the same size, and at the same distance from the eye, and are, therefore, precisely in the same circumstances as the moon in the three positions already mentioned. If we now contemplate them in the stereoscope, we shall see the circular summit of the hollow cone the *largest*, like the *horizontal* moon, because it seems at the *greatest* distance from the eye; the circular summit of the *raised* cone the *smallest*, because it appears at the *least* distance, like the *zenith* moon; and the circular summit of the cones on each of an *intermediate* size, like the moon at an altitude of 45°, because their distance from the eye is intermediate. In the accompanying model, this effect will be distinctly seen, by placing three small wafers of the same size and colour on the square summits of the drawings of the cones or four-sided pyramids. No change is produced in the apparent magnitude of these circles by making one or more of them less bright than the rest, and hence we see the incorrectness of the explanation of the size of the horizontal moon, as given by Dr Berkeley.†

When the observer fails to see the object in relief from the cause already mentioned, but sees only the *two* drawings, if there are *two*, or the *three* drawings, if there are *three*, the plane of the drawings appears *deeply hollow*; and, what is very

---

* In place of using semilenses, as I at first did, I now use quarters of lenses, which answer the purpose equally well. With a single lens, therefore, we can construct two stereoscopes of exactly the same power. This is the first time that a quadrant of a lens has been used in optics. The eye-end of the stereoscope should consist of two short tubes, with the lenses at their extremities.

† Berkeley's *Works*, p. 98; Essay on the Theory of Vision, § 67–78. Lond., 1837.

remarkable, if we look with the eccentric lenses at a flat table from above, it also appears deeply hollow, and if we touch it with the palm of our hand, *it is felt as hollow*, while we are looking at it, but the sensation of hollowness disappears upon shutting our eyes. The sense of sight, therefore, instead of being the pupil of the sense of touch, as Berkeley and others have believed, is, in this as in other cases, its teacher and its guide.*

2. *The Total-Reflexion Telescope.*

This form of the stereocope is a very interesting one, and possesses valuable properties. It requires only a small prism and *one* diagram, or picture of the solid, as seen by one eye, the other diagram, or picture which is to be combined with it, being created by total reflexion from the base of the prism. This instrument is shewn in Fig. 5, where D is the picture of a cone as seen by the left eye L, and ABC a prism, whose base BC is so large, that when the eye is placed close to it, it may see, by reflexion, the whole of the diagram D. The angles ABC, ACB must be equal, but may be of any magnitude. Great accuracy in the equality of the angles is not necessary, and a prism constructed by a lapidary out of a fragment of thick plate glass, the face BC being one of the surfaces of the plate, will answer the purpose.† When the prism is placed at *abc*, Fig. 6, at one end of a conical tube LD, and the diagram D, at the other end, in a cap which can be turned round so as to have the line *mn*, which passes through the centre of the base and summit of the cone parallel to the line joining the two eyes, the instrument is ready for use. The observer places his left eye at L, and views with it the picture D, as seen by total reflexion from the base BC or *bc* of the prism, Figs. 5 and 6, while with his right eye R, Fig. 5, he views the same picture directly. The first of these pictures being the reverse of the second D, like all pictures formed by one reflexion, we thus combine two dissimilar pictures into a *raised* cone as in the figure, or into a *hollow* one, if the picture at D is turned round 180°. If we place two diagrams, one like one of those at A, Fig. 4, and the other like the other at A, Fig. 4, vertically above one another, we shall then see, at the same time, the *raised* and the *hollow* cone as produced in the lenticular stereoscope by the three diagrams in Fig. 4, at C. When the prism is good, the dissimilar image produced by the two refractions at B and C, and the one reflexion at E, is, of course, more accurate than if it had been drawn by the most skilful artist, and therefore this form of the stereoscope has, in this respect, an advantage over every other in which two dissimilar figures, executed by art, are necessary. In consequence of the length of the reflected pencil DB + BE + EC + CL being a little greater than the direct pencil of rays DR, the two images combined have not exactly the same apparent magnitude; but

* See *Edinburgh Transactions*, vol xv., p. 672.

† In this case the prism may have the form B*cd* C, Fig. 5, the parallel sides BC, *cd* being the original faces of the piece of the plate-glass, and the inclined faces B*c*, C*d* only, the work of the lapidary.

the difference is not perceptible to the eye, and a remedy could easily be provided were it required.

If the conical tube LD is held in the left hand, the left eye must be used, and if in the right hand, the right eye must be used, so that the hand may not obstruct the direct vision of the drawing by the eye which does not look through the prism. The cone LD must be turned round slightly in the hand till the line *mn* joining the centre and apex of the figure is parallel to the line joining the two eyes. The same line must be parallel to the plane of reflexion from the prism, but this parallelism is secured by fixing the prism and the drawing.

It is scarcely necessary to state, that this stereoscope is applicable only to those diagrams and forms where the one image is the reflected picture of the other.

If we wish to make a microscopic stereoscope of this form, or to magnify the drawings, we have only to cement planoconvex lenses, of the requisite focal length, upon the faces AB, AC of the prism, or, what is simpler still, to use a section of a deeply convex lens ABC, Fig. 7, and apply the other half of the lens to the right eye, the face BC having been previously ground flat and polished for the prismatic lens. By using a lens of larger focus for the right eye, we may correct, if required, the imperfection arising from the difference of paths in the reflected and direct pencils. This difference is so trivial that it might be corrected by applying to the right eye the central portion of the same lens whose margin is used for the prism.

3. The Single Prismatic Stereoscope.

The prismatic stereoscope, represented in Fig. 8, consists of a single prism P, with a small refracting angle, capable of refracting the image of the figure A, so as just to combine it with the dissimilar figure B, seen directly by the right eye. The second picture should be placed close to A, in order that they may be united by a prism with the smallest refracting angle. There is a slight degree of colour in the refracted image, but it does not injure the general effect. The prism, therefore, should not be made of flint-glass, or any glass with a high dispersive power. A single face ground by a lapidary upon one of the faces of a morsel of plate-glass, the size of the pupil of the eye, will give a prism sufficient for every ordinary purpose. Any person may make one for himself by placing a little bit of window-glass upon another piece inclined to it, and inserting in the angle between them a drop of water. When the figures are small and near one another, a water prism with the requisite angle will scarcely produce any perceptible colour.*

If we make a double prism, as shewn at PP′, Fig. 9, and apply it to the two dissimilar figures A, B, so that with the left eye L looking through the prism P, we may place the refracted image of B upon A, as seen by the right eye R, we shall see

---

* Professor Wheatstone has, we believe, used *two* achromatic prisms, but they are not necessary.

a *hollow* cone; and if with the left eye L′, looking through the other prism P′, we place the refracted image of A upon B, as seen with the right eye R′, we shall see a *raised* cone.

4. *The Singly-Reflecting Stereoscope.*

A very simple stereoscope may be constructed as in Fig. 10, by using a small piece of black glass, or plate glass with one side covered with black wax. This piece of glass MN reflects to the left eye L a reverted image of the figure B, which, when seen in the direction LCA, and combined with the figure A, seen directly by the right eye R, gives a raised cone. The cone will be seen hollow by reversing the figures A, B. As BC + CL is greater than AR, the reflected image of B will be slightly less than A, but the difference is so little, that it does not affect the appearance of the *hollow* or the *raised* cone. By bringing B a little nearer the reflector MN, the two pictures may be made exactly the same. The small reflector and the dissimilar figures may be fitted up in a conical tube, like that shewn in Fig. 6, the tube having an elliptical section to accommodate *two* figures at its farther end, the major axis of the ellipse being parallel to the line joining the two eyes.

5. *The Double Reflecting Stereoscope.*

In this form of the instrument a second reflector is added for the right eye, as shewn at M′N′, Fig. 11, and the effect of this is to exhibit at the same instant the *raised* and the *hollow* cone. The image of B seen by reflection from MN at the point C, is combined with the direct picture of A, seen by the right eye, and forms a hollow cone, while the image of A seen by reflexion from M′N′ at the point C′, is combined with the direct picture of B, seen by the left eye. These reflectors may be placed in an elliptical tube, with an opening near the end AB to illuminate the figures A, B, or we may dispense with an opening, by having the figures drawn upon thin or transparent paper. When the figures are drawn in transparent lines on a ground of opaque varnish, like the diagrams in the magic lantern, the effect is very fine.

Another form of the double reflecting stereoscope is shewn in Fig. 12, which differs from that shewn in Fig. 11, in the position of the two reflectors, and of the figures to be united. The reflecting faces of the mirrors are turned outwards, their distance being less than the distance between the eyes, and the effect of this is to unite into a *hollow* cone the same figures which the other form in Fig. 11 unite into a *raised* one. The superiority of this position of the reflectors is, that they are more easily enclosed in a tube, and that the instrument is more portable.

In describing these various forms of the stereoscope, by which the instrument may not only be rendered portable, but may be constructed out of materials which

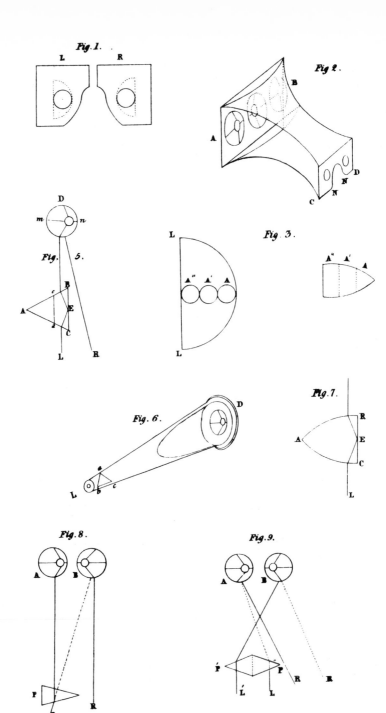

Fig. 1.

Fig. 2.

Fig. 3.

Fig. 5.

Fig. 6.

Fig. 7.

Fig. 8.

Fig. 9.

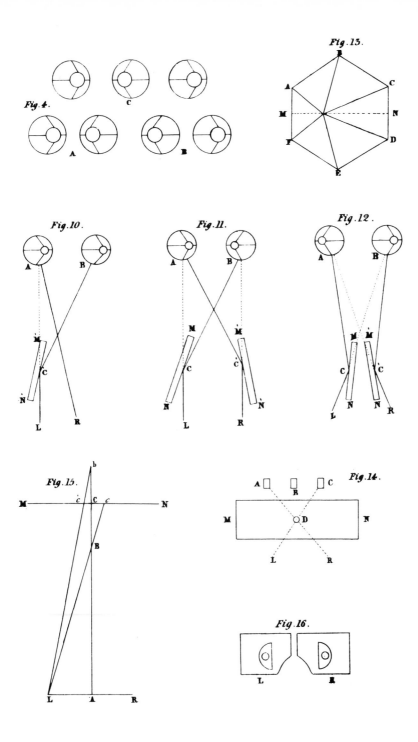

Fig. 4.

Fig. 13.

Fig. 10.

Fig. 11.

Fig. 12.

Fig. 15.

Fig. 14.

Fig. 16.

every person possesses, and without the aid of an optician, we have supposed the two dissimilar figures to be those of the frustum of a cone as seen by each eye separately, the large circle being the representation of the base of the cone, and the small circle the representation of its truncated summit. If we join similar points of these two circles by lines, as is done in the figures, the conical figure will be more distinct.

If we take the drawing of a six-sided pyramid as seen by the right eye, as shewn in Fig. 13, and place it in the total-reflexion stereoscope at D, Fig. 5, so that the line MN coincides with *mn* and is parallel to the line joining the eyes of the observer, we shall perceive a perfect raised pyramid of a given height, the reflected image of CD, Fig. 13, being combined with AF seen directly. If we now turn the figure round 30°, CD will come into the position AB, and unite with AB, and we shall still perceive a raised pyramid, with less height and less symmetry. If we turn it round 30° more, CD will be combined with BC, and we shall still perceive a raised pyramid with still less height, and still less symmetry. When the figure is turned round other 30°, or 90° from its first position, CD will coincide with CD seen directly, and the combined figures will be perfectly flat. If we continue the rotation through other 30°, CD will coincide with DE, and a slightly hollow, but not very symmetrical, pyramid will be seen. A rotation of other 30° will bring CD into coalescence with EF, and we shall see a still more hollow and more symmetrical pyramid. A farther rotation of other 30°, making 180° from the commencement, will bring CD into union with AF, and we shall have a perfectly symmetrical hollow pyramid of still greater depth, and the exact counterpart of the raised pyramid which was seen before the rotation of the figure commenced. If the pyramid had been square, the *raised* would have passed into the *hollow* pyramid by rotations of 45° each. If it had been rectangular, the change would have been effected by rotations of 90°. If the space between the two circular sections of the cone in Fig. 12 had been uniformly shaded, or if lines had been drawn from every degree of the one circle to every corresponding degree in the other, in place of from every 90th degree, as in the figure, the raised cone would have gradually diminished in height by the rotation of the figure till it became flat, after a rotation of 90°; – and by continuing the rotation, it would have become hollow, and gradually reached its maximum depth, after a revolution of 180°.

There are two classes of phenomena of a very interesting kind, to which the stereoscope is not properly applicable, namely, those where it is required to unite a great number of similar and equidistant patterns, such as those which compose paper-hangings, carpets, and the openings in the cane bottoms of chairs, and those in which we binocularly unite, and give a new position to, lines meeting at, or converging to, a point, the eye being placed at different heights above the plane of the paper, and at different distances from the angular point.* In studying these

---

* These two classes of phenomena are described in my paper "On the Knowledge of Distance given by Binocular Vision," published in the *Edinburgh Transactions*, vol. xv., p. 663.

phenomena, we produce the required union by straining the eyes, or by contemplating the objects while the eyes are directed to a point either nearer to or farther from them. The power of doing this with facility is possessed by very few persons, and it is therefore necessary to have a simple and infallible method of effecting the union of such objects without instrumental assistance. The following method, when practised for a short time, will answer this purpose.

6. *Method of uniting Similar or Dissimilar Figures.*

Upon a piece of glass MN, Fig. 14, place a very small circle of white paper D, and let A, B, C, be similar patterns which we wish to unite, A with C, or A with B. Hold the piece of glass MN in both hands, and at such a distance from the eyes that, when with the left eye L, and shutting the right eye, we see the circle D covering C, we also, upon opening the right eye B, see with it the circle D covering A. By continuing for a short time to look at the circle D with both eyes open, we shall see the patterns all united, and the wall or plane which contains them situated at the same distance from the eye as the circle D. If there are one or more intermediate patterns, such as B, the piece of glass MN must be held farther from the eyes in order to unite A with B, instead of A with C. Those who acquire, in this way, the art of uniting dissimilar and similar figures, will not require, in any case, the aid of the stereoscope, unless when there is only one figure or object; in which case, they must have recourse to the total-reflexion stereoscope, in order to convert the single figure into a solid, by creating and uniting with it its opposite or reflected image.

7. *Method of Drawing on a Plane the Dissimilar Representations of Solids for the Stereoscope.*

Let L, R, Fig. 15, be the left and right eye, and A the middle point between them. Let MN be the plane on which an object or solid, whose height is CB, is to be drawn. Through B draw LB, meeting MN in c; then, if the object is a solid, with its apex at B, Cc will be the distance of its apex from the centre C of its base, as seen by the left eye. As seen by the right eye R, Cc' will have the same value, but c' will lie on the left side of C. Calling E the distance between the two eyes and h, the height B C of the solid, we shall have

$$AB:h = \frac{E}{2}:Cc \text{ and } Cc = \frac{hE}{2\,AB}$$

which will give us the results in the following Table, AC being = 8 and E = 2½ inches: –

Height.

BC	h		AB		Cc
1		....	7	....	0·279 inches.
2		....	6	....	0·4166 ....
3		....	5	....	0·75 .....
4		....	4	....	1.25 ....
5		....	3	....	2·088 .....
6		....	2	....	3·75 .....
7		....	1	....	8.75 ....
8		....	0	....	Infinite.

If we now wish, by directing the axes of the eyes beyond MN to b, to ascertain the value of Cc', which will give different depths d of the *hollow* solids corresponding to different values of Cb, we shall have

$$Ab:\frac{E}{2} = d:Cc' \text{ and } Cc' = \frac{dE}{2\,Ab}$$

which, making AC 8 inches as before, will give the following results:

Depth.

$Cb = d$		Ab		Cc'
1	....	9	....	0·139 inches.
2	....	10	....	0·25 ......
3	....	11	....	0·34 ......
4	....	12	....	0·4166 ....
5	....	13	....	0·48 ......
6	....	14	....	0·535 ......
7	....	15	....	0·58 ......
8	....	16	....	0·625 ......
9	....	17	....	0·663 ......
10	....	18	....	0·696 ......
11	....	19	....	0·723 ......
12	....	20	....	0·75 ......

The values of h and d, when the excentricities Cc, Cc', as we may call them, are known, will be found by the formulæ

$$h = \frac{Cc\,E}{2\,AB} \text{ and } d = \frac{Cc'E}{2\,Ab}.$$

As Cc is always equal to Cc' in each pair of figures or dissimilar pictures, the depth of the *hollow* solid will always appear much greater than the height of the *raised* solid one. When Cc and Cc' are both 0·75 $h:d = 3:12$, and when they are both 0·4166, $h:d = 2:4$, and when they are both 0·139 $h:d = 0·8:1·0$.

2.10. Wheatstone: "Contributions to the physiology of vision – Part the second. On some remarkable, and hitherto unobserved, phenomena of binocular vision". *Philosophical Transactions of the Royal Society*, 1852, 1–17.

§ 17.

In § 3. of the first part of my "Contributions to the Physiology of Vision," published in the Philosophical Transactions for 1838, speaking of the stereoscope, I stated,

> The pictures will indeed coincide when the sliding pannels are in a variety of different positions, and consequently when viewed under different inclinations of the optic axes; but there is only one position in which the binocular image will be immediately seen single, of its proper magnitude, and without fatigue to the eyes, because in this position only the ordinary relations between the magnitude of the pictures on the retina, the inclination of the optic axes, and the adaptation of the eye to distinct vision at different distances, are preserved. The alteration in the apparent magnitude of the binocular images, when these usual relations are disturbed, will be discussed in another paper of this series, with a variety of remarkable phenomena depending thereon.

In 1833, five years before the publication of the memoir just mentioned, these yet unpublished investigations were announced in the third edition of Herbert Mayo's "Outlines of Human Physiology" in the following words: –

> Mr. Wheatstone has shown, in a paper he is about to publish, that if by artificial means the usual relations which subsist between the degree of inclination of the optic axes and the visual angle which the object subtends on the retina be disturbed, some extraordinary illusions may be produced. Thus, the magnitude of the image remaining constant on the retina, its apparent size may be made to vary with every alteration of the angular inclination of the optic axes.

I shall resume the consideration of the phenomena of binocular vision with this subject, because the facts I have ascertained regarding it are necessary to be understood before entering on the new experiments relating to stereoscopic appearances which I intend to bring forward on the present occasion.

Under the ordinary conditions of vision, when an object is placed at a certain distance before the eyes, several concurring circumstances remain constant, and they always vary in the same order when the distance of the object is changed. Thus, as we approach the object, or as it is brought nearer to us, the magnitude of the picture on the retina increases; the inclination of the optic axes, required to cause the pictures to fall on corresponding places of the retinæ, becomes greater; the divergence of the rays of light proceeding from each point of the object, and which determines the adaptation of the eyes to distinct vision of that point, increases; and the dissimilarity of the two pictures projected on the retinæ also becomes greater. It is important to ascertain in what manner our perception of the magnitude and distance of objects depends on these various circumstances, and to inquire which are the most, and which the least influential in the judgements we form. To advance this inquiry beyond the point to which it has hitherto been brought, it is not sufficient to content ourselves with drawing conclusions from observations on the circumstances under which vision naturally occurs, as preceding writers on this subject mostly have done, but it is necessary to have more extended recourse to the methods so successfully employed in experimental philosophy, and to endeavour, wherever it be possible, not only to analyse the elements of vision, but also to recombine them in unusual manners, so that they may be associated under circumstances that never naturally occur.

The instrument I shall proceed to describe enables these abnormal combinations to be made in a very simple and effectual manner. Its principal object is to cause the binocular pictures to coincide, with any inclination of the optic axes, while their magnitudes on the retinæ remain the same; or inversely, while the optic axes remain at the same angle, to cause the size of the pictures on the retinæ to vary in any manner.

Two plane mirrors inclined 90° to each other are placed together and fixed vertically upon a horizontal board. Two wooden arms move round a common centre situated on this board in the vertical plane which bisects the angle of the mirrors, and about 1½ inch beyond their line of junction. Upon each of these arms is placed an upright pannel, at right angles thereto, for the purpose of receiving its appropriate picture, and each pannel is made to slide to and from the opposite mirror. The eyes being placed before the mirrors, the right eye to the right mirror and the left eye to the left mirror, and the pannels being adjusted to the same distances, however the arms be moved round their centre, the distance of the reflected image of each picture from the eye will remain exactly the same, and consequently its retinal magnitude will be unchanged. But as the two reflected images do not occupy the same place when the pictures are in different positions, to cause the former to coincide the optic axes must converge differently. When the arms are in the same straight line, the images coincide while the optic axes are parallel; and as they form a less angle with each other, the optic axes converge more to occasion the coincidence. When the arms remain in the same positions, while the pannels slide towards or from the mirrors, the convergence of the optic axes remains the same, but the magnitude of the pictures on the retinæ increases as the distance decreases. By the arrangement described, and which is represented by Figs. 1 and 2, the reflected pictures are always perpendicular to the optic axes, and the corresponding points of the pictures, when they are exactly similar, fall upon corresponding points of the retinæ. The instrument has an adjustment for otherwise inclining them if it be required.

Let us now attend to the effects produced. The pictures being fixed at the same distance from the mirrors, there is a certain adjustment of the arms at which the

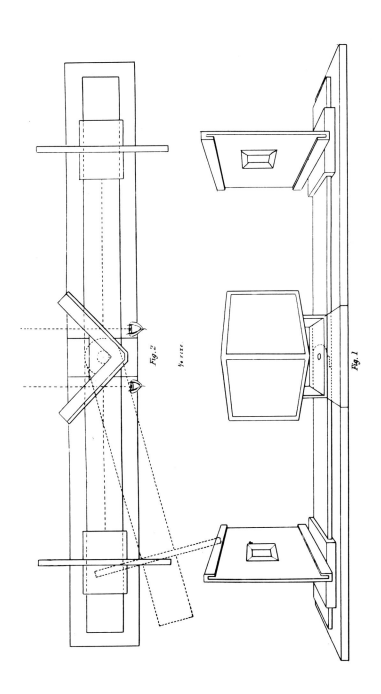

Fig. 2

⅓ size.

Fig. 1

binocular image will appear of its natural size, that is, the size we judge the picture itself to be when we look at it directly; in this case the magnitude of the pictures on the retinæ and the inclination of the optic axes preserve their usual relation to each other. If now the arms be moved back, so as to cause a less convergence of the axes, the image will appear to increase in magnitude until the arms are in a straight line and the optic axes are parallel; and, on the other hand, if the arms be moved forwards, so as to form a less angle, the optic axes will converge more, and the image will appear gradually smaller. In this manner, while the retinal magnitude remains the same, the perceived magnitude of the binocular object varies through a very considerable range.

The instrument being again adjusted so that the image shall be seen of its natural size; on sliding the pictures nearer the mirrors its perceived magnitude will be augmented, and on sliding them from the mirrors it will appear diminished in size. During these variations of magnitude the inclination of the optic axes remains the same.

The perceived magnitude of an object, therefore, diminishes as the inclination of the axes becomes greater, while the distance remains the same; and it increases, when the inclination of the axes remains the same, while the distance diminishes. When both these conditions vary inversely, as they do in ordinary vision when the distance of an object changes, the perceived magnitude remains the same.*

Before I proceed further it will be proper to explain the meaning of some of the terms I employ. I call the magnitude of the object itself, the real or objective magnitude; the magnitude of the picture on the retina, the retinal magnitude; and the magnitude we estimate the object to be from its retinal magnitude and the inclination of the optic axes conjointly, I name the perceived magnitude. I do not use the term apparent magnitude, because, according to its ordinary acceptation, it sometimes means what I call retinal, and at other times what I name perceived magnitude.

We have seen in what manner our perception of magnitude is modified by the new associations which this instrument enables us to form; let us now examine how our perception of distance is affected by them. If we continue to observe the binocular picture whilst it apparently increases or decreases, in consequence of the inclination of the optic axes varying while the magnitude of the impressions on the retinæ remains the same, it does not appear either to approach or to recede; and yet if we attentively regard it in any fixed position, it is perceived to be at a different distance. On the other hand, if we continue to regard the binocular picture, enlarging and diminishing in consequence of the change of retinal

* Several cases of the alteration of the perceived magnitude of objects are mentioned by Dr. R. Smith (Complete System of Opticks, 1738, vol. ii. p. 388, and rem. 526 and 532); and Dr. R. Darwin (Philosophical Transactions, vol. lxxvi. p. 313) observed that when an ocular spectrum was impressed on both eyes it appeared magnified when they were directed to a wall at a considerable distance. The facts noticed by these authors are satisfactorily explained by the above considerations.

magnitude while the convergence of the axes remains the same, we perceive it to approach or recede in the most evident manner; but on fixing the attention to it, when it is stationary, at any instant, it appears to be at the same distance at one time as it is at another.

Convergence of the optic axes therefore suggests fixed distance to the mind; variation of retinal magnitude suggests change of distance. We may, as I have above shown, perceive an object approach or recede without appearing to change its distance, and an object to be at a different distance, without appearing to approach or recede; the paradoxical effects render it difficult, until the phenomena are well apprehended, to know, or to express, what we actually do perceive.

It is the prevalent opinion that the sensation which accompanies the inclination of the optic axes immediately suggests distance, and that the perceived magnitude of an object is a judgement arising from our consciousness of its distance and of the magnitude of its picture on the retina. From the experiments I have brought forward, it rather appears to me that what the sensation which is connected with the convergence of the axes immediately suggests is a correction of the retinal magnitude to make it agree with the real magnitude of the object, and that distance, instead of being a simple perception, is a judgement arising from a comparison of the retinal and perceived magnitudes. However this may be, unless other signs accompany this sensation the notion of distance we thence derive is uncertain and obscure, whereas the perception of the change of magnitude it occasions is obvious and unmistakeable.

To see, in their full extent, the variations of magnitude exhibited by the instrument I have described, it is necessary to attend to the following observations.

As the inclination of the optic axes corresponding to a different distance is habitually, under ordinary circumstances, accompanied with the particular adaptation of the eyes required for distinct vision at that distance, it is difficult to disassociate these two conditions so as to see with equal distinctness the binocular picture when the optic axes are parallel, and when they converge greatly, although the pictures remain, in both cases, at the same distance from the eyes. The adaptation is, therefore, not entirely dependent on the divergence of the rays of light which proceed from the object regarded, but also, in some degree, on the inclination of the optic axes. I have acquired by practice considerable power of adjustment, or rather disadjustment, of the eyes, and can, without having recourse to artificial means, see the binocular picture distinctly when its perceived magnitude is widely different. Those to whom such an effort is painful may employ short-sighted spectacles to see the binocular picture when the eyes converge within the limit of distinct vision for the distance at which the pictures are placed; and long-sighted spectacles when the eyes converge beyond that limit, or become parallel.

There is a means of avoiding to a very considerable extent the influence of the adjustment of the eyes, and thereby enabling the pictures to be seen distinctly within the entire range of the inclination of the optic axes. This is by looking at the reflected images in the mirrors through two very minute apertures, not larger than fine pin-holes, placed near each eye, and illuminating the pictures by a very strong light; sunshine in the middle of the day answers the purpose very well. By this expedient the divergence of the rays of light is greatly diminished, and the adaptation of the eyes does not materially influence the result.

§ 18.

Leaving this subject, I will now revert to the stereoscope and its effects.

Since 1838 numerous modifications of the stereoscope have occurred to me, and several ingenious arrangements have also been proposed by Sir David Brewster and Prof. Dove; but there is no form of the instrument which has so many advantages for investigating the phenomena of binocular vision as the original reflecting stereoscope. Pictures of any size may be placed in it, and it admits of every kind of adjustment.

I have constructed a very portable reflecting stereoscope which is represented at Fig. 3. The sides fold over the mirrors, and the mirrors then fold into a box, which is not larger than 6 inches in any of its dimensions. To avoid the second feeble reflection from the anterior surface of the silvered glass, which has a bad effect when the attention is attracted to it, I have sometimes employed reflecting prisms. The reflecting surfaces of the prisms should be silvered in order to obviate the unequal brightness of the field of view on each side of the limit of total

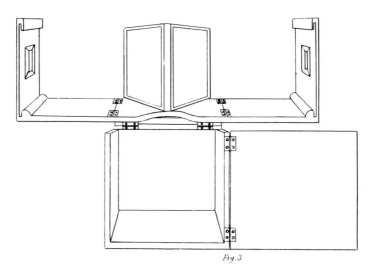

Fig. 3

reflection; and as it would be too costly to employ very large prisms, they should have an adjustment to accommodate their distance to the width between the eyes of the observer.

I have, for many years past, employed also another means to occasion, without any straining of the eyes, the coincidence of the pictures so that the image in relief shall appear of the same magnitude and at the same distance as the object which they represent would do if it were itself directly regarded. In this apparatus, prisms being employed to deflect the rays of light proceeding from the pictures, so as to make them appear to occupy the same place, I have called it the refracting stereoscope.

It is represented by Fig. 4. It consists of a base 6 inches long and 4 inches broad, upon which stands an upright partition, 5 inches high, dividing it equally; this partition is capable of extension by means of a slide to double the length, and carries at its upper extremity a board placed parallel to the base, and of the same dimensions. In this upper board there are two apertures an inch square, one on each side of the partition, the centres of which are 2½ inches from each other; in these apertures are fixed a pair of glass prisms having their faces inclined 15°, and their refractive angles turned towards each other. The stereoscope pictures are to be placed on the base, and their centres ought not to exceed the distance of 2½ inches.

A pair of plate-glass prisms, their faces making with each other an angle of 12°, will bring two pictures, the corresponding points of which are 2½ inches apart, to coincidence at a distance of 12 inches, and a pair with an angle of 15° will occasion coincidence at 8 inches.

The refracting stereoscope has the advantage of portability, but it is limited to pictures of small dimensions. It is well suited for Daguerreotypes, which are usually of small size, and, on account of the nature of their reflecting surface, must be viewed in a particular direction with respect to the light which falls upon them; whereas in the reflecting stereoscope it is somewhat difficult to render the

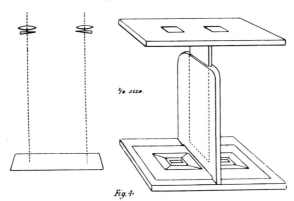

¼ size.

Fig. 4.

two Daguerreotypes equally visible. For drawings and Talbotypes it however offers no advantages, though it is equally well suited for them when their dimensions are small.

Stereoscopic drawings afford a means of illustrating works with figures of three dimensions, instead of with mere plane representations. Works on crystallography, solid geometry, spherical trigonometry, architecture, machinery, &c., might be thus rendered more instructive, from the perfect counterpart of the solid figure seen from a single point of view being represented, instead of merely one of its plane projections. For this purpose the corresponding binocular figures must be engraved in parallel vertical columns, and their coalescence may be effected by viewing them through a pair of prisms, similar to those employed in the refracting stereoscope, placed in a frame at the proper distance from each other. If the engravings should be less than 2½ inches apart, the prisms may be dispensed with by persons who have command over the adaptation of their eyes, particularly if they be short-sighted.

§ 19.

At the date of the publication of my experiments on binocular vision, the brilliant photographic discoveries of Talbot, Niepce and Daguerre, had not been announced to the world. To illustrate the phenomena of the stereoscope I could therefore, at that time, only employ drawings made by the hands of an artist. Mere outline figures, or even shaded perspective drawings of simple objects, do not present much difficulty; but it is evidently impossible for the most accurate and accomplished artist to delineate, by the sole aid of his eye, the two projections necessary to form the stereoscopic relief of objects as they exist in nature with their delicate differences of outline, light and shade. What the hand of the artist was unable to accomplish, the chemical action of light, directed by the camera, has enabled us to effect.

It was at the beginning of 1839, about six months after the appearance of my memoir in the Philosophical Transactions, that the photographic art became known, and soon after, at my request, Mr. Talbot, the inventor, and Mr. Collen (one of the first cultivators of the art) obligingly prepared for me stereoscopic Talbotypes of full-sized statues, buildings, and even portraits of living persons. M. Quetelet, to whom I communicated this application and sent specimens, made mention of it in the Bulletins of the Brussels Academy of October 1841. To M. Fizeau and M. Claudet I was indebted for the first Daguerreotypes executed for the stereoscope. The beautiful stereoscopic representations of statuary, architecture, machinery, natural history specimens, portraits of living persons, single and in groups, &c., which have recently been produced by M. Soleil and M. Claudet, are now too well known to the public to need more than a slight reference to them.

With respect to the means of preparing the binocular photographs (and in this general term I include both Talbotypes and Daguerreotypes), little requires to be said beyond a few directions as to the proper positions in which it is necessary to place the camera in order to obtain the two required projections.

We will suppose that the binocular pictures are required to be seen in the stereoscope at a distance of 8 inches before the eyes, in which case the convergence of the optic axes is about 18°. To obtain the proper projections for this distance, the camera must be placed, with its lens accurately directed towards the object, successively in two points of the circumference of a circle of which the object is the centre, and the points at which the camera is so placed must have the angular distance of 18° from each other, exactly that of the optic axes in the stereoscope. The distance of the camera from the object may be taken arbitrarily, for, so long as the same angle is employed, whatever that distance may be, the pictures will exhibit in the stereoscope the same relief, and be seen at the same distance of 8 inches, only the magnitude of the picture will appear different. Miniature stereoscopic representations of buildings and full-sized statues are therefore obtained merely by taking the two projections of the object from a considerable distance, but at the same angle as if the object were only 8 inches distant, that is, at an angle of 18°.

To produce the best effect, it is necessary that the pictures be so placed in the stereoscope that each eye shall see its respective picture at the proper point of sight: if this condition be not attended to, the binocular perspective will be incorrect.

For obtaining binocular photographic portraits, it has been found advantageous to employ, simultaneously, two cameras fixed at the proper angular positions.

I subjoin a Table of the inclinations of the optic axes which correspond to different distances; it also shows the angular positions of the camera required to obtain binocular pictures which shall appear at a given distance in the stereoscope in their true relief.

Inclination of the optic axes	2°	4°	6°	8°	10°	12°	14°	16°	18°	20°	22°	24°	26°	28°	30°
Distance in inches	71·5	35·7	23·8	17·8	13·2	11·8	10·1	8·8	7·8	7·0	6·4	5·8	5·4	5·0	4·6

The distance is equal to $\frac{a}{2}$ cotang $\frac{\theta}{2}$; a denoting the distance between the two eyes, and θ the inclination of the optic axes.

§ 20.

As the inclination of the optic axes diminishes by the removal of an object to which they are directed to a greater distance, not only does the magnitude of the pictures projected by it on the retinæ proportionately diminish, but the dissimilarity of the pictures becomes less. The difference of distance between any two points of each of the pictures will diminish until the projections become sensibly similar. Under the usual circumstances attending the vision of a solid object placed at a given distance, a particular inclination of the axes is invariably accompanied by a specific pair of dissimilar projections; and if the distance be changed, a different inclination of the axes is accompanied by another pair of projections; but, by means of the stereoscope, we have it within our power to associate these circumstances abnormally, and to cause any degree of inclination of the axes to coexist with any dissimilarity of the two pictures. To ascertain experimentally what takes place under these circumstances M. Claudet prepared for me a number of Daguerreotypes of the same bust, taken at a variety of different angles, so that I was enabled to place in the stereoscope two pictures taken at any angular distance from 2° to 18°, the former corresponding with a distance of about 6 feet, and the latter with a distance of about 8 inches. The effect of a pair of near projections seen with a distant convergence of the optic axes, is to give an undue elongation to lines joining two unequally distant points, so that all the features of a bust appear to be exaggerated in depth. The effect, on the contrary, of a pair of distant projections, seen with a *near* convergence of the axes, is to give an undue shortening to the same lines, so that the appearance of a bas-relief is obtained from the two projections of the bust. The apparent dimensions in breadth and height remain in both cases the same.

§ 21.

To reproduce the conditions of the binocular vision of a solid object as completely as possible by means of its two plane projections, it is necessary, as I have before stated, that the projections shall be such as correspond exactly with the inclination of the optic axes under which they are viewed. I have already shown in § 20 what takes place when this condition is not strictly observed, and I may add that the mind is not unpleasantly affected by a considerable incongruity in this respect; on the contrary, the effect in many cases seems heightened by viewing the solid appearance, intended for a determinate degree of inclination of the axes, under an angle several degrees less; the reality is as it were exaggerated. When the optic axes are parallel, in strictness there should be no difference between the pictures presented to each eye, and in this case there would be no binocular relief; but I find that an excellent effect is produced when the axes are nearly parallel by pictures taken at an inclination of 7° or 8°, and even a difference of 16° or 17° has no decidedly bad effect.

This circumstance enables us to combine the ideal amplification arising from viewing pictures placed near the eyes under a small inclination, or even parallelism, of the optic axes mentioned in § 17, with the perception of solidity arising from the dissimilarity of the projections; for this purpose, the pictures in the refracting stereoscope, or their reflected images in the reflecting instrument, must be viewed through lenses the focal distance of which is equal to the distance between them and the pictures; the perceived magnitude of the binocular image will increase with the nearness of the pictures, and depends almost entirely on the disassociation of the retinal magnitude from its usually accompanying inclination of the optic axes, the actual magnifying power of the lenses having a very small influence.

The sole use of the lenses is to render the rays of light parallel, which it is necessary they should be for distinct vision when the optic axes are parallel. When the reflecting stereoscope is employed, this means of magnifying the effect is not of much utility, as pictures of any size may be adapted to that instrument. But in the case of the refracting stereoscope it may be advantageously made use of. By combining lenses with the refracting stereoscope, described in § 18, Daguerreotypes somewhat wider than the width between the eyes may be employed. Sir David Brewster has used, to effect the same purpose, semi-lenses with their edges directed towards each other, which serve at the same time to render the rays less convergent and slightly to displace the pictures towards each other. Two corresponding Daguerreotypes, each not exceeding in breadth the width between the eyes, being placed close to each other, and viewed with lenses of short focal distance, will even without the aid of the prisms give an apparently highly magnified binocular image in bold relief.

There is a peculiarity in such images worthy of remark; although the optic axes are parallel, or nearly so, the image does not appear to be referred to the distance we should, from this circumstance, suppose it to be, but it is perceived to be much nearer, and indeed more so, as the pictures are nearer the eyes, though the inclination of the optic axes remains the same, and should therefore suggest the same distance; it seems as if the dissimilarity of the projections, corresponding as they do to a nearer distance than that which would be suggested by the former circumstance alone, alters in some degree the perception of distance.

I recommend, as a convenient arrangement of a refracting stereoscope for viewing Daguerreotypes of small dimensions, the instrument represented, Fig. 4, shortened in its length from 8 inches to 5, and lenses of 5 inches focal distance placed before and close to the prisms.

§ 22.

I now proceed to another subject – to the consideration of those phenomena which I have termed Conversions of Relief.

In § 5 of my first memoir I noticed the remarkable circumstance, that when the drawing intended to be seen by the right eye is presented to the left eye in the stereoscope, and *vice versâ*, a totally different solid figure is perceived to that seen before the transposition. I called this the converse figure, and showed that it differs from the normal figure in the circumstance, that those points which appear the most distant in the latter, appear the nearest in the former.

The pictures being, in the first place, presented directly to their corresponding eyes, as in the refracting stereoscope, and exhibiting therefore the resultant image in its normal relief, the conversion of the relief may be effected in three different ways, – 1st, by transposing the pictures from one eye to the other, as mentioned above; 2ndly, by reflecting the pictures, while they remain presented to the same eye, as in the reflecting stereoscope; and 3rdly, by inverting the position of the pictures without transposing them.

The following considerations will explain the cause of the conversion of relief in the preceding cases.

If two different objects, or parts of an object (Fig. 5a), have a greater lateral distance between them on the right-hand picture than that which they have on the left-hand picture, the optic axes must converge more to make the left-hand than to make the right-hand objects coincide, and the left-hand object will appear the nearest.

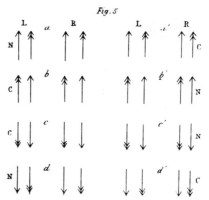

Fig. 5

If the pictures be now transposed from one eye to the other (Fig. 5a'), the greatest distance will be between the corresponding points of the picture presented to the left eye; the optic axes must therefore converge less to make the left-hand objects coincide, and the right-hand object will appear the nearest.

If the pictures, remaining untransposed, be each separately reflected (Fig. 5b), the relative distances of the corresponding objects remain the same to each eye, and the left-hand object will still appear nearest; but in consequence of the lateral inversion of the objects in each picture by reflexion, that which was previously on the left will now be on the right, and therefore, the object which before appeared nearest, will now appear farthest.

When the pictures are turned upside down, still remaining untransposed (Fig. 5c), the objects are reversed with respect to the right and left, in the same manner as they are when reflected, and the lateral distances between the objects remaining the same to each eye, precisely the same conversion of relief is produced as in the preceding case, except that the resultant image is inverted. The diagram (Fig. 5) represents all the possible changes of the two binocular pictures; those marked N show the normal relief, and those marked C the converse relief.

But it may be asked why, if the reflection or inversion of the binocular pictures of an object gives rise to the mental idea of the converse relief, the same converse relief is not observed when the object itself is reflected in a mirror, or inverted. The reason is this; that in the former cases the projections to each eye are separately reflected or inverted, still remaining presented to the same eye, whereas, by the reflection or inversion of the object itself, not only are the projections reflected or inverted, but they are also transposed from one eye to the other; and these circumstances occurring simultaneously reproduce the normal relief.

Figure 6 will render this evident in the case of reflexion: A is the object, B its reflexion in the mirror CD; RB and LB are the directions in which the right and left eyes view the reflected image respectively, and lA and rA the directions in which the eyes would view the corresponding face of the object directly.

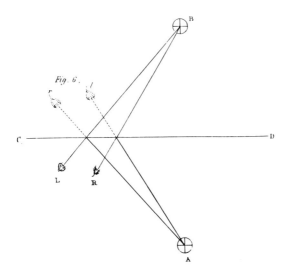

Fig. 6.

In the case of an inverted object, it is obvious that that projection which was before seen by the right eye must be seen by the left eye, and the contrary.

It is possible to make this normal or converse relief appear while one of the pictures remains constantly presented to the same eye. This result may be thus obtained. Having taken a photograph of the object, which should be one the converse of which has a meaning, take two others at the same angular distance (say 18°), one on the right side, the other on the left side of the original. Of the three pictures thus taken, if the middle one be presented to the right eye, and the left picture to the left eye, a normal relief will be seen; but if the right picture be presented to the left eye, the other remaining unchanged, a converse relief will be seen. In like manner, if the middle picture be presented to the left eye, and the right picture to the right eye, a normal relief will appear; but if the left picture be presented to the right eye, the converse relief will present itself. It must be observed, that the normal and converse reliefs, when the same picture remains presented to the same eye, belong to two different positions of the object.

§ 23.

Hitherto I have taken into consideration only those cases of the conversion of relief which are exhibited by binocular pictures in the stereoscope, when they are transposed, reflected or inverted; I shall now proceed to show how phenomena of the same kind may be elicited by regarding objects themselves, by means of an instrument adapted for the purpose. As this instrument conveys to the mind false perceptions of all external objects, I have called it the Pseudoscope. It is represented by Fig. 7, and is thus constructed: two rectangular prisms of flint glass, the faces of which are 1·2 inch square, are placed in a frame with their hypothenuses parallel, and 2·1 inches from each other; each prism has a motion on an axis corresponding with the angle nearest the eyes, so that they may be adjusted that their bases may have any inclination towards each other; and the frame itself is adjustable by a hinge at *a*, in order to bring the prisms nearer each other to suit the eyes of the observer.

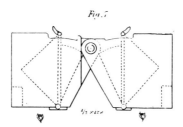

Fig. 7

The instrument being held to the eyes, and adjusted to an object, so that it shall appear single, each eye will see a reflected image of that projection of the object which would be seen by the same eye without the pseudoscope. This is exactly the contrary of what occurs when the eyes regard the reflected image of an object in a looking-glass; the left eye then sees the reflected image of the right-hand projection, and the right eye the reflected image of the left projection, as shown by Fig. 6.

Plane mirrors cannot be substituted for the reflecting prisms, for this reason; the refraction of the rays of light at the incident and emergent surfaces of the prisms enables the reflexion of an object to be seen when the object is even

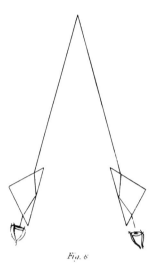

Fig. 8

behind the prolongation of the reflecting surface, as shown at Fig. 8, and thus the reflected binocular image may be seen in the same place as the object itself, whereas the images cannot be made by means of plane mirrors thus to coincide.

When the pseudoscope is so adjusted as to see a near object while the optic axes are parallel, to view a more distant object with the same adjustment, the axes must converge, and the more so as the object is more distant; all nearer objects than that seen when the axes are parallel, will appear double, because the optic axes can never be simultaneously directed to them. If this instrument be so adjusted that very distant objects are seen single when the eyes are parallel, *all* nearer objects will appear double, because the optic axes can never converge to make their binocular images coincide. If the attention is required to be directed to an object at a particular distance, the best mode of viewing it with the pseudo-scope is to adjust the instrument so that the object shall appear at the proper distance and of its natural size. In this case the more distant objects will appear nearer and smaller, and the nearer objects will appear more distant and larger.

In ordinary vision, whenever the distance of an object varies, the magnitude of the picture on the retina, and the degree of convergence of the optic axes, always maintain a constant relation to each other, both increasing or decreasing to-gether; and the perceived magnitude, suggesting to the mind the real magnitude of the object, in consequence thereof remains the same. The instrument I described in § 17 shows what illusions arise when the usual relations of these elements of our perceptions are disturbed, by causing one to remain constant while the other varies. The pseudoscope exhibits the still more curious illusions, which results from combining these elements inversely, so that as an object becomes nearer, its larger picture on the retina is accompanied by a less convergence of the optic axes. With the pseudoscope we have a glance, as it were, into another visible world, in which external objects and our internal perceptions have no longer their habitual relation with each other.

I will now proceed to describe some of the illusions produced by the aid of this instrument. Those which may be strictly designated conversions of relief, in which the illusive appearance has the same relation to that of the real object as a cast to a mould, or a mould to a cast, are very readily perceived. I must however remark, that it is necessary to illuminate the object equally, so as to allow no lights or shades to appear upon them, for their presence has a considerable influence on the judgement, and is one of the principal causes of the perception of the proper relief when a single eye is employed.

The inside of a tea-cup appears as a solid convex body; the effect is more striking if there are painted figures within the cup.

A china vase, ornamented with coloured flowers in relief, presents a very remarkable appearance; we apparently see a vertical section of the interior of the vase, with painted hollow impressions of the flowers.

A small terrestrial globe appears as a concave hemisphere; on turning it round on its axis, it was curious to see different portions of the spherical map appear and disappear in a manner that nothing in external nature can imitate.

A bust regarded in front becomes a deep hollow mask; the appearance when regarded in profile is equally striking.

A framed picture hanging against a wall, appears as if imbedded in a cavity made in the wall.

A medal, or the impression of a seal, is perfectly converted into a representation of the die from which it has been struck; and, on the other hand, the mould or die of a medal, or an engraved seal, becomes a *fac-simile* of the medal or raised impression. It will also be observed, that if the medal be placed on a flat surface, as a sheet of paper, it will appear sunk beneath the surface; and if it be placed in a hollow of the same size, it will appear to stand above the surface as much as it actually is below it.

These appearances are not always immediately perceived; and some much more readily present themselves than others. Those converse forms which have a meaning, and resemble real forms we have been accustomed to see, are those which are the most easily apprehended. Viewed with the pseudoscope, notwithstanding the inversion of the pictures on the retina, the natural appearance of the object continues to intrude itself, when sometimes suddenly, and at other times gradually, the converse occupies its place. The reason of this is, that the relief and distance of objects is not suggested to the mind solely by the binocular pictures and the convergence of the optic axes, but also by other signs, which are perceived by means of each eye singly; among which the most effective are the distributions of light and shade and the perspective forms which we have been accustomed to see accompany these appearances. One idea being therefore suggested to the mind by one set of signs, and another totally incompatible idea by another set, according as the mental attention is directed to the one and abstracted from the other, the normal form or its converse is perceived. This mental attention is involuntary; no immediate effort of the will can call up one idea while the other continues to present itself, though the transition may be facilitated by intentionally removing some of the signs which suggest the preponderating idea; thus the converse form being perceived, closing either eye will most frequently cause an instant reversion to the normal form; and always, if the monocular signs of relief are sufficiently suggestive.

I know of nothing more wonderful, among the phenomena of perception, than the spontaneous successive occurrence of these two very different ideas in the mind, while all external circumstances remain precisely the same. Thus a small statuary group, an elegant and beautiful object, without any apparent cause becomes converted into another totally dissimilar object uncouth in appearance, and which gives rise to no agreeable emotions in the mind; yet in both cases all the sensations that intervene between objective reality and ideal conception continue unchanged.

The effects of the pseudoscope I have already mentioned, may be strictly called conversions of relief, because the illusive appearance is in each case the converse impression of the relief of the real object. If, however, the object consists of parts detached from and behind each other, the preceding term is inappropriate to denote the effects which result, but the more general expression conversion or inversion of distance may be employed to designate them. I proceed to call attention to a few such effects.

Skeleton figures of geometrical solids, as cubes, pyramids, &c., readily show their converse.

Two objects at different distances, being simultaneously regarded, the most remote will appear the nearest and the nearest the most remote.

An ivory foot rule, held immediately before the eyes a little inclined to the horizon with its remote end elevated, appears inclined in the opposite way, its nearer end elevated, and as if the observer were looking at its lower surface. Its form also undergoes a change. Since the nearest end, the retinal magnitude of which is the largest, appears farthest from the eyes, and the nearest end, the retinal magnitude of which is greatest, appears near the eyes, the rule will no longer be perceived to be rectangular, but trapezoidal. If the rule be placed horizontally, and it be regarded with the pseudoscope at an angle of 45°, it will appear with the form just described standing vertically.

Any object placed before the wall of a room will appear behind the wall, and as if an aperture of the proper dimensions had been made in the wall to allow it to be seen; if the object be illuminated by a candle, its shadow will appear as far before the object as in reality it is behind.

The appearance of a plant is very remarkable; as the branches which are farthest from the eye are perceived to be the nearest, those parts which are actually obscured by the branches before them, appear broken away and allow the parts apparently behind them to be seen. A flowering shrub before a hedge appears to be transferred behind it; and a tree standing outside a window may be brought visibly within the room in which the observer is standing.

I have before observed that the transition from the normal to the converse perception is often gradual; I will give one instance of this as an illustration. The object was a page of medallions embossed on card-board, and the raised impressions were protected from injury by a thick piece of mill-board having apertures in it made to correspond to each medallion. The page was placed horizontally, illuminated by a candle placed beyond it, and looked at through the pseudoscope at an angle of 45°; for the first moment the page appeared as it would have done without the instrument; soon after the medallions appeared level with the upper surface, and the shadows on the upper parts of the circular apertures were converted into deep depressions as if cut out with a tool; they next, from horizontal, became vertical, each standing erect on the horizontal plane, and immediately afterwards the reliefs were all changed into hollows; finally, the page itself stood vertical, but with that change of form which I indicated in the case of the rule, the upper edge appearing much shorter than the lower edge: the series of changes being now complete, the final form remained constant as long as the object was regarded.

In endeavouring to analyse the phenomena of converse perception, it must be borne in mind that the transposition of distances has reference only to distances from the retinæ, not to absolute horizontal distances in space. Thus, if a straight ruler be held in the vertical plane perpendicular to the optic base, and also inclined 45° to the horizon so that its upper end shall be the most distant, when the eyes are directed horizontally towards it, the rule will appear exactly in the converse position. If the rule be now removed lower down in the same vertical plane, its inclination remaining unchanged, so that to look upon it the plane of the optic axes must be inclined 45°, it will appear unaltered in position, because its two pictures are parallel on the retinæ, and the optic axes would require the same convergence to make the upper and lower ends coalesce. The rule being removed still lower down, instead of its position being apparently reversed, it will appear to have a greater inclination on the same side than the object itself has. In the first case the more distant end is actually farthest from the eyes; in the second the near and remote ends are equally distant; and in the third the nearest end is most distant.

Attention to what I have just stated will explain many anomalous circumstances which occur when the eyes are differently directed towards the same object. It may also be necessary to remark, that the conversion of distance takes place only within those limits in which the optic axes sensibly converge, or the pictures projected on the retinæ are sensibly dissimilar. Beyond this range there is no mutual transposition of the apparent distances of objects with the pseudoscope; a distant view therefore appears unchanged.

Some very paradoxical results are obtained when objects in motion are viewed through the pseudoscope. When an object approaches, the magnitude of its picture on the retinæ increases as in ordinary vision, but the inclination of the optic axes, instead of increasing, becomes less, as I have already explained. Now an enlargement of the picture on the retina invariably suggests approach, and a less convergence of the optic axes indicates that the object is at a greater distance; and we have thus two contradictory suggestions. Hence, if two objects be placed side by side at a certain distance before the eyes, and one of them be moved forwards, so as to vary its distance from the other, its continually enlarging picture on the retina makes it appear to come towards the eyes, as it actually does, while at the same time it appears at every step at a greater distance beyond the fixed object; from one suggestion the object appears to approach, from the other to have receded. I again observe that retinal magnitude does not itself suggest distance, but from its changes we infer changes of distance.

I have hitherto only described the pseudoscope constructed with two reflecting prisms. This is the most convenient apparatus for effecting the conversion of distance and relief that has occurred to me; but other means may be employed, which I will briefly mention.

1st. Two plane mirrors are placed together so as to form a very obtuse angle towards the eyes of the observer; immediately before them the object is to be placed at such distance that a reflected image shall appear in each mirror. The eyes being placed before and a little above the object, must be caused to converge to a point between the object and the mirrors; the right-hand image of the left-eye will then unite with the left-hand image of the right eye, and the converse relief will be perceived. The disadvantages of this method are that only particular objects can be examined, and it requires a painful adaptation of the eye to distinct vision.

2ndly. Place between the object and each eye a lens of small focal distance, and adjust the distances of the object and the lenses so that distinct inverted images of the object shall be seen by each eye; on directing the eyes to the place of the object the two images will unite, and the converse relief be perceived. As the rays of light proceeding from the images have a greater divergence than those which would proceed from the point to which the optic axes are directed, long-sighted persons will see the binocular image more distinctly by wearing a pair of short-sighted spectacles. In this experiment the field of view is very small on account of the distance at which it is necessary to place the lenses from the eyes; but I have been enabled in this manner to see beautifully the converse relief of a small ivory bust and of other small objects, which however should be inverted in order to see them direct.

3rdly. The inverted images of the lenses, instead of being received immediately by the eyes as just described, may be thrown on a plate of ground glass as in the case of the ordinary camera-obscura, and may be then caused to unite by the means employed in any form of the refracting stereoscope.

§ 24.

The cases of the conversion of relief when the object is regarded with one eye only, some of which were known more than a century ago, were taken into consideration and endeavoured to be explained by me in § 11 of the first part of this memoir, and Sir David Brewster* has published some interesting and instructive observations on the same subject; I will therefore not revert to this matter here, but only to say that I have myself never observed the conversion of relief when looking with both eyes immediately on a solid object, and if it has been observed by others under such circumstances, I should be inclined to attribute the effect to an inequality in the impressions on the two eyes so that one only is attended to. But the plane shaded representation of a solid object, the relief of which is not very deep, may easily be made to appear at will either as the solid which it is intended to represent or as its converse, even when both eyes are employed. This effect is strikingly observed in the glyptographic engravings of medals of low relief, and depends entirely on whether the light is so placed that it would cast the same shadows on the real object as are represented in the picture, or that it would cast shadows in the opposite direction. In the former case the picture appears with the relief it was intended to suggest; in the latter with the converse relief. I have observed similar effects with Daguerreotypes of medallions and cameos, and with carefully shaded drawings of simple objects.

2.11. **Wheatstone**: "On the binocular microscope, and on stereoscopic pictures of microscopic objects". *Transactions of the Microscopical Society of London*, 1853, **1**, 99–102.

In Section 11 of my first Memoir on Binocular Vision, published in the Philosophical Transactions for 1838, I have alluded to the illusions to which microscopic observers are liable, from their inability to judge correctly the relief of objects when one eye only is employed. This indetermination of the judgment exists whenever a shadowless object is regarded with a single eye. Frequently an elevation appears as a depression, a cameo as an intaglio, a hollow pyramid (as a crystal of muriate of soda) as a pyramid in relief, &c., and *vice versâ*; but this indecision is entirely removed when the object is viewed with both eyes

* Transactions of the Royal Society of Edinburgh, vol. xv. p. 365 and 657.

simultaneously. No mistake, if the object be a near one, can then be made with regard to its relief; and the relative positions of every point, in depth as well as in length and breadth, can be correctly determined.

The stereoscope affords a convincing proof that the two projections of an object presented to the two eyes, suggest the real object far more effectively to the mind than a single projection to one eye does; and those who have paid much attention to the appearance of binocular pictures in the stereoscope, will not have failed to remark, that not only is double vision of importance to enable us more accurately to judge of the relief of bodies, but it also occasions us to perceive things which pass entirely unnoticed when monocular pictures alone are regarded.

Fully impressed with these views, and convinced, from the reasons above stated, that a binocular microscope would possess great advantages over the present monocular instrument, I, shortly after the publication of my first memoir, called the attention both of Mr. Ross and Mr. Powell to this subject, and strongly recommended them to make an instrument to realize the anticipated effect; their occupations, however, prevented either of these artists from taking the matter up. The year before last, previous to the publication of my second memoir, I again urged Mr. Ross, and subsequently Mr. Beck, to attempt its construction, and for a short time they interested themselves in the matter, but ultimately relinquished it for want of time, and in my opinion over-estimating the difficulties of the undertaking.

It appears, however, from a communication in the 'American Journal of Science' of January, 1853, which has been reprinted in the last number of the 'Microscopical Journal', that such an instrument has been actually constructed by Professor J. L. Riddell of New Orleans, and the results expected have been obtained. The method Mr. Riddell employs is similar to the one I recommended to Mr. Beck. After the rays from the object pass through the compound object-glass is the usual manner, he deflects them by means of a system of rectangular prisms into two directions parallel to the original, and sufficiently separated for the images to be seen by each eye. As in this arrangement there must be a considerable loss of light, I have proposed another which will not have this disadvantage, and which I will shortly submit to the Society.

A binocular microscope is, however, by no means a novelty, and its invention dates nearly two centuries back. I have found, in the library of the Royal Society, a work entitled 'La Vision parfaite, ou les Concours des deux Axes de la Vision, en un seul point de l'Objet. Par le P. Cherubin d'Orléans, Capucin.' This work was published at Paris in 1677, and in it eight chapters and a plate are devoted to a minute description of the instrument, which he informs us he constructed, and presented to the Dauphin. The following is an extract from the Preface: –

> Some years ago I resolved to effect what I had long before premeditated, to make a microscope to see the smallest objects with the two eyes conjointly; and this project

has succeeded even beyond my expectation, with advantages above the single instrument so extraordinary, and so surprising, that every intelligent person to whom I have shown the effect has assured me that inquiring philosophers will be highly pleased with the communication. For this reason I have determined to make it the principal subject of the present work.

And the second part, which contains a description of the instrument, is thus headed: –

Section the first, in which is taught the method of constructing a newly-invented microscope to see the smallest objects very agreeably and conveniently, represented entire to the two eyes conjointly, with a magnitude and distinctness which surpasses everything which has been hitherto seen in this kind of instrument.

In the Père d'Orléans' binocular microscope, two object-glasses have their lateral portions cut away so as to allow of close juxta-position, and these nearly semi-lenses are so arranged, that their axes correspond with the two optic axes passing through the tubes containing the eye-pieces. The author's aim in its construction was solely the reinforcement of the impression by presenting an image to each eye, for he assumes, according to the then prevalent error, that vision by the two organs conjointly is naturally and necessarily unique, from the perfect conformity of all the homonymous parts of the two images of the object on the two retinæ. The real advantage of such an instrument entirely escaped his attention; viz., that of presenting to the two eyes the two *dissimilar* microscopic images of an object, under precisely the same circumstances as the two unlike images of any usual object is presented to them when no instrument is employed, by which simultaneous presentment the same accurate judgment as to its real solid form, and the relative distances of all its points, can be as readily determined in the former case as in the latter.

In the construction of a binocular microscope there is one thing especially to be attended to – viz., that the images be both direct, for in this case only a true stereoscopic representation will be obtained. If the images, on the contrary, be inverted, a pseudoscopic effect would be produced which will give a very erroneous idea of the real form. The reason of these effects is fully explained in Sections 5, 10, 22, 23, of my Memoirs. The reversal of the images by reflection from mirrors or reflecting prisms, will produce the same result as to the stereoscopic and pseudoscopic appearances as their inversion by lenses. The binocular microscope constructed by the Père d'Orleans was pseudoscopic, though he describes one which, had it been made, would have been stereoscopic; he was, however, quite unaware that there would be any difference of this kind between them. The pseudoscopic effects when inverted images are presented, and the natural appearances when erecting eye-pieces are employed, have not escaped the observation of Mr. Riddell.

Besides actual inspection by means of the binocular microscope, there is another way in which the advantages of binocular vision may be applied to microscopic objects. The beautiful specimens of photography, reproducing the highly magnified images of objects, inserted in a recent number of the Micro-scopic Journal, makes one regret that they were not accompanied by their stereoscopic complements. A very simple modification of the usual microscope would fit it for producing the two pictures at the proper angles; all that is necessary is to cause the tube of the microscope to move independently of the fixed stand round an axis, the imaginary prolongation of which should pass through the object. A motion of 15° would include every difference of relief which it would be desirable to have, and it is indifferent in what direction this motion is made in respect to the stand. The pair of stereoscopic pictures may be obtained by a still simpler method, which requires no alteration in the microscope; the object itself may be turned round on an imaginary axis within itself, from 7° to 15°. But this method is inapplicable unless the light be perfectly diffused and uniform so as to avoid all shadows, the presence of which would give rise to false stereoscopic appearances. In the former case, where the object remains stationary and the tube moves independently of the frame, the arrangement of the light so as to cast single shadows might be an advantage, and assist the visual judgment.

2.12. Correspondence between Brewster and Wheatstone regarding the invention of the stereoscope, published in *The Times*, 17, 20, 25, 31 October and 5, 15 November, 1856.

Sir, – M. Faye, a distinguished astronomer, and member of the Academy of Sciences in Paris, communicated to that body, on the 6th of October, an account of a new and simple stereoscope, of which the Abbé Moigno has given the following description in his *Cosmos* of the 12th of October: –

M. Faye presented a new stereoscope, of his invention, of extreme simplicity. It is indeed a simple piece of cardboard or paper, in which are pierced two holes, whose centres are on the same horizontal line, and at the distance which separates the two eyes of the person who uses it. In looking through these two holes, about 12 millimetres wide (less than half an inch), at a stereoscopic slide, we see but one image, and for that reason we see it as much in relief as in the reflecting or refracting stereoscope. This is certainly a happy idea.

The paper or the cardboard of M. Faye has the effect of making the optic axes rigorously parallel, as if they were directed to a point situated at an infinite distance. It is for this reason, and not, as Mr. Grove maintains, by crossing the optic axes by a forced and voluntary squinting, that the two images are superimposed.

In reference to this last remark, involving the theory of M. Faye's stereoscope, I may observe, in passing, that if Mr. Grove means that the optic axes are crossed, or converged to a point, in order to superimpose the images, he is unquestionably right, for the axes must be crossed at a point beyond the binocular slide. If he means that the axes are crossed at a point between the slide and the observer, he is wrong.

My object, however, is not to discuss the theory of the instrument, but to state the fact that it is not new, and has been long known and used in England. It is the invention of Mr. James Elliot, teacher of mathematics in Edinburgh, who contrived it in 1834, but did not execute it till 1839. Mr. Wheatstone had previously published the same principle in 1838 (*Phil. Trans.*, 1838, p. 373.), but he used two separate tubes in place of the two holes employed by Mr. Elliot and M. Faye, and he directed the tubes to a point of convergence beyond the binocular pictures. It is well known that M. Claudet and others have the facility of converging their optical axes beyond the binocular pictures, and thus doing exactly what is done by Mr. Wheatstone's tubes, and Mr. Elliot's and M. Faye's holes; so that we can only consider these tubes and holes as auxiliaries to our natural vision.

In M. Faye's stereoscope the effect produced does not depend upon the holes: it is produced by the opaque card between them simply eclipsing one of the pictures from each eye – the left hand picture from the right eye, and the right hand picture from the left eye. Here we have a still simpler stereoscope. Hold up between the eyes and the pictures two or three fingers, and looking past the left side of them with the left eye, and past the right side of them with the right eye, so that each eye sees only one picture, you will see the two superimposed, and the relief perfect. A piece of card of less width will answer better than the fingers, but the fingers are always at hand.

A short-sighted person, or a person wearing very deep convex glasses, may, upon bringing the pictures close to his face, unite them into stereoscopic relief without the aid of holes, tubes, or fingers.

I am, Sir, yours, &c.,

October 15th   A.

Sir, – Allow me to make a few remarks on a letter which appeared in your columns yesterday, relating to the invention of the stereoscope.

In my memoir "on some remarkable and hitherto unobserved phenomena of binocular vision," which was presented to the Royal Society in June, 1838, and published in the Philosophical Transactions of that year, I described, besides the more perfect instrument to which I gave the name of "stereoscope," the only two methods by which binocular drawings might be seen in stereoscopic relief, without employing any optical appliances. In one, the pictures were placed beyond the intersection of the optic axis, in the other they were placed before it.

The latter is the method subsequently adopted by Mr. Elliot and M. Faye.

I should not, however, have thought it of sufficient importance to trouble you with this explanation alone, but your correspondent "A," by exclusively adopting the dates and statements put forward in various publications by Sir D. Brewster, with the intention of proving that Mr. Elliot had conceived the idea of a stereoscope before I had, has given the extensive circulation of *The Times* to these imperfect allegations, and I wish to shew by sufficient facts that the claim thus supported is untenable.

The first public announcement of the principles of this invention appeared in the third edition of Professor Herbert Mayo's *Outlines of Human Physiology*, published in 1833. In giving a short notice of my then unpublished experiments, the author says (p. 288): –

> One of the most remarkable results of Mr. Wheatstone's investigations respecting binocular vision is the following: – A solid object being placed so as to be regarded by both eyes, projects a different perspective figure on each retina; now, if these two perspectives be actually copied on paper, and presented one to each eye so as to fall on corresponding parts, the original solid figure will be apparently re-produced in such a manner that no effort of the imagination can make it appear as a representation on a plane surface. This and numerous other experiments explain the cause of the inadequacy of painting to represent the relief of objects, and indicate a means of representing external nature with more truth and fidelity than have yet been obtained. It would require too much space to enter upon the physiological views to which these experiments have led their author.

Shortly after the publication of my completed memoir, I gave a brief account of it at the meeting of the British Association, which was held at Newcastle, in September, 1838. The great interest excited when the stereoscope was on that occasion brought forward, may be seen by referring to the contemporaneous accounts of the proceedings of that body in the *Athenæum* and *Literary Gazette*.

Sir D. Brewster and your correspondent, in accordance with him, represent Mr. Elliot as having conceived the idea of a stereoscope in 1834, and as having realized his conception in 1839. Admitting these dates, the first is the year after my experiments had been announced in a work of standard authority, and the latter date is the year after my instrument had been completely described, and had become extensively known. It moreover appears that Mr. Elliot made no public announcement of what he is stated to have done until 18 years after the public were informed of my results.

These are surely insufficient grounds to dispute the originality of an invention, and Sir David is the last person who ought to have advanced them, since I can shew, from our correspondence, that he was aware, so early as 1832, that at that time I was preparing for publication my memoir on the subject.

                    I am, sir, your obedient servant,

Athenæum, Oct. 18   C. WHEATSTONE.

Sir, – In the notice of Mr. Faye's stereoscope which I sent you under the signature "A," not thinking it of sufficient importance to add my name, I claimed the invention of it for Mr. Wheatstone as well as for Mr. Elliot, referring distinctly to Mr. Wheatstone's paper, as published in 1838, and to the later date of 1839, when Mr. Elliot executed his instrument. I therefore gave to Mr. Wheatstone all the originality, which he claims from prior publication. But, as I had undoubted evidence that Mr. Elliot invented the stereoscope in 1834, and as his form of the instrument was exactly the same as Mr. Faye's, while Mr. Wheatstone's, though equally ingenious, was different, I placed Mr. Elliot's claim before Mr. Wheatstone's. I believe, therefore, that Mr. Elliot and Mr. Wheatstone are independent inventors of an instrument, or method, for uniting two dissimilar pictures, and thus producing relief, but that neither of them discovered the principle of the stereoscope. Mr. Elliot lays no claim to such a discovery. Mr. Wheatstone does, on the following grounds. After quoting a curious experiment on binocular vision, in which Leonardo da Vinci was on the eve of inventing the stereoscope, he makes the following observations: –

> Had Leonardo da Vinci taken, instead of a sphere, a less simple figure for the purpose of his illustration, he would not only have observed that the object obscured from each eye a different part of the more distant field of view, but the fact would also, perhaps, have forced itself upon his attention that the object itself presented a different appearance to each eye. He failed to do this, and no subsequent writer within my knowledge has supplied the omission; the projection of two obviously dissimilar pictures on the two *retinæ* when a single object is viewed, while the optic axes converge, must, therefore, be regarded as a new fact in the theory of vision. – *Philosophical Transactions*, 1838, pp. 372–3.

Now, this claim to the fundamental principle of the stereoscope is groundless – Euclid knew it; Galen knew it, and explained it. Baptista Porta quoted Galen's explanation, and illustrates it with a figure. Aguilonius, in various parts of his *Optics*, does the same; and, in his chapter on the vision of solids (τα στερεα, *ta sterea*), he is puzzled in explaining how the two dissimilar pictures give a distinct image in relief. Early in 1852, and more recently, in my *Treatise on the Stereoscope*, I have quoted the passage from these authors to prove their knowledge of the principle in question, and Mr. Wheatstone has made no reply to the statement. It is, doubtless, strange that he was not acquainted with the researches of Galen, Porta, and Aguilonius, for he tells us (*Phil. Trans.* 1838, page 372) that, "after looking over the works of many authors who might be expected to have made some remarks relating to this subject, he was able to find but one, which is in the *Trattato della Pittura*, of Leonardo da Vinci." Among these works were those of Porta and Aguilonius, for he has, more than once, quoted both of them (pages 388, 390, 391, 393); but, though I make this remark, I do not mean to insinuate, nor do I believe, that Mr. Wheatstone saw the passages to which I have referred.

In the extract from Mayo's *Outlines*, &c., from which it is evident that Mr. Wheatstone was acquainted with the principle of the stereoscope in 1833, and therefore earlier than Mr. Elliot, there is no mention whatever of any instrument or method of combining the pictures. It affords no proof that the reflecting stereoscope was then in existence; that he did combine them is obvious, and, if he had assured us that he did it by means of the reflecting instrument, I should have placed implicit confidence in the statement.

In concluding his letter, Mr. Wheatstone remarks that I was the last person to have disputed the originality of his invention, as he can shew, from his correspondence with me in 1832, "that I was aware that at that time he was preparing for publication his memoir on the subject."

I therefore call upon Mr. Wheatstone to publish this letter, or any part of it that has the least reference to the stereoscope. If it has, I pledge myself in future to place his claims above those of Mr. Elliot, whenever I have occasion to write or speak on the subject. Mr. Wheatstone's memoir is entitled *Contributions to the Physiology of Vision,* and I may well have known that he was preparing it for publication without the slightest knowledge that the stereoscope was to be one of the various subjects of which it treats.

As priority of publication is held by Mr. Wheatstone to establish the "originality of an invention," it may be sufficient to state to English readers that if this doctrine be admitted Sir Isaac Newton has no claim to be the inventor of Fluxions; Leibnitz published the method before him, but there is ample proof that Newton was the earliest inventor.

In the preceding observations I have avoided the offensive personalities with which this subject has been noticed in a silly article in the *Westminster Review.* I have no personal feelings to gratify in giving an opinion on this question. As the inventor of the lenticular stereoscope now in universal use, and of other forms of the instrument, I, of course, feel an interest in the subject, and involving as it does nice questions in the theory of vision, that interest has been greatly increased. In preparing lectures on the philosophy of the senses, I had occasion to study the department of binocular vision, and in the *Edinburgh Transactions* for 1843 I have given the true and demonstrable theory of the stereoscope, after Mr. Wheatstone had wholly failed and acknowledged his failure. (*Phil. Trans.* 1838, p. 360.) That theory has now been before the scientific world for nearly 14 years, and has never been controverted. When the paper which contains it was written, I believed that Mr. Wheatstone was the sole inventor of the principle of the stereoscope, as well as of the reflecting instrument, and I never failed to give him the credit of both. He himself knows how I was compelled to investigate the subject, and to establish the claims of others – of ancient authors to the principle, and of Mr. Elliot to an instrument for exhibiting it.

I am, Sir, your obedient servant,

St. Leonard's College,   D. BREWSTER.
St. Andrew's, Oct. 22nd

Sir, – It is difficult to deal with Sir David Brewster's reasoning. I have proved by incontrovertible dates my priority both in the discovery of the principle of the stereoscope and in the invention of the instrument. Sir David, in his reply, fully admits these dates, and says, "it is evident that Mr. Wheatstone was acquainted with the principles of the stereoscope in 1833, and therefore earlier than Mr. Elliot;" yet he announces that unless additional evidence be brought forward he will continue to place that gentleman's claims above mine whenever he has occasion to write or speak on the subject; and he further requires a proof of my having constructed a stereoscope at the time my discovery was first announced. I cannot conceive why such a proof should be thought necessary, but I trust that the following evidence of Mr. Murray, of the firm of Murray and Heath, opticians in Piccadilly, will be deemed conclusive as to this point: –

"43, *Piccadilly, Oct. 27th.*

Sir, – From an examination of the accounts furnished to you by Mr. Newman, of Regent-street, during the time I was in his establishment, and which were prepared by myself, I am able to assign the date of my first knowledge of your stereoscopes, both with reflecting mirrors and refracting prisms, to the latter part of 1832.

I am, Sir, yours faithfully,

"R. MURRAY.

"Professor Wheatstone."

The undue prominence given to Mr. Elliot's single experiment may lead some persons to imagine that the results he obtained were at least as perfect as those which I had previously produced; but it appears he did not proceed so far as to give the representation in relief of any solid body whatever. His attempt, as described by Sir D. Brewster in his recent work, was limited to represent three different flat distances, to either of which the eyes might be converged at will. The name "stereoscope" is quite inappropriate to an instrument exhibiting this effect alone.

Sir D. Brewster calls upon me to publish the letter I alluded to in my former communication, or "any part of it that has the least reference to the stereoscope." The correspondence, consisting of my letter and Sir David's reply to it (dated November 3rd, 1832), would be too long for insertion here. From the former I extract the following passage: –

I propose in the ensuing session of the Royal Society to present two papers – one on the acoustic figures of which I gave a short account at the meeting at Oxford, and the other on binocular vision, in which I shall describe a series of very curious optical illusions, which I believe to be perfectly original.

But Sir D. Brewster, not content with disputing my claim to be considered the inventor of the stereoscope, denies, even if that were to be admitted, my claim to the discovery of the principle upon which it is founded. The real fundamental principle of the stereoscope is that clearly stated in my earliest announcement –

namely, the apparent reproduction of a solid object by simultaneously presenting its two perspective projections, artificially delineated, one to each eye. I have yet to learn that any philosopher, either ancient or modern, had made this discovery before me, or had even nearly approached it. What Sir D. Brewster assumes to be the principle of the stereoscope is very different to this, and his endeavour to shew that the facts he has alluded to were already known to Euclid, Galen, Porta, and Aguilonius does not at all affect the point at issue. I shall not enter into any discussion on this collateral and comparatively unimportant subject, but proceed to shew that Sir David, when he was uninfluenced by his present feelings, took a very different view of the originality of the principle in question, even when generalized so as to include the phenomena of the binocular vision of real objects, than he now does.

In the *Transactions of the Royal Society of Edinburgh*, vol. xv., part 3, 1843, he says: –

> In prosecuting this subject, my attention has been particularly fixed upon the interesting paper of my distinguished friend, Professor Wheatstone, on some remarkable and hitherto unobserved phenomena of binocular vision. It is impossible to over-estimate the importance of this paper, or to admire too highly the value and beauty of the leading discovery which it describes – namely, the perception of an object of three dimensions by the union of the two dissimilar pictures formed on the retinæ.

When the originality of an invention of Sir D. Brewster's was formerly disputed, on somewhat similar grounds to those on which he has now impugned mine, he said, in words which have some present applicability –

> It has always been the fate of new inventions to have their origin referred to some remote period; and those who labour to enlarge the boundaries of science, or to multiply the means of improvement, are destined to learn, at a very early period of their career, that the desire of doing justice to the living is a much less powerful principle than that of being generous to the dead. – *Treatise on the Kaleidoscope*, p. 137.

A public journal is not the proper place to enter into a public controversy on points of scientific theory, but I cannot allow Sir D. Brewster's assertion, that he has "given the true and demonstrable theory of the stereoscope, after Mr. Wheatstone had wholly failed and acknowledged his failure," to remain unnoticed. It is true that I have stated, and still believe, that there are some points requiring further investigation; but I venture to affirm that Sir D. Brewster has done nothing to advance our previous theoretical knowledge of the subject; and many of the views he has brought forward regarding the philosophy of vision I hold to be manifestly erroneous. In his recent work, and elsewhere, he misrepresents my facts and conclusions in a most extraordinary manner; and he attributes to me, without the slightest foundation, an hypothesis which I never for a moment maintained, and which I utterly repudiate. He makes no mention of some of my most important results, and, when he does borrow from my memoirs, unless he has a depreciating remark to make, he omits all mention of my name; and further, he entirely ignores the memoirs of those eminent writers who, since my first publication, have treated of the stereoscopic phenomena; and the names of Bruecke, Tourtual, Prevost, Moser, Volkmann, Dove, Rogers, Serre, &c., who have all brought much thought to bear upon the subject, are not even once mentioned in his pages.

I am, Sir, your obedient Servant.

C. WHEATSTONE.

Athenæum, Oct. 29th.

Sir, – If you can spare me a few lines to correct some of Mr. Wheatstone's very incorrect statements, and also to add some new information on the history of the stereoscope, I shall not again trespass on your columns.

1. In his first letter in *The Times* Mr. Wheatstone refers to my correspondence with him in 1832, as proving that I then knew that he had invented the stereoscope. Knowing that I never heard of the stereoscope till 1838. I challenged him to publish the letter, or any part of it that mentioned the instrument. He has declined to do this, and has substituted a paragraph of his letter to me which neither alludes to the stereoscope nor anything that has the least resemblance to it. My answer to that letter, which I again call upon him to publish, could, therefore, contain nothing on the subject.

2. Mr. Wheatstone asserts that I announced, "that unless additional evidence were brought forward, I would continue to place Mr. Elliot's claim above his," and that I further required a proof that he had constructed a stereoscope at a particular time. I deny that I made any such announcement, or any such requisition; I consider Mr. Elliot as an independent inventor and constructor of the stereoscope. I believed, on the authority of his letters, that he had anticipated Mr. Wheatstone in the conception of the instrument, till I read the passage from Mayo, and I think your readers will share with me in the surprise that so remarkable an invention as the stereoscope, if actually constructed and exhibited in 1832, should have remained six years in Mr. Wheatstone's desk, and make its appearance before the public only in 1838!

3. In reference to the theory or explanation of stereoscopic phenomena which I published in 1843 in refutation of Mr. Wheatstone's views, I have only to state that it has remained for thirteen years unopposed by himself or any other person; that he had annual opportunities of discussing the question with me before distinguished members of the British Association; and that in 1852, when he was specially bound to defend himself, in his second paper on the stereoscope, in the *Philosophical Transactions* for that year, he was silent on the subject. In 1843 I

demonstrated the laws of visible direction, visible position, and visible distance, and I assert that "by means of these laws all the phenomena of erect vision from an inverted image of the single vision of points, of the vision of plane surfaces and solids, and of the conversion of two plane pictures into solids or objects in relief, may be calculated with as much accuracy as we can compute the positions of the heavenly bodies" (*Life of Newton,* vol i., p. 235), and I challenge Mr. Wheatstone to discuss these or any other points to which he has referred in the philosophical journals of the day. I call upon him also to defend the method of taking binocular pictures which he has sanctioned, and which I have proved to be as erroneous in science as it is truthless in art.

4. I have stated, and Mr. Wheatstone denies, that Aguilonius and others anticipated him in the principle of the stereoscope. The principle of the stereoscope consists of two facts, – the one, that the pictures in each eye are dissimilar; and the other, that when two objects or points upon a plane surface are united by squinting, that is by looking at a point nearer the eyes, they are seen as one object or point at the place of convergence of the optic axes; or, to express it differently, that difference of distance from the eye, or relief, is obtained and measured by the different distances of objects or points united by squinting, or any other process. The first of these facts Mr. Wheatstone claimed as his own discovery; but I have proved, and he does not now deny it, that Aguilonius and others had anticipated him in this discovery. With respect to the second fact, it is distinctly established by Dr. Smith, of Cambridge, in his *Optics.* (Rem. vol. ii., p. 86, fig. 161.) He places two candles at the distance of two or three feet from the eyes, and after uniting them he sees a single candle nearer his eyes. If the two candles are made to approach one another, the single candle recedes from him, and if they are made to recede from one another, the single candle approaches to him. He makes the same experiment with the same result, with the points of a pair of compasses, thus demonstrating by direct experiment the second principle of the stereoscope, that the different distances of similar points in binocular pictures give, when united, different distances from the eye of relief. Dr. Smith (*Id.* vol. ii. sec. 977), has proved the same thing, when the eyes are converged to a point beyond the points of the compasses, as in M. Faye's stereoscope. In place of taking compass points, Mr. Elliot took two moons at a certain distance from each other, and two crosses at a different distance, and two spots of water at a third distance, and he united those, as Dr. Smith did, and thus saw the three objects in relief forming a rude landscape, decidedly the first landscape seen in relief by any stereoscope.

5. Another candidate for stereoscopic discovery, (or bathoscopic, as the author calls them, from βαθοζ depth), has appeared in Canada. In the *Toronto Times,* of October 8, sent me by Mr. George Maynard, he claims to be the first person who published anything on the peculiar phenomena of binocular vision and the principles of the stereoscope.

"In the year 1838," he says,

(If I mistake not) at a meeting of the British Association, the attention of philosophers on the continent of Europe was invited by Professor Wheatstone to some remarkable phenomena of vision with two eyes; and a small apparatus, the stereoscope, was presented in illustration of his experiments.

It did so happen, however, that in the year 1836 (two years previous to the period afore-mentioned) a protracted article signed "Theophilus," and involving a detailed enunciation of binocular phenomena, with their bathoscopical results, was published by me in the *Royal Standard*, daily paper, at Toronto, and such is (in my opinion) the misapprehension generally existing on this interesting subject, that (even after twenty years of additional information) I am encouraged to hope that the remarks then published, with a little amplification, will not prove unacceptable to the generality of your readers.

Such is the commencement of a long and very interesting article, occupying a whole page of the newspaper, and shewing, if the paper by 'Theophilus' contains the same truths, that Mr. Maynard was, in 1836, possessed of the true principles of the stereoscope, and had produced relief by uniting objects at different distances on a plane surface. His observations on the vision of points are admirable, and in entire harmony with the views which I have published.

I am, Sir, your most obedient servant,

D. BREWSTER.

St. Leonard's College, St. Andrew's,
Nov. 1

Sir, – The following observations, in reply to Sir D. Brewster's third letter, will, I trust, close the discussion which he has opened in your columns: –

1. Sir. D. Brewster, who, to distract attention from the real questions at issue, seems desirous to involve me in a contest of mere words, misrepresents what I said respecting our correspondence in 1832, when he asserts that I referred to his correspondence with me as proving that he then knew that I had "invented the stereoscope." What I actually stated in my first letter to *The Times* was, that I could "show from our correspondence that he was aware, so early as 1832, that at that time I was preparing for publication my memoir on the subject." In my second communication I justified this statement, by giving an extract from a letter sent by me to him, the receipt of which letter was acknowledged in a reply, dated November 3, 1832. In the passage quoted, I stated my intention of presenting to the Royal Society a paper "on binocular vision," in which I said "I shall describe a series of very curious optical illusions, which I believe to be perfectly original." The memoir thus announced to Sir David subsequently appeared in the *Philosophical Transactions of the Royal Society*, under the title, "On some remarkable and hitherto unobserved phenomena of binocular vision," and it contained a full description of the curious optical illusions exhibited by the stereoscope. Sir D. Brewster was therefore certainly aware, in 1832, that I was then preparing my memoir on the phenomena of binocular vision, however afterwards he might have

forgotten the circumstance.

2. Notwithstanding Sir D. Brewster's denial of his requiring a proof that I had constructed a stereoscope in 1832, he still affects to doubt its existence at that time. "I think," says he, "your readers will share with me in the surprise that so remarkable an invention as the stereoscope, if actually constructed and exhibited in 1832, should have remained in Mr. Wheatstone's desk, and make its appearance before the public only in 1838!" If any justification of the delay in publishing my complete results, after I had announced the general facts, be necessary, it may be found in the following circumstances. Between the periods referred to, I published, in 1833, my memoir "on the figures of vibrating surfaces," and, in 1834, my memoir "on the velocity of electricity and the duration of electric light," which gained for me admission to the French Academy of Sciences; from 1834 to 1838 I was engrossingly engaged in those experiments relating to electrical phenomena to which my last investigations had led me, and from which resulted all my inventions connected with the electric telegraph. It is not much to be wondered at, that, during this interval I was obliged to defer to a future time the consideration of subjects of less immediate interest, some of which I have not even yet had the opportunity of resuming.

3. I have hitherto avoided entangling myself in the meshes of controversy with so disputatious an antagonist as Sir D. Brewster. I have always thought myself more usefully employed in investigating new facts, than in contending respecting errors which time will inevitably correct. I deny Sir David's right to challenge me to a combative discussion; but since nothing else will satisfy him, I accept his defiance, and will undertake to point out in the pages of the *Philosophical Magazine*, the numerous misapprehensions and misrepresentations he has made with regard to my researches on the subject of binocular vision, and the errors into which, I conceive, he has himself fallen.*

I was far from thinking, when answering an anonymous letter in the columns of *The Times*, that it had emanated from the same source from which had proceeded all the attacks which have, with reference to this matter, during the last four years been directed against me; but I cannot regret the opportunity which that circumstance has afforded me to correct, in the most efficacious manner, a few of the most prominent of the mis-statements made. I have limited my replies to those points only which Sir David has brought forward on the present occasion; others of equal importance, remain to be considered elsewhere.

4. Sir D. Brewster still insists that Aguilonius and others have anticipated me in the principle of the stereoscope. None of the particular facts which Sir David has brought forward, constitute, either taken by themselves or together, the principle of this invention, which I maintain to be what I stated in my last letter. No invention ever has been made, nor any invention ever will be made, with respect to which something involved in it has not been said or done previously;

---

* No subsequent article by Wheatstone on binocular vision appeared in the *Philosophical Magazine*. (Ed.)

but it is uncandid to allege that such or such a thing is the principle of a discovery, leaving out of consideration those superadded ideas which, in combination with what has been previously known, constitute its originality.

But even with regard to the fact that when an object of three dimensions is viewed while the optic axes converge, two obviously dissimilar pictures are projected on the two retinæ, however strange it may now appear that it should ever have been overlooked. I have not yet been able to find a distinct enunciation of it in any author before the date of my first memoir. Euclid, and the subsequent writers alluded to by Sir D. Brewster, merely show that when a solid body, as a sphere or a cylinder, is seen with both eyes, under certain circumstances, a little more of its right side is seen by the right eye, and a little more of its left side by the left eye.

Sir D. Brewster, indeed, endeavours to prove that Aguilonius was perfectly acquainted with the fact that dissimilar pictures or perspective projections of an object are seen by the two eyes; but he completely misrepresents what this author says. In the chapter alluded to by Sir David in his second letter, and more fully referred to in his work on the stereoscope, (pp. 11–13,) the purpose of Aguilonius is to show that when the optic axes are directed towards an object obliquely, the visual rays proceeding from the object to the centres of the eyes, make, in consequence of the unequal length of the axes, a greater angle to one eye than they do to the other, so that the object is seen of a different magnitude by each eye; and he endeavours to explain the cause of distinct single vision in the case of the dissimilar magnitude to each eye of an object, when viewed obliquely, by assuming a corrective power to exist in the mind. Aguilonius does not in any way refer to dissimilar figures, and he expressly says that in the direct view – that is, when the eyes look immediately forward, and the optic axes are equal in length – the optical pyramids formed by the visual rays are similar.

Sir D. Brewster's assertions that Aguilonius in this chapter was treating of "the union of dissimilar pictures in each eye by which a solid body is seen," and was endeavouring to explain "why two dissimilar pictures of a solid, seen by each eye, do not, when united, give a confused and imperfect view of it," are therefore quite erroneous. The passages, even as quoted by Sir David Brewster, would be alone sufficient to show this; but he has rendered them unintelligible by interpolating references to a diagram which the author does not give, and which is incompatible with his text. Besides this, Sir David misleads the reader by stating that the passages he quotes occur in the first (second) book of the learned Jesuit's work "where he is treating of the vision of solids of all forms (*de genere illorum quæ τὰ στέρεα nuncupantur*)." Now the title of the book is *De Radio Optico et Horoptere*, and it does not in any part treat of the subject Sir David names; the sentence above quoted only incidentally occurs in the course of a proposition, and τὰ στέρεα, instead of signifying solid bodies, means, as Aguilonius himself explains, certain hypothetical forms, which he elsewhere calls optical pyramids, having the vertices of their angles in the eye, and their bases on the surfaces of the objects; and he further says that this form (*corporea forma*) is a cone when the base is a circle, and a pyramid when the base is a triangle, a square, or a polygon.

It is evident that Sir David has looked upon Aguilonius through a pseudoscope.

5. With reference to the new candidate whom Sir D. Brewster has brought forward, it is sufficient to observe that the date given is three years subsequent to the public announcement of my discovery. There is nothing in the article in the *Toronto Times* which enables me to distinguish what the author now additionally puts forward from what he originally published. But still I can see nothing in the experiments related, which is not to be found in the works of Bishop Berkeley and Dr. Smith, who both wrote more than a century ago. But since the Canadian author makes no allusion to the facts and conclusions of these eminent writers, he must, I suppose, according to the law which Sir D. Brewster would enforce, be considered, "in the history of science", as their independent discoverer.

I am, Sir, your obedient servant,
C. WHEATSTONE.

Athenæum, Nov. 11

2.13. Brewster: "Notice respecting the invention of the stereoscope in the sixteenth century, and of binocular drawings, by Jacopo Chimenti da Empoli, a Florentine artist". *The Photographic Journal*, 1860, 6, 232–233.

Having had occasion to inquire into the history of the stereoscope, I found, contrary to the general opinion, that its fundamental principle was well known even to Euclid; that it was distinctly described by Galen 1500 years ago, and that Baptista Porta had, in 1593, given such a complete drawing of the two separate pictures as seen by each eye, and of the combined picture placed between them, that we recognize in it not only the principle, but the construction of the stereoscope.

Still, however, we had no proof that any person had drawn a *right*- and *left*-eye picture of any object and united them either by the eye or by an instrument; and it was hardly to be expected that any such discovery should be made.

Last summer, however, when Mr. Alexander Crum Brown and his brother Dr. John Brown were visiting the Musée Wicar at Lille, Mr. Brown observed two drawings placed side by side, and so perfectly similar that he could account for the fact only by supposing that they were binocular pictures intended to be combined into relief either by the eye or by an instrument.

The following is the account of these pictures which he communicated to Principal Forbes, who brought it under my notice: –

In the Musée Wicar at Lille there are two drawings, with a pen and in water colours (viz. No. 215, 216), of a young man sitting upon a bank and drawing with a pair of compasses. These two drawings are by Jacopo Chimenti da Empoli, a painter of the Florentine school, who was born at Empoli, near Florence, in 1554, and died in 1640.

They are drawings of the same object, from points of view slightly different. That on the right hand is from a point of view slightly to the left of that on the left hand.

They are so exactly on the same scale, that, by converging the optic axes, I succeeded in uniting the two so as to produce an image in relief. They united so

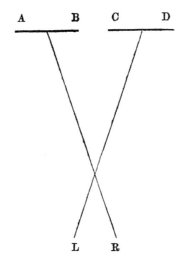

easily and completely that I could not help thinking that they had been drawn for the purpose of being looked at in that way. The figure has one arm extended towards the spectator, and with the other has drawn a line upon the floor almost at right angles with the plane of the picture. The arm and the line stand out most remarkably in relief when the two pictures are united. As far as I could judge, the difference between the two pictures was greater than would be produced by a change of the position of a spectator equal to the distance between the two eyes, so that the stereoscopic effect was somewhat exaggerated.

It was best seen at the distance of four or five yards. The height of each picture is given in the catalogue as 0·297, and the breadth as 0·216, in parts of a metre (12 inches and 8½ inches). I think, if we had a photograph of the pictures, it would be much easier to prove the stereoscopic character than merely by referring to them; and if the photographs were of such a size that they could be transposed and put into the stereoscope, any one could see it.

This account of the two drawings is so distinct and evinces such a knowledge of the subject, that we cannot for a moment doubt that they are binocular drawings intended by the artist to be united into relief either by the eye or by an instrument.

This conclusion is the more probable as the drawings must have been executed before 1640, the year in which Chimenti died at the age of eighty-six; and it is highly probable that they were executed soon after 1593, when Baptista Porta had published the Theory of the Stereoscope, and when Chimenti was in his fortieth year.

The curious discovery of these pictures, thus made by Mr. Brown, seemed to me so interesting and important, that I wrote to Mr. Delezenne, a Corresponding Member of the Institute of France, residing near Lille, and requested him to obtain for me photographs of the pictures.

In his reply to this letter, M. Delezenne informed me that the Director of the Musée Wicar, in consequence of certain abuses having taken place, had resolved not to allow any copies to be taken of the pictures and drawings. An exception, however, was made in favour of Prince Albert, who had employed Mr. Bingham to take photographs of the most important of them. I have no doubt that, through the kindness of His Royal Highness, photographic copies of the binocular pictures of Chimenti will be obtained for publication.

2.14. Brewster: "On the stereoscopic pictures executed in the 16th century". *The Photographic Journal*, 1862, **8**, 9–12.

In 1859, when Dr. John Brown and his brother Dr. Alexander Crum Brown were visiting the Museum of Wica at Lille, their attention was called to two pictures of a man sitting upon a low stool, and holding in his left hand a pair of compasses, and in his right hand a line reaching the ground. These two pictures appeared to be exactly the same, as if the one had been copied from the other. They were each about *twelve* inches high and *eight and a half* broad, and were placed close to one another like the pictures in a stereoscopic slide. Dr. A. Crum Brown, on his return to England, sent me, through Principal Forbes, the following account of these two pictures, which I think was read in his presence at a former meeting of this Society.*

"These two drawings," he says,

> are by Jacopo Chimenti da Empoli, a painter of the Florentine school, who was born in 1554, and who died in 1640. They are drawings of the same person from points of view slightly different. That on the right hand is from a point of view slightly to the left of that on the left hand. They are so exactly on the same scale, that by converging the optic axes I succeeded in uniting the two so as to produce *an image in relief*. They united so easily and completely, that I could not help thinking that they had been drawn for the purpose of being looked at in that way. So far as I could judge, the difference between the pictures was greater than would be produced by a change of the position of a spectator equal to the distance between the two eyes; so that *the*

* See, 'The Photographic Journal,' May 15, 1860, vol. vi. p. 232.

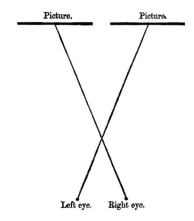

stereoscopic effect was somewhat exaggerated. I think, if we had a photograph of the pictures it would be much easier to prove their stereoscopic character than merely by referring to them; and if the photographs were of such a size that they could be *transposed* and put in the stereoscope, any one could see it.

I had no sooner received this very interesting communication from Dr. Crum Brown, than I took measures for obtaining a photograph of this stereoscopic picture. I wrote to M. Delezenne, a corresponding Member of the Academy of Sciences, requesting him to have such a photograph executed at my expense. In replying to my letter, he told me that photographs were not permitted to be taken of the objects in the Museum, but that Mr. Bingham was engaged in taking photographs of them for the Prince Consort, who alone had received this privilege from the trustees of the Museum.

Upon receiving this information, I applied to the Prince Consort, through Sir Charles Phipps, for a copy of the photograph of the stereoscopic picture, and explaining the high interest which attached to it as a great fact in the history of binocular vision and the stereoscope. In answer to this application, I learned that though the Prince had not the slightest wish to confine these photographs to himself, yet His Royal Highness did not think that he had any power to give permission for additional copies to be taken, though he had certainly no objection to this being done.

When I received this letter, I was writing the article "STEREOSCOPE" for the 'Encyclopædia Britannica,' and I inserted in it the remarkable discovery made by Dr. Crum Brown. I had previously shown, in my Treatise on the Stereoscope, that Galen had, 1500 years ago, proved that in looking at solid bodies the pictures given by each eye were dissimilar, and that with both eyes we saw these two pictures combined. In illustrating these views of Galen, Baptista Porta gives a figure, in which we not only see the principle of the Stereoscope, but a virtual representation of the binocular slide by three circles, two of them indicating the right- and left-eye pictures, and the middle one the other two united by the eyes and producing the figure in relief which we actually see.

The work of Baptista Porta, containing this diagram, was published in 1593, and Jacopo Chimenti lived 47 years after its publication. It was therefore probable, as I stated, that in executing the stereoscopic picture Chimenti was illustrating the binocular diagram of the Neapolitan philosopher, and was the true inventor of the Ocular Stereoscope, that is, of the method of obtaining a solid representation of any object by uniting right- and left-eye pictures of it by converging the optic axes to a point nearer the observer than the pictures.

This opinion was founded on the supposition that Chimenti's figures were truly stereoscopic; and as I knew that Dr. Crum Brown was thoroughly acquainted with the subject of binocular vision and the theory of the Stereoscope, I had no doubt that he had seen a figure in perfect relief by uniting the two plane pictures of it.

Having failed in procuring a copy of these pictures, I had no means of testing the accuracy of Dr. Brown's experiment; but it appears that, in June 1860, Mr. Wheatstone applied to Prof. Kuhlmann of Lille, and obtained from him a photograph of Chimenti's drawings. In the letter which accompanied it Prof. Kuhlmann states "that the copy has been taken of such a size as to be suitable for examination *in the stereoscope*," and he adds "that, at the first sight of it, and without the aid of any instrument, it would be seen that the two pictures were *not stereoscopic*."

The photograph, thus described, was accordingly placed in the stereoscope by Mr. Wheatstone and his friends in London, and they all found it *not to be stereoscopic*.

Copies of the photograph were also sent to Paris with the same result, as will be seen from the following extract from the 'British Journal of Photography' for August 1860: –

It will, doubtless, be in the recollection of our readers that lately an intimation was thrown out by Sir David Brewster relative to the supposed antiquity of the knowledge of stereoscopic principles, the supposition arising from the fact that an artist, named Jacopo Chimenti, who lived in the 16th century, had executed a pair of pictures, which are at present preserved in the Museum at Lille, and which, it was alleged, on being viewed in such a manner as to allow each eye to see only one of the designs, presented a stereoscopic effect. It is very unfortunate that when an announcement of any supposed fact is once made, and subsequently proved to be erroneous, it is almost impossible to correct the false impression as thoroughly as is desirable, because there must always exist many persons who read the assertion but not the contradiction, while those who see the contradiction without the previous erroneous statement can play but a very unimportant part in its rectification. Under these circumstances we conceive it to be advisable to draw special attention to a paragraph in the letter of our Paris correspondent, M. Ernest Lacan, which was published in our last number, and from which we learn that, in order to settle the question satisfactorily, our countryman, Mr. Bingham, who is a resident in Paris, took photographic copies of the alleged pair of stereographs, and laid them before the members of the French Photographic Society at the July meeting.

When placed in the stereoscope, the two pictures united perfectly, but did not present the smallest effect of relief.

We think it is fair, therefore, to presume that, whatever may have been the object proposed by the artist in executing the two similar pictures, it was certainly not from any knowledge of the stereoscopic phenomenon, and that Sir David Brewster was in this instance wrong in his conjecture. It is but right to add that Sir David had not had ocular demonstration of the alleged fact when he threw out the suggestion.

The following is the letter of M. Ernest Lacan, the editor of 'La Lumière,' above referred to: –

The letter in which Sir David Brewster spoke of the two drawings of Chimenti existing in the Lille Museum, and presenting, according to the illustrious savant, the stereoscopic relief, has been reprinted in the 'Lumière' and other special journals. We were all asking whether the invention which so greatly honours Wheatstone and Brewster really dated from the 16th century. Mr. Bingham, who has just returned from Lille, conceived the happy idea of reproducing the two designs in question, to offer them to the French Photographic Society. We all examined them with care, but no one detected in them the slightest difference. They appeared to all perfectly identical. In the stereoscope they are superposed, but without any effect of relief. For the present, then, we must be permitted to doubt that they were intended for the application Sir David attributes to them.

Upon authorities so high, Dr. Brown's observations of the stereoscopic effect of the pictures was pronounced incorrect; and though I was utterly ignorant of the existence of the photograph in England, excepting in the collection of the Prince Consort, and had never either seen it or heard of it, I have been charged by Mr. Wheatstone's friends with *dishonesty* in not having retracted the opinion which I had merely published, not as my own, but on the authority of Dr. Brown, who alone was bound to retract it, if erroneous.

This charge, and others equally false and groundless, have been publicly urged against me by Dr. W. B. Carpenter, F.R.S., Registrar to the University of London, and that, too, in language so malignant and libellous, that I shall probably be advised by my friends to seek redress in a Court of Law.

In reply to such a charge, I had no other defence than that I had not only never seen the photographs in question, but had never heard, directly nor indirectly, any other opinion about them than that of a competent judge who found them to be stereoscopic; and I added that as the evidence of Mr. Wheatstone and his friends, who were interested parties, was comparatively of little value, *I still believed that the pictures were truly stereoscopic.*

The paper on which this opinion was printed was hardly dry from the press, when I received, through the kindness of Professor Kuhlmann, the photograph which had excited so much interest, and which I now submit to the inspection of the Society. As in all stereoscopic pictures, it is difficult by a casual inspection of them to perceive any difference between the right- and left-eye picture, when they are taken at the proper angle; but when they are combined by converging the optic axes to a point between the pictures and the eye, as done by Dr. Brown, *their stereoscopic character is instantly seen*. As very few persons, however, are able to unite the pictures in this way, I had a copy of them taken by Mr. Moffat, and the pictures transposed, in order to be viewed in the stereoscope. This photograph, with the pictures transposed, is now before the Society; and I have no doubt that every person that looks at it in the stereoscope will see the figure in relief, though it is more distinct when seen by the convergency of the optic axes, as Chimenti of course intended it to be seen. As the photograph now before us has been reduced to about *one-fourth* of the original, the stereoscopic relief observed by Dr. Brown in the Museum at Lille must have been more distinct than in a reduced copy taken photographically.

It is hardly necessary to observe that a stereoscopic picture executed by the hand must be very imperfect compared with those obtained by the binocular camera. The artist fixes only certain points in his copy of the original drawing, and joins these points as skilfully as he can; but if the original is stippled, or drawn only in points, and if, with his compasses, he places these points, in his twin copy, at the proper binocular distances from the same points on the original, which may be easily calculated, the stereoscopic relief will be as perfect as if the two pictures had been taken in the binocular camera. I hope to be able to show such a stereoscopic picture to the Society, and also copies of Chimenti's drawings of the same size as the original, and with all the lines, points, and shades more distinctly separated than they can possibly be in the best reduced photograph.

Some of those persons who have not seen the stereoscopic effect of Chimenti's drawings, in consequence of *not knowing how to see it*, have been surprised at finding two perfectly similar drawings, as they believed them to be, placed side by side, and have been led to conjecture that one of them may have been a copy by a pupil of the Florentine artist. Both the figures, however, bear the name of Chimenti; and, as we have seen, the one is as essentially different from the other as the binocular views of a solid statue.

[N.B. The full stereoscopic relief of Chimenti's pictures was seen and acknowledged by all the Members of the Society.]

Professor Archer remarked, as an interesting fact in connexion with what Sir David had now brought under their notice, that just before leaving Liverpool, in a turn-out of the Museum there, what appeared to be a stereoscope was found, bearing the date of 1670. Being out of order, it was laid aside at the time, and probably had not been touched since. It appeared to be of Roman manufacture; and he suggested that an attempt should be made to get it for examination, as having an important bearing on the subject before the Society.

The thanks of the Meeting were voted to Sir David for his paper, and the trouble he had taken in procuring the photograph of Chimenti's drawing.

2.15. Brewster: "On the stereoscopic relief in the Chimenti pictures". *London, Edinburgh and Dublin Philosophical Magazine and Journal of Science*, 1864, **27**, 1–3.

To William Francis, Esq., Ph.D.

DEAR SIR,

My attention has just been called to the following statement by Professor Edwin Emerson, of Troy University, U.S., published in the Philosophical Magazine for February 1863.

> To *prove* this [that the stereoscopic qualities of the Chimenti pictures are 'evidently accidental'], let anyone execute a pen-and-ink sketch, and then let him make as perfect a copy of it as he can without careful measurements: now place these two drawings in the stereoscope, and *you get the same kind of effect seen in the Chimenti drawings, and for the same reason.*

This appeal to *any one* for a scientific truth is rather an unusual mode of ascertaining it. Has Professor Emerson himself executed and copied any such sketch, and obtained the result which he assumes; and if he has, why has he not distinctly published the fact, and stated the nature of the sketch, and the precise *kind of relief* which he obtained. Had he done this, we might have challenged the accuracy of his experiment, and suggested a better mode of arriving at the truth.

In the absence of this information, however, we beg to ask him if he made a correct copy of *one* or *other* of the Chimenti drawings; and if he did, why he did not advise *any one* to do the same in order to obtain the only satisfactory *proof* of his assertion, that the relief in the Chimenti pictures is accidental.

Now we beg to tell Professor Emerson that we took this very method, and the only judicious one, of arriving at the truth. We went to one of the masters of the School of Art under the Board of Trustees in Edinburgh, with whom we were not personally acquainted, and requested him to obtain from his pupils copies of each of the Chimenti drawings. We were thus furnished with *six* copies of one of the Chimenti figures by a pupil* of the School, which could not produce, by any combination of them in the stereoscope, the effect of the Chimenti drawings. This was the opinion of Professor Tait, who mentions the experiment in the

---

* We had the sketches made by a pupil, to meet the gratuitous statement that one of the Chimenti figures *might have been* a copy by one of his pupils. It certainly might have been; but the drawings have been handed down to us as Chimenti's, and we are not entitled to assume, for any particular purpose, that *one* of them is the work of a pupil. The existence of two such drawings exactly similar to the eye, and placed as they are, is a circumstance so remarkable, that we venture to say that no similar pair of figures will be found, either in juxtaposition or singly, among the thousands of drawings left by ancient and modern artists.

Number of the Photographic Journal referred to by Professor Emerson, who ought in fairness to have told his readers that the very experiment which he maintained could be made by *any one* with *a certain result*, had been already carefully made with *the very opposite result*.

If Professor Emerson made the experiment himself, or had it made by others, why has he not told us the *precise effect* that was produced? If it was only "*the same kind of effect*," as in the Chimenti drawings, and not the *same degree of effect*, the experiment was worthless. It might have been a stereoscopic leg, or a stereoscopic arm, or a stereoscopic shoulder, or a stereoscopic knee, or any other "kind of stereoscopic effect," without having any resemblance to the *actual degree of stereoscopic effect* produced by the Chimenti drawings.

As this question must be decided by experiment, we defy Professor Emerson to produce *one* result in a *hundred* sketches by different individuals in which the stereoscopic relief exists at all, instead of being as perfect as in the drawings alluded to; and if he could produce this miraculous sketch, it would merely prove that it was 99 chances to 1 that the stereoscopic relief produced by Chimenti was *not accidental*.

But if Professor Emerson were to obtain many examples of the production of relief by blunders in copying a drawing, this would only prove that the relief we have been considering *might be* thus produced, not that *it was* thus produced. An important question in the history of science is not to be settled by such poor logic as this. Many points must be considered before it is proved that what *might be* produced actually *was* produced.

The stereoscopic pictures have been preserved as the work of Chimenti himself, and the historian of science will naturally ask what led so eminent an artist to make so uninteresting a sketch as that of a man sitting upon a stool with a pair of compasses in one hand and a string in the other. He will ask what led him to make a copy of it of the very same size, and without any change or improvement whatever. He will ask what led him to preserve such uninteresting sketches; but, above all, he will ask, with a peculiar interest, what led him *to place these two figures side by side*, and in such a manner that the instant they were seen by an intelligent traveller, Dr. Crum Brown, he conceived that they were intended to be brought into relief by binocular vision, and actually brought them into stereoscopic relief by retiring and combining the two separate pictures. The historian of science will not be satisfied even with the obvious answer to these questions. He will inquire into the *date* of these drawings, and he will be struck with the fact that they were executed at the time when Baptista Porta had called the attention of philosophers to the subject of binocular vision, and had shown in a diagram so far resembling a stereoscope slide, that external objects, that is objects in relief, were seen binocularly by the combination of a right- and left-eye picture of them. He will also connect with these facts, though he may not yet give it much weight, the statement of Professor Archer, the distinguished Director of the Industrial

Museum of Scotland, "that just before he left Liverpool, in a turn-out of the Museum there, *what appeared to be a stereoscope was found*, bearing the date of 1670. Being out of order," he adds, "it was laid aside at the time, and probably had not been touched since. It appeared, he said, to be of *Roman* manufacture; and he suggested that an attempt should be made to get it for examination, as having an important bearing on the subject before the Society",* namely the subject of Chimenti's stereoscopic figures.

In forming his opinion from these various considerations, the historian of science will not fail to notice that the binocular theory of Baptista Porta was published in *Italy* in 1593; that the stereoscopic drawings which so wonderfully illustrate it were also made in *Italy* some time after this, between 1620 and 1640, and that the probable stereoscope in Liverpool, with the date of 1670, is considered to be of *Italian* origin.

I am, ever most truly yours,

D. Brewster.

Allerly, November 27, 1863.

---

* Photographic Journal, vol. viii. p. 12.

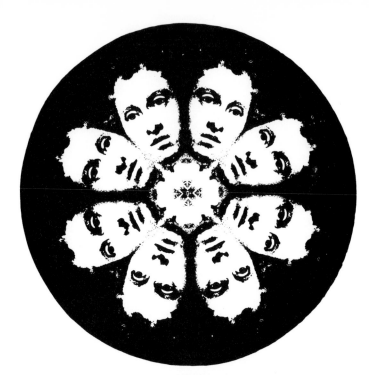

Kaleidoscopic image of Brewster.

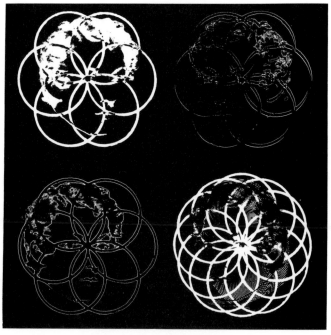

Kaleidophonic images of Wheatstone.

3. Inventions

3.1. Introduction

The reflecting and lenticular stereoscopes constitute the major inventions of Wheatstone and Brewster in the field of vision, but they were not the only ones. Many years earlier, Brewster had fascinated the public with his "philosophical toy", the kaleidoscope. The initial material reprinted in this chapter (3.2) is the introduction to Brewster's *Treatise on the Kaleidoscope*, published in 1819. He described the manner of its invention and the optical principles involved in its construction. An illustration of a simple kaleidoscope is shown in Fig. 1. The kaleidoscope was phenomenally popular, the demand often outstripping their

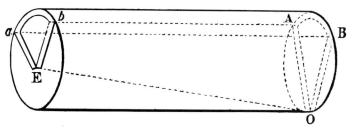

Fig. 1. The simple kaleidoscope, as illustrated in Brewster's *Treatise on the Kaleidoscope* (1819, Plate II, Fig. 13).

manufacture by numerous opticians. Indeed, Brewster was exceedingly bitter about what he considered as infringements of his patent, not the least because of the loss of revenue at a time when his financial position was not secure (see Morrison-Low, 1983). It would appear, however, that his patent was mishandled, as is indicated in a letter written to his wife from London in May 1818:

> I dine to-morrow with the Royal Society Club, and in the evening I undergo the ceremony of being admitted a member, which is a more formal business than I had supposed. I called yesterday at Sir Joseph Banks', and met Sir Everard Home, and other wise men there. Both of these gentlemen assured me that had I managed my patent rightly, I would have made one hundred thousand pounds by it! This is the

universal opinion, and therefore the mortification is very great. You can form no conception of the effect which the instrument excited in London; all that you have heard falls infinitely short of the reality. No book and no instrument in the memory of man ever produced such a singular effect. They are exhibited publicly on the streets for a penny, and I had the pleasure of paying this sum yesterday; These are about two feet long and foot wide. Infants are seen carrying them in their hands, and the coachmen on their boxes are busy using them, and thousands of poor people make their bread by making and selling them (Gordon, 1870, p. 99).

The problems of the kaleidoscope were not confined to its patent and production. Within the scientific community there was considerable debate concerning its originality. Various contenders were proposed by anonymous correspondents to the *Annals of Philosophy*, shortly after the details of the kaleidoscope were made public. These included Porta (1558), who arranged two plane mirrors like a book, so that the angle between them could be changed and the multiple reflections varied. Kircher (1646) described a similar arrangement and specified the relationship between the inclination of the mirrors and the number of images formed. Bradley (1717), Professor of Botany in the University of Cambridge, adopted a similar system for the design of garden plots and fortifications, and described it in his book *New Improvements in Planting and Garden*. In the eighteenth century, some popular instruments, like the Debusscope and the polyscope, were made, which multiplied designs placed between two angled, plane mirrors. There were, however, some voices raised in Brewster's defense. One of these was Roget* (1818), who later gave the following assessment in his entry on the Kaleidoscope for the *Encyclopaedia Britannica*:

> The particular application of this principle in the case where the two reflectors are inclined to one another at a small angle, so as to form a series of symmetric images, distinctly visible only in a particular position of the eye, was a discovery reserved for Dr. Brewster (Roget, 1824, p. 163).

Brewster also defended the originality of his design in the final chapter of his treatise, and appended the opinions of four authorities – John Wood, James Watt, John Playfair and M. A. Pictet – to this end.

It is ironical to note how aggrieved and affronted Brewster felt when his own creativity was questioned, and yet later he did not hesitate to doubt that of Wheatstone regarding the stereoscope.

The kaleidoscope was among the first philosophical toys that had a widespread appeal to a public increasingly fascinated by the marvels of the machine age. Many of those that followed were dependent upon visual persistence, and they incorporated some element of movement in their operation. However, there was

* Peter Mark Roget (1779–1869) entered the University of Edinburgh in the same year as Brewster, 1793, but Roget read medicine. He was regarded as an authority on the senses, and he gave a course of lectures on "The Physiology of the Senses" at the Royal Institution in 1836. He was Secretary of the Royal Society for over 20 years, during which time he was instrumental in introducing Cooke to Wheatstone. It was not until Roget was in his retirement that he completed his *Thesaurus*.

one feature they shared with the kaleidoscope, namely, disputes over the priority of invention.

In 1825, Dr. J. A. Paris demonstrated his thaumatrope, or wonder turner, to his scientific acquaintances in London. It consisted of a circular piece of card with designs drawn on both sides, and strings attached to opposite sides so that it could be twirled by hand. During rotation both designs were seen superimposed. For example, a bird could be caged when the thaumatrope was turning, but free when it was stationary. A wide range of designs, often incorporating visual or verbal puns, was used and the device was described more fully in Paris's *Philosophy in Sport made Science in Earnest* (1827). Babbage, in his autobiographical sketch, claimed that the effect was first noticed by Herschel:

> One day Herschel, sitting with me after dinner, amusing himself by spinning a pear upon the table, suddenly asked me whether I could show him the two sides of a shilling at the same moment. I took out of my pocket a shilling, and holding it up before the looking glass, pointed out *my* method. "No", said my friend, "that won't do;" then spinning my shilling upon the table, he pointed out *his* method of seeing both sides at once (Babbage, 1864, p. 189).

Babbage said that a friend, Dr. Fitton, made a device like the thaumatrope before Dr. Paris's novelty appeared. Faraday* (1831) was even more dismissive, and referred to "the schoolboy experiment of seeing both sides of a whirling halfpenny at the same moment" (p. 211).

In the early years of the next decade, Plateau and Stampfer independently invented rotating discs that could provide the visual impression of movement. The discs had a sequence of systematically changing designs on one side, and a similar sequence of slits around the circumference. The discs were rotated in front of a mirror and the reflected images were viewed successively through the slits. With suitable drawings a convincing impression of motion could be seen. Plateau's (1832) device was called a phenakistoscope or fantascope and Stampfer (1833) coined the term stroboscopic disc. In the following year, Horner (1834) devised an even more convenient contrivance that enabled a number of people to see the movement at the same time. Horner's daedeleum consisted of a cylinder mounted on a vertical spindle so that it could spin round. Vertical slits in the cylinder exposed designs printed on the inner surface of the opposite side. In spite of these advantages the daedeleum was not manufactured until the 1860s, when it was renamed the zoetrope.

* Michael Faraday (1791–1867) was a close friend of Wheatstone's from the late 1820s until his death. He must have been very familiar with Wheatstone's research, because he delivered many of Wheatstone's papers to learned societies. Faraday revelled in the art that Wheatstone abhorred – lecturing. It is stated of Faraday (in *Chambers's Encyclopaedia* of 1862) that "His manner, his unvarying success in illustration, and his felicitous choice of expression, though the subjects are often of the most obscure nature, are such as to charm and attract all classes of hearers". Faraday was fascinated by Wheatstone's researches in both acoustics and electricity, and was a frequent visitor to Wheatstone's laboratory in King's College. It was in the related areas of electromagnetic induction and electrolysis that Faraday achieved eminence.

Both Plateau and Stampfer were stimulated to make their discs after reading an article by Faraday (1831). Faraday described an optical deception upon viewing two counter-rotating cog-wheels: sighting "through" the spaces between the cogs gave the impression of twice as many stationary cogs. In order to examine this phenomenon in more detail he constructed a simple device, consisting of two cardboard discs with sectors removed, that could be rotated in opposite directions. Faraday related the phenomenon to one that had been reported earlier by Roget (1825), and it is highly likely that Wheatstone's developing interest in visual persistence was an influence upon him too. Wheatstone's initial venture into vision was to describe a device of his construction that rendered visible the paths followed by rapidly vibrating rods, due to the reflection of light from glass beads attached to their extremities (see Article 3.3). This instrument he called the kaleidophone, or phonic kaleidoscope, because in creating beautiful forms it "resembles the celebrated invention of Dr. Brewster". Because the paths were traced so rapidly they were within the "duration of the visual impression" and hence visible simultaneously. Rods of different cross-section and shape were employed, and illustrations of the paths traced were given. Of greater significance to the philosophical toys described several years later was the optical contrivance mentioned in the last section of Article 3.3. This consisted of a stationary glass plate on which a design was painted; in front of it was a rotatable metal disc with an open sector so that light could be projected through the part of the design corresponding to the open sector. If the metal disc was rotated at a suitable speed then the whole pattern was rendered visible. Wheatstone continued developing novel devices to display the "durations of impressions" and these would have been known to his close associate, Faraday. Indeed, Faraday mentioned the kaleidophone in his article on optical deceptions.

Yet another claimant for the original invention of the stroboscopic disc was Roget. In his *Bridgewater Treatise* (1834) he argued that he made a device like the phenakistoscope in 1831. Earlier, in 1825, he had published an insightful account of the curved appearance of moving wheelspokes when observed through railings. His interests in these phenomena were also rekindled by Faraday's (1831) article.

> This again directed my attention to the subject, and led me to the invention of an instrument which has since been introduced into notice under the name of the Phantasmascope or Phenakistoscope. I constructed several of these at that period (in the spring of 1831) which I showed to many of my friends; but in consequence of occupations and cares of a more serious kind, I did not publish any account of this invention, which was reproduced on the continent in the year 1833 (Roget, 1834, p. 466).

Wheatstone did not use his disc to measure the duration of impressions at that time, but the suitability of his contrivances for so doing was not lost on him. Indeed, a report in *The Athenaeum* (16 March, 1833) of a talk by Wheatstone (perhaps one of the few he delivered himself) was entitled "On the duration of luminous impressions on the organ of vision". In it he described some experiments by Plateau on coloured sensations as well as some of his own observations.

> Mr. W. then proceeded to establish, by some experiments of his own, that the intensity of the line described by the motion of a luminous point, diminishes, as the velocity of the motion increases, and increases with the frequency of recurrence of the generating point; when a luminous point continues to describe the same curve, variations of velocity occasion no alteration in the brightness of the images, as these two effects exactly compensate each other. To illustrate these principles, Mr. W. exhibited a little instrument, which, when at rest, showed a number of luminous points, arranged on a small wheel, half an inch in diameter; and putting this into rapid motion, by means of a train of wheels immediately connected with it, each point appeared to expand in a different line, and the symmetrical arrangement of these lines, formed a beautiful and brilliant figure . . . Numerous illusions, occasioned by the duration of luminous impressions, were afterwards shown and explained . . ., Mr. W. concluded, by observing that the experiments he had brought forward this evening, proved that an affection of vision, to which hitherto very little attention had been paid, might be usefully employed in investigations concerning physical phenomena, with which, at first thought, it might not appear to have the most remote connexion (1833, pp. 170–171).

The physical phenomena to which Wheatstone was alluding were those of electricity, and it was with the aid of a system not dissimilar to the apparatus described above that he was shortly to measure the velocity of electricity (Wheatstone, 1834). Wheatstone passed a current through half a mile of insulated copper wire, with spark gaps at each end and at the centre, arranged side by side. The sparks were observed by means of a rapidly rotating mirror, the angular velocity of which could be measured. Wheatstone observed the reflections of the sparks, which could be seen simultaneously due to the persistence of vision. However, the images of the spark from the central gap was displaced with respect to those from the extremities of the wire. By determining the degree of displacement visually, Wheatstone was able to determine the velocity of electricity because the length of wire and the angular velocity of the mirror were known (see Bowers, 1975). These initial experiments were conducted in the Adelaide Gallery, London, where Claudet was later to set up his photographic studio. Wheatstone continued his experiments, with greater lengths of wire and more refined observational techniques, at King's College.

Knowledge of the velocity of electricity was considered essential for the development of the electric telegraph. A practical electric telegraph was achieved through the collaboration of Wheatstone with Cooke, and they took out their initial patents in 1837 and 1840 (see Bowers, 1975; Wheatstone, 1840b). One of the many offshoots from the electric telegraph was the electro-magnetic chronoscope. Initially it was used for determining the velocity of projectiles, but it is also of interest to psychology because it became the standard means for precise laboratory measurement of reaction times. The chronoscopes used for this purpose were modified slightly by a German watchmaker, Mathias Hipp (see Edgell and Symes, 1906). The article reprinted here (3.4) is a translation from the French in which it was originally written (Wheatstone, 1845). An article in *Comptes Rendus* earlier in 1845 suggested that the principles and operation of the electro-magnetic chronoscope were due, in the main, to Breguet and Konstantinoff. The purpose of Wheatstone's note was to establish his priority, as well as pointing to the advantages of his apparatus over that of Breguet.

The binocular camera was first described at the same meeting of the British Association as that at which the lenticular stereoscope was announced (see Brewster, 1849). The principles employed in the camera were virtually the same as those for the lenticular stereoscope. A single lens was halved, and the semi-lenses were mounted in the camera at the interocular separation of 2½ inches. A longer report was published in the *Transactions of the Royal Scottish Society of Arts* and this is reprinted in Article 3.5. Because no illustration of the camera was given in the article, a diagram of it (taken from *The Stereoscope*) is shown here (Fig. 2).

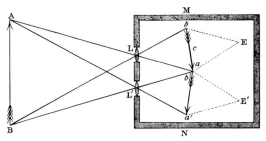

Fig. 2. The binocular camera as illustrated in Brewster's *The Stereoscope* (1856, p. 146).

It might seem from the stereoscopic photographs included in the article that Brewster did construct a binocular camera. However, he met similar difficulties in persuading optical instrument makers to produce his binocular camera to those encountered with the lenticular stereoscope. Indeed, they were perhaps greater, because he had lost favour with Lowdon the Dundee optician who had made the first stereoscopes. Lowdon made many single-lensed cameras, but there is no record of him producing binocular cameras (see Millar, 1925; Morrison-Low, 1983). The stereoscopic photographs could equally well have been taken with a normal camera. The binocular photographs of Dr. Adamson (see Fig. 3, p. 38) appear to be separate pictures taken successively from different positions. Dr. Adamson's stereoscopic portrait was taken by Brewster to Paris in 1850, together with the stereoscope made by Lowdon. Brewster (1852) did not report taking a binocular camera with him, although he did describe its construction and operation to the Abbé Moigno, Soleil and Duboscq. One possible consequence of this was that a Parisian photographer, Quinet, made a binocular camera of similar design to Brewster's, and called it the Quinetoscope. As Moigno and Brewster later pointed out, this must have been an instrument for seeing Quinet!

A small number of binocular cameras, incorporating semi-lenses, were made by a Mr. Slater, a London optician, but these were sent to America (see Brewster, 1852). However, far more intricate models were designed and manufactured by the Manchester optician, Dancer,* and they were generally available from 1856. Brewster had demonstrated his stereoscope to Dancer, personally, although it is not apparent that Dancer was shown a binocular camera. He made a preliminary model of a twin-lensed camera in 1853, and patented a more sophisticated version in 1856. Not only did the camera utilize complete rather than semi-lenses, but it was the first practical magazine camera (see Coe, 1978). Dancer corresponded with Brewster on the appropriate separation of lenses for stereo-scopic photographs, and both championed the interocular distance against the varied and larger separations proposed by Wheatstone.

Brewster's binocular camera cannot be considered a success, despite some of the grandiose claims he made for it. He argued that his semi-lens system, while requiring longer exposures because of the loss of light, *"will give better binocular pictures than two whole lenses whose focal length is exactly the same, if two such lenses could be made"* (1852, p. 181). Even Dancer's refined models, and the many that followed, did not entirely supplant the use of single or paired cameras for taking stereoscopic pictures. The latter gave photographers the flexibility to vary the inter-lens separation according to the distance of the objects to be pictured. This was necessary if any dissimilarity between the paired pictures was to be recorded, as Wheatstone had foreseen. Brewster's prediction of the enduring popularity of stereoscopic photography was also unrealistic:

> The Photographers, both Daguerreotypists and Talbotypists now take Binocular portraits, to be thrown into relief by the Stereoscope, as an important branch of their profession, and we have no doubt that the time is near at hand when no other portraits will be taken (1852, p. 177).

---

* John Benjamin Dancer (1812–1885) is best known for his pioneering work on microscopic photographs, using the wet-plate collodion process. Brewster was so impressed with these micro-graphs that he took examples with him to France and Italy in 1856. In the next year Brewster suggested to Dancer that micrographs of finely ruled gratings would prove of great assistance for diffraction experiments, and for incorporation in the micrometers of telescopes and microscopes (see the letters enclosed with Dancer's autobiographical notes, published in 1964).

3.2. Brewster: "Circumstances which led to the invention of the Kaleidoscope". From *A Treatise on the Kaleidoscope*, 1819.

The name KALEIDOSCOPE, which I have given to a new Optical Instrument, for creating and exhibiting beautiful forms, is derived from the Greek words χαλοξ, *beautiful*; ειδοξ, *a form*; and εχοπεω, to see.

The first idea of this instrument presented itself to me in the year 1814, in the course of a series of experiments on the polarisation of light by successive reflections between plates of glass, which were published in the Philosophical Transactions for 1815, and which the Royal Society did me the honour to distinguish by the adjudication of the Copley Medal. In these experiments, the reflecting plates were necessarily inclined to each other, during the operation of placing their surfaces in parallel planes; and I was therefore led to remark the circular arrangement of the images of a candle round a centre, and the multiplication of the sectors found by the extremities of the plates and glass. In consequence, however, of the distance of the candles, &c. from the ends of the reflectors, their arrangement was so destitute of symmetry, that I was not induced to give any farther attention to the subject.

On the 7th of February 1815, when I discovered the development of the complementary colours, by the successive reflections of polarised light between two plates of gold and silver, the effects of the Kaleidoscope, though rudely exhibited, were again forced upon my notice; the multiplied images were, however, coloured with the most splendid tints; and the whole effect, though inconceivably inferior to the creations of the Kaleidoscope, was still far superior to any thing that I had previously witnessed.

In giving an account of these experiments to M. Biot, on the 6th of March 1815, I remarked to him,

> that when the angle of incidence (on the plates of silver) was about 85° or 86°, and the plates almost in contact, and inclined at a very small angle, the two series of reflected images appeared at once in the form of two curves; and that the succession of splendid colours formed a phenomenon which I had no doubt would be considered, by every person who saw it to advantage, as one of the most beautiful in optics.

These experiments were afterwards repeated with more perfectly polished plates of different metals, and the effects were proportionally more brilliant; but notwithstanding the beauty arising from the multiplication of the images, and the additional splendour which was communicated to the picture by the richness of the polarised tints, it was wholly destitute of symmetry; as I was then ignorant of those positions for the eye and the objects, which are absolutely necessary to produce that magical union of parts, and that mathematical symmetry throughout the whole picture, which, independently of all colouring, give to the visions of the Kaleidoscope that peculiar charm which distinguishes them from all artificial creations.*

Although I had thus combined two plain mirrors, so as to produce highly pleasing effects, from the multiplication and circular arrangement of the images of objects placed at a distance from their extremities, yet I had scarcely made a step towards the invention of the Kaleidoscope. The effects, however, which I had observed, were sufficient to prepare me for taking advantage of any suggestion which experiment might afterwards throw in the way.

In repeating, at a subsequent period, the very beautiful experiments of M. Biot, on the action of homogeneous fluids upon polarised light, and in extending them to other fluids which he had not tried, I found it most convenient to place them in a triangular trough, formed by two plates of glass cemented together by two of their sides, so as to form an acute angle. The ends being closed up with pieces of plate glass cemented to the other plates, the trough was fixed horizontally, for the reception of the fluids. The eye being necessarily placed without the trough, and at one end, some of the cement, which had been pressed through between the plates at the object end of the trough, appeared to be arranged in a manner far more regular and symmetrical than I had before observed when the objects, in my early experiments, were situated at a distance from the reflectors. From the approximation to perfect symmetry which the figure now displayed, compared with the great deviation from symmetry which I had formerly observed, it was obvious that the progression from the one effect to the other must take place during the passage of the object from the one position to the other; and it became highly probable, that a position would be found where the symmetry was mathematically perfect. By investigating this subject optically, I discovered the leading principles of the Kaleidoscope, in so far as the inclination of the reflectors, the position of the object, and the position of the eye, were concerned. I found, that in order to produce perfectly beautiful and symmetrical forms, three conditions were necessary:

1. That the reflectors should be placed at an angle, which was an *even* or an *odd* aliquot part of a circle, when the object was regular, and similarly situated with respect to both the mirrors; or the *even* aliquot part of a circle when the object was irregular, and had any position whatever.

2. That out of an infinite number of positions for the object, both within and without the reflectors, there was *only one* where perfect symmetry could be obtained, namely, when the object was placed in contact with the ends of the reflectors.

---

* The experiments above alluded to have not yet been published, but an account of them has been given in the *Analyse des Travaux de la Classe des Sciences Mathématiques et Physiques de l'Institut Royal de France, pendant l'année* 1815, par M. le Chev. Delambre, p. 29, &c.

3. That out of an infinite number of positions for the eye, there was *only one* where the symmetry was perfect, namely, as near as possible to the angular point, so that the circular field could be distinctly seen; and that this point was the *only one* out of an infinite number at which the uniformity of the light of the circular field was a maximum, and from which the direct and the reflected images had the same form and the same magnitude, in consequence of being placed at the same distance from the eye.

Upon these principles I constructed an instrument, in which I fixed *permanently*, across the ends of the reflectors, pieces of coloured glass, and other irregular objects; and I shewed the instrument in this state to some Members of the Royal Society of Edinburgh, who were much struck with the beauty of its effects. In this case, however, the forms were nearly permanent, and a slight variation was produced by varying the position of the instrument with respect to the light.

The great step, however, towards the completion of the instrument, remained yet to be made; and it was not till some time afterwards that the idea occurred to me *of giving motion to objects, such as pieces of coloured glass, &c. which were either fixed or placed loosely in a cell at the end of the instrument.* When this idea was carried into execution, and the reflectors placed in a tube, and fitted up on the preceding principles, the Kaleidoscope, in its *simple form*, was completed.

In this form, however, the Kaleidoscope could not be considered as a general philosophical instrument of universal application. The least deviation of the object from the position of symmetry at the end of the reflectors, produced a deviation from beauty and symmetry in the figure, and this deviation increased with the distance of the object. The use of the instrument was therefore limited to objects held close to the reflectors, and consequently to objects whose magnitudes were less than its triangular aperture.

The next, and by far the most important step of the invention, was to remove this limitation, and to extend indefinitely the use and application of the instrument. This effect was obtained by employing a draw tube, containing a convex lens of such a focal length, that the images of objects, of all magnitudes and at all distances, might be distinctly formed at the end of the reflectors, and introduced into the pictures created by the instrument in the same manner as if they had been reduced in size, and placed in the true position of symmetry.

When the Kaleidoscope was brought to this degree of perfection, it was impossible not to perceive that it would prove of the highest service in all the ornamental arts, and would, at the same time, become a popular instrument for the purposes of rational amusement. With these views I thought it adviseable to secure the exclusive property of it by a Patent; but in consequence of one of the Patent instruments having been exhibited to some of the London opticians, the remarkable properties of the Kaleidoscope became known, before any number of them could be prepared for sale. The sensation excited in London by this

premature exhibition of its effects is incapable of description, and can be conceived only by those who witnesssed it. It may be sufficient to remark, that,
according to the computation of those who were best able to form an opinion on
the subject, no fewer than two hundred thousand instruments have been sold in
London and Paris during three months. Out of this immense number there is
perhaps not one thousand constructed upon scientific principles, and capable of
giving any thing like a correct idea of the power of the Kaleidoscope; and of the
millions who have witnessed its effects, there is perhaps not an hundred who have
any idea of the principles upon which it is constructed, who are capable of
distinguishing the spurious from the real instrument, or who have sufficient
knowledge of its principles for applying it to the numerous branches of the useful
and ornamental arts.

Under these circumstances I have thought it necessary to draw up the following short treatise, for the purpose of explaining, in as popular a manner as I could,
the principles and construction of the Kaleidoscope; of describing the different
forms in which it is fitted up; of pointing out the various methods of using it as an
instrument of recreation; and of instructing the artist how to employ it in the
numerous branches of the useful and ornamental arts to which it is applicable.

3.3. Wheatstone: "Description of the kaleidophone, or phonic kaleidoscope; A
new philosophical toy, for the illustration of several interesting and amusing
acoustical and optical phenomena". *Quarterly Journal of Science, Literature and
Art*, 1827, **23**, 344–351.

The application of the principles of science to ornamental and amusing purposes
contributes, in a great degree, to render them extensively popular; for the
exhibition of striking experiments induces the observer to investigate their causes
with additional interest, and enables him more permanently to remember their
effects. I shall not, therefore, need an apology for presenting the tyro in science
with another combination of philosophy with amusement, in addition to those
already extant.

But this instrument possesses higher claims to attention; for it exemplifies an
interesting series of natural phenomena, and renders obvious to the common
observer what has hitherto been confined to the calculations of the
mathematician; it presents another proof, that however remote from common
observation the operations of nature may be, the most beautiful order and
symmetry prevail through all.

In the property of "creating beautiful forms," the Kaleidophone resembles the
celebrated invention of Dr. Brewster, from which its name is modified; but to the
instrument itself, and its mode of action, it is almost superfluous to say there is no

similarity. Previously to entering into an explanation of its construction and effects, the following brief summary may suffice to give a general idea of the nature of the experiments it is intended to illustrate.

These experiments principally consist in subjecting to ocular demonstration the orbits or paths described by the points of greatest excursion in vibrating rods, which in the most frequent cases, those of the combinations of different modes of vibration, assume the most diversified and elegant curvilinear forms.* The entire track of each orbit is rendered simultaneously visible by causing it to be delineated by a brilliantly luminous point, and the figure being completed in less time than the duration of the visual impression, the whole orbit appears as a continuous line of light. As besides the changes which result from the combinations of the primitive with the higher modes of vibration, the figures of the orbits are affected by the form of the rod, by the extent of the excursions of the vibrations, by the mode of producing the motions, and by many other circumstances, a great variety of pleasing and regular forms is obtained. This variety is also enhanced by giving the same motions to a number of symmetrically disposed luminous points, the mutual intersections of the orbits of which produce innumerable elegant forms; and the appearances may be still more variegated by occasionally causing these points to reflect differently-coloured lights.

The apparatus for exhibiting these experiments consists of a circular board about nine inches in diameter, into which are perpendicularly fixed, at equal distances from the circumference and from each other, three steel rods each about a foot in length. The first rod is cylindrical, about 1–10th of an inch in diameter, and is surmounted by a spherical bead† which concentrates and reflects the light which falls upon it. The second is a similar rod, upon the upper

---

* We are indebted to Dr. T. Young for the first observation of these phenomena; the following account of his experiments is quoted from the *Philosophical Transactions* for 1800. "Take one of the lowest strings of a square piano-forte, round which a fine silvered wire is wound in a spiral form; contract the light of a window, so that when the eye is placed in a proper position, the image of the light may appear small, bright, and well defined, on each of the convolutions of the wire. Let the chord be now made to vibrate, and the luminous point will delineate its path like a burning coal whirled round, and will present to the eye a line of light, which, by the assistance of a microscope, may be very accurately observed. According to the different ways by which the wire is put in motion, the form of this path is no less diversified and amusing than the multifarious forms of the quiescent lines of vibrating plates discovered by Professor Chladni; and it is, indeed, in one respect even more interesting, as it appears to be more within the reach of mathematical calculation to determine it."

The extremely limited extent of the excursions of a vibrating chord prevents its motions from being distinctly observed by the naked eye, but as the rods employed in the present experiments can extend their excursions to nearly two inches, and as the means employed greatly increase the intensity of the light, the phenomena are exhibited in a far more evident manner.

† The only beads well adapted for this purpose are made of extremely thin glass silvered on the interior surface, and about one-sixth of an inch in diameter; they are to be obtained at the shops under the name of steel beads. The protuberances at the apertures must be removed or blackened, otherwise the reflections from them will render the images confused. To produce the coloured tracks, these beads must be coated with transparent colours, such as are ordinarily used for painting on glass;

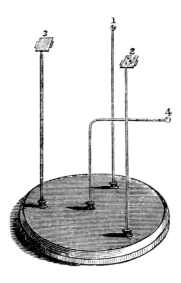

extremity of which is placed a plate moving on a joint, so that its plane may be rendered either horizontal, oblique, or perpendicular; this plate is adapted to the reception of the objects, which consist of beads differently coloured and arranged on pieces of black card in symmetrical forms. The third is a four-sided prismatic rod, and a similar plate is attached to its extremity for the reception of the same objects. Another rod is fixed at the centre of the board; this is bent to a right angle, and is furnished with a bead similarly to the first-mentioned rod. A small nut and screw is fixed to the board near the lower end of the first rod, in order by pressing upon it to render occasionally its rigidity unequal. A hammer, softened by a leather covering, is employed to strike the rods; and a violin-bow is necessary to produce some varieties of effect.

I shall now proceed to describe the different appearances which the rods present when in action, and to give directions for the production of the different effects, following the order in which the rods have been previously mentioned.

No. 1. On causing the entire rod to vibrate, so that its lowest sound be produced,* as it is seldom that the motions of a cylindrical rod can be confined to

---

the light will then be reflected through the coloured surface; but in beads made of coloured glass, the reflection being made from the external surface, shows only white light. The bead is cemented into small brass cup screwed to the top of the wire.

* The most simple mode of vibration of a rod vibrating transversely, when one of its extremities is fixed and the other is free, is that in which the entire rod makes its vibrations alternately on each side of the axis, which is nowhere intersected by the curve, but only touched at the fixed end. This gives the gravest sound which can be produced from the rod. In the other modes of vibration, the axis is intersected by the curve 1, 2, 3, or more times. The best means to command the production of these

a plane, the vibrations will almost always be combined with a circular motion. When the pressure on the fixed end is exerted on to opposite points, and the rod put in motion in the direction of the pressure, the following progression in the changes of form will be distinctly observed: the track will commence as a line, and almost immediately open into an ellipse, the lesser axis of which will gradually extend as the larger axis diminishes, until it becomes a circle; what was before the lesser will then become the larger axis, and thus the motions will alternate until, from their decreasing magnitudes, they cease to be visible. In the case just described the ellipses make a right angle with each other; but by altering the direction of the motion, so as to render it oblique to the direction of the pressure, they may be made to intersect under any required angle, and when this angle $= 0$ the motion will be merely vibratory.

Every single sound formed by the subdivisions of the rod will present similar appearances, but the excursions will be smaller as the sound is higher, or, which is the same thing, as the number of the vibrations increases.

In the most simple case of the co-existence of two sounds, shown by putting the entire rod in motion, and producing also a higher sound by the friction of a bow; the original figure will appear waved or indented, and as unity is to the number of indentations, so will the number of vibrations in the lower sound be to the number in the higher sound. On varying the mode of excitation, by striking the rod in different parts and with different forces, very complicated and beautiful curvilinear forms may be obtained: some of these are represented by the opposite figures.

---

sounds is to touch a node of vibration lightly with the finger, and to put a vibrating part in motion by a violin-bow. In the second sound, the number of vibrations is to that of the first, as $5^2:2^2$, or as $25:4$; the difference of the sound is, therefore, two octaves and an augmented fifth. Separating the first sound from the series, the number of the vibrations of all the others will be to one another as the squares of the numbers 3, 5, 7, 9, &c.; the third, in which there are three nodes, will therefore exceed the second by an octave and an augmented fourth; in the fourth, the acuteness will be augmented by nearly an octave; in the fifth, by nearly a major sixth, &c. To reduce to the same pitch all the proportions of the sounds which such a rod is capable of producing, I shall regard the sound corresponding with the most simple motion as the C one octave lower than the lowest of the piano-forte; the proportions of the sounds will then be –

Numbers of nodes	0	1	2	3	4	5
Sounds......................	$\overline{\text{C}}$	G ♯²	D⁴	D⁵–	B ♭⁵	F⁸+
Numbers, the squares of which correspond with these sounds .... }	(2)	(5) 3	5	7	9	11

The possible series of sounds, regarding the fundamental as unity, will therefore be – 1, $6^{1}/_{4}$, $17^{13}/_{36}$, $34^{1}/_{36}$, $56^{1}/_{4}$, &c.; or expressed in integral numbers – 36, 225, 625, 1225, 2025, &c. – Chladni, *Traité d'Acoustique*, P. 91.

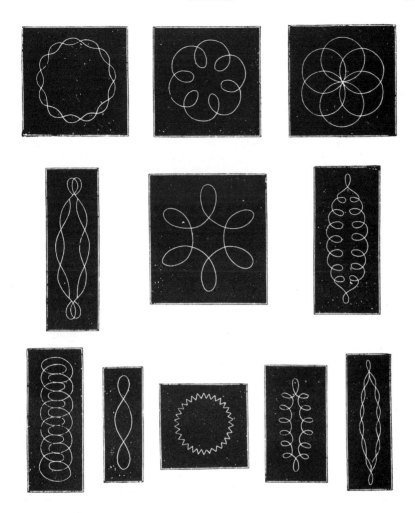

Placing the hand on the lower part of the rod, below the place at which it is excited, the excursions of the motions will rapidly decrease and exhibit spiral figures.

To obtain the figures with brilliancy and distinctness, a single light only should be employed, as that of the sun, a lamp, or a candle; rays of light proceeding from several points, as from a number of candles, or from the reflection of the clouds, occasion the track to be broad and indistinct; but double lights may be employed with effect, provided they be of equal intensity and symmetrically placed; each bead will then describe two similar figures. The appearances, in a bright sunshine, are remarkably vivid and brilliant.

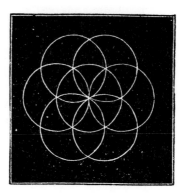

No. 2. Although very beautiful and varied forms may be produced from the motion of a single point, yet the compound figures which are presented by objects, formed by a number of points, offer appearances still more pleasing to the eye.

An object being placed horizontally on the plate, and the rod being put in motion, the mutual intersections of the points, each describing a similar figure, present to the eye complicated, yet symmetrical figures, resembling elegant specimens of engine-turning.

When the plate is horizontal, the figures are all in one plane, but if it be inclined or perpendicular, the curves being then made in parallel planes, gives the idea of a solid figure, and in some cases the appearances are particularly striking.

Complementary colours alone should be employed in the objects; for these harmonising together, give greater pleasure to the eye than an injudicious combination of discordant tints: the intensities should be occasionally varied, and colourless light intermingled with the different shades.

No. 3. When this prismatic rod is put in motion, in the direction of either of its sides, the points move only rectilineally, but when the motion is applied in an oblique direction, a variety of compound curves is shown: this rod is principally employed to exhibit the optical phenomena, which will be afterwards mentioned.

No. 4. When a rod is straight, the curve produced by any point describing its motion, is always in the same plane; but in a rod bent to any angle, the two parts moving most frequently in different directions, curves are produced whose parts do not lie in the same plane. A few trials will soon indicate the best way of applying the motion, so as to cause the two parts to vibrate in different directions.

Before the conclusion of this subject, I will avail myself of the opportunity of observing, that the application of this mode of experimenting may be extended to the delineation of every description of curvilinear and angular motion, when the amplitudes of the tracks are not too great; and by this means, it is not improbable that the experimental knowledge of many interesting principles in science may be facilitated.

On the Duplication and Multiplication of Objects.

When dark objects are substituted for luminous ones, their tracks become nearly invisible, and from the longer duration of visual impression at the limits of vibration, the images are multiplied in proportion to the number of points at which they are retarded. Place horizontally on the rod No. 2, a word printed or written on a piece of card; in the lowest mode of vibration, at the opposite limits of the excursions, two legible images of the word will be distinctly seen, and but an indistinct shade, occasioned by the tracks of the letters, will appear in the intermediate space: the vibratory motion is imperceptible to the eye; the images will, therefore, appear stationary in this respect, but the diminution of the excursions will cause them to approximate very slowly and gradually towards the centre: this diminution operates so gradually, as to allow the images to superpose each other completely at each recurring vibration, without producing any intermingling or confusion.

On placing the object perpendicularly, the two images will appear in parallel planes, the furthest image appearing through the first apparent surface. Small pictures have a singular effect applied in this manner.

When other sounds co-exist with the fundamental, the images are multiplied, but they become fainter as their number increases: these multiplied images are equally visible, whether the vibrations be rectilineal, elliptical, or circular.

A New Optical Experiment.

As that property of vision which occasions the apparent duration in the same places of visible images, after the objects which excite them have changed their positions,* has enabled us to submit to inspection the phenomena above described, it may not be irrelevant to subjoin a description on an apparatus which illustrates the transient duration of the impressions of light in a very evident manner.

At the back of a wooden frame, about six inches in height and breadth, and from one to three inches or more in depth, a circular plate of glass is placed, upon which a design is painted with transparent colours; at the front, is placed, parallel to the glass, a circle of tin, covered on its exterior surface with white paper, and having the space between two adjacent radii cut out. This circle moves freely on

* It has been proved by the Chevalier d'Arcy, from the only experiments approaching to accuracy which have been made on this subject, that the extent of this duration is eight thirds. See his "Memoire sur la durée de la sensation de la vue:" Hist. de l'Acad. An. 1765.

its centre round an axis, supported by a bar in front, and is put into rapid and regular motion by the application of any mechanical principle proper for the purpose; and a catch is so placed, that when the motion ceases, the aperture shall be concealed by the bar which supports the axis.

If a light be placed behind the transparent painting, and still better if it be concentrated by a lens, on making the circle revolve with rapidity, the whole of the picture will be rendered visible at one view, although but very limited portions are successively presented to the eye.

The intensity will differ in proportion to the excess of the transmitted light above that which falls in front of the circle; it will, therefore, increase the distinctness of the picture, to darken the latter as much as possible.

3.4. Wheatstone: "Note on the electro-magnetic chronoscope". *Walker's Electrical Magazine*, 1845, 2, 86–93.

I perceive, in the *Comptes Rendus de l'Académie des Sciences*, that, at the sitting of Jan. 20, a communication was read from M. Breguet, in which he attributes to Captain Konstantinoff and to himself the invention of the electro-magnetic chronoscope, an instrument which I had myself invented and completed several years previously, for the purpose of measuring rapid motions, and especially the velocity of projectiles.

It was in the commencement of 1840 that I invented this instrument. My chronoscope was then composed of the clock-movement, acting on an index-needle, which moved on or stopped, according as an electro-magnet acted on a piece of soft iron, attracting it when a current traversed the helix of the magnet, and abandoning it to itself when the current ceased, as in my electro-magnetic telegraph, of which this invention may be considered as one of the derivations. The duration of the current was thus measured by the extent of the circle traversed by the hand of the chronoscope.

A relation was established between the duration of the current, and that of the movement of the projectile by the following means: a wooden ring embraced the mouth of a loaded gun, and a stretched wire connected the two opposite sides of this ring, thus passing in front of the mouth of the gun. At a proper distance, the target was erected, and so arranged that the least motion given to it would establish a permanent contact between a little metal spring and another piece of metal. One of the extremities of the wire of the electro-magnet was attached to one of the poles of a small voltaic battery; to the other extremity of the electro-magnet were attached two wires, one of which communicated with the little spring of the target, and the other with one of the ends of the wire stretched before the mouth of the gun; from the other extremity of the voltaic battery two wires were also given off, one of which came to the piece of metal affixed to the target, and the other to the opposite extremity of the wire that passed in front of the gun. Thus, antecedently to the explosion of the gun, there was established between the gun and the target an uninterrupted circuit of wire, and of which the wire in front of the gun formed part. When once the target was struck by the bullet, the second circuit was complete; but during the passage of the projectile through the air, and during this time alone, both circuits were interrupted; and the duration of this interruption was indicated by the chronoscope.

I had already demonstrated, by my electro-magnetic telegraph, that when the magnets are properly arranged, they may be brought into action by a very feeble battery, even though the wires should describe a circuit of several miles. Consequently, the gun, the target, and the chronoscope, may be placed at any required distances from each other. On account of the very great rapidity with which electricity is propagated, as was proved by my experiments, published in the *Philosophical Transactions* of 1834, no sensible error can result from its successive transmission.

During a visit which I paid to Brussels in the month of September, 1840, I described this apparatus to my friend M. Quetelet, who made it known on the 7th of October, to the Academy of Sciences of that town, – a communication mentioned in the bulletin of that sitting.*

In a visit which I afterwards paid to Paris (May 1841), I explained this apparatus, and showed the drawings to several members of the Academy of Sciences of Paris, who came to see me at the *Collège de France*; where, thanks to the kindness of M. Regnault, I had an opportunity of repeating before them several of my electro-magnetic experiments. Among the persons present was M. Pouillet, who asked of me permission to copy my drawings, to which I willingly consented. I learned from him, in December last, that these drawings were still in his possession.

On my return to England, my friend Captain Chapman,† of the Royal Artillery, convinced of the utility of this instrument, was very desirous that it should be introduced in the practice of the Artillery at Woolwich; and he took much pains to accomplish this. We had an interview on this subject with the late Lord Vivian, then Master General of the Ordnance; and on July 17, 1841, I explained at the Institution of the Royal Artillery, the construction of the instrument and its different applications. Twenty-two officers assisted at this meeting; in the report of it (a report, of which I possess a copy) it is said that my chronoscope "indicated

* Vide *Elec. Mag.* Vol. I. p. 611.

† I had for a long time kept up a correspondence with Captain Chapman on this subject. In one of his letters of August 27, 1840, after having communicated to me his views on the manner of conducting his experiments, he says: – "We shall thus obtain the velocity of a projectile in each of the sections of its course; and I am bold to believe that we shall arrive at a knowledge of the effect of gravitation on the projectile, much more satisfactory than all that has been hitherto obtained."

$^1/_{7300}$ of a second," and that my object was to "show its application to the practical uses of artillery," namely, to determine the time employed by a projectile in passing over the different sections of its course, as well as its initial velocity. At the same meeting, I showed a "chronoscope intended to measure the velocity of lights, such as those produced by the ignition of powder." This instrument, the only one that M. Breguet attributes to me, had, however, nothing in common with electric currents, as he supposes; it was simply a series of wheels, carrying on their axes three light paper discs, of about an inch in diameter. The times of their respective revolutions were as 1, 10, and 100; the disc, whose movement was the most rapid, made 200 revolutions per second; on each disc was traced a radius: when they were illuminated by an electric spark all the radii appeared at rest, on account of the excessively small duration of that kind of light (as is explained in my memoir, *On the Velocity of Electricity and on the duration of the Electric Light*, published in the *Philosophical Transactions* of 1834); but when they were illuminated by a light of a duration of the two-hundredth part of a second, the third disc appeared uniformly tinted, while the second disc showed a shaded section of 36°. When the light lasted only the two-thousandth part of a second, a similar section appeared on the third disc.

For several reasons, the experiments with my electro-magnetic chronoscope were not pursued at Woolwich. In 1842, I became acquainted with M. de Konstantinoff, captain of Artillery in the Imperial Guard of his Majesty the Emperor of Russia, and attaché to the staff of General de Winspaer; he took much interest in this affair, expressed a great desire to have a complete apparatus, in order to undertake himself, on his return to Russia, a series of experiments such as those which I had in view. As I had not myself the time to follow out these experiments, and as no one in England, more skilful and better circumstanced for this, showed the desire to following them out, I willingly yielded to his demand, in the hope that some important results to science might be obtained. The only condition that I attached to my consent was that M. de Konstantinoff should not publish any description of the instrument until I myself had done so. The instrument that I furnished to M. Konstantinoff, and which was directed to him at Paris, in January, 1843, was differently constructed from that previously described, although essentially the same in principle.

I had found, by experience, that when a piece of soft iron had been attracted by an electro-magnet, and the current was then made to cease, although the iron appeared to fall immediately, its contact was maintained for a time which was frequently equal to a considerable fraction of a second. The duration of this adherence increased with the energy of the voltaic current, and with the weakness of the reacting spring. To reduce it to a minimum, it was necessary to employ a very feeble current, and to augment the resistance of the circuit until the attractive force of the magnet was reduced so as to exceed the reacting force of the spring by a very feeble quantity; but then the magnet had no longer sufficient force to attract the iron, when the projectile struck the target. However, I surmounted this difficulty in the following manner: – I arranged the wires of the circuit in such a manner that, before the bullet left the gun, the current of a single element of very small dimensions, and reduced to a suitable degree by means of a rheostat,* also interposed in the circuit, acted on the electro-magnet; but when the ball arrived at the target, six elements, without the resistance of the rheostat, acted simultaneously upon the magnet. But even with these precautions, which are efficacious to a certain degree, there is still some time lost during the attraction of the iron by the magnet, as well as during its adherence after the current had ceased. The difference of these two errors would render approximations such as the $^1/_{500}$ or $^1/_{1000}$ of a second altogether uncertain. However, the error arising from this source may be easily reduced to at least $^1/_{60}$ or $^1/_{100}$ of a second; and, in my opinion, a chronoscope which divides the second into sixty parts, and which may be proved never to give rise to an error exceeding a single one of these divisions, is preferable to an instrument presenting more minute divisions, and which would give rise to errors embracing a good number of these divisions. Guided by these experiments, I was in a condition to construct a very simple and very efficacious chronoscope. A very simple escapement was put in motion by a weight suspended to the end of a thread wound, in a hollow helix, round a cylinder fixed on the axis of an escapement wheel. On this axis was also adapted an index, which consequently advanced one division for every escapement. When it was necessary to prolong the time of the experiment, the escapement wheel and the cylinder were established on different axes, and their inter-communication was brought about by means of a wheel and pinion; in this case two hands were employed. By means of this construction we avoid the acceleration of motion that might take place if there were no escapement; and the index passes over each division in the same time. The weight was so arranged as to be able to regulate itself; and the value of a single division was obtained by dividing the time of the entire fall by the number of divisions passed over in this interval; but methods still more exact may be employed.

By means of this instrument, I have measured the time occupied by a pistol ball in traversing different ranges, with different charges of powder. The repetition of these experiments gave out results that were very constant, rarely presenting a difference of more than one division of the chronoscope.† I also measured the fall of a ball from different heights; and the law of accelerated velocities was obtained with mathematical rigour. With the apparatus that I employed for this latter experiment, I could measure the fall of a ball from the height of an inch. It would

---

* An explanation of this instrument will be found in my *Account of several new Instruments and Processes for determining the Constants of a Voltaic Circuit*, published in the *Philosophical Transactions* of 1843, 2nd part; and translated into the *Annales de Chim. et de Phys.* – Vide *Elec. Mag.*, Vol. I., p. 203.

† These experiments, in which I was assisted by Sir James South and Mr. Purday, the celebrated gunsmith, took place in October, 1842, in the grounds belonging to the observatory at Camden Hill.

be difficult, without the assistance of drawings, to give an idea of the different arrangements that I have adopted to render the instrument applicable to different series of experiments; but I may mention that, among the applications, I propose to employ it for measuring the velocity of sound through air, water, and masses of rock, with an approximation that has never been obtained heretofore.

Independently of the instrument which I furnished to M. de Konstantinoff, in April, 1843, Prof. Christie deposited one in the Museum of Natural Philosophy of the Military Academy at Woolwich; and another was made for Mr. R. Addams, who has since constantly used it in his lectures at the United Service Museum* and elsewhere.

I will mention a modification of the instrument that is important for certain series of experiments: – instead of breaking the continuity of the circuit, and re-establishing it immediately, as we have hitherto said, the electro-magnet is maintained in equilibrio by means of two equal and opposite currents; on interrupting the first circuit the equilibrium is destroyed, and on interrupting the second the current occasioned by the interruption of the equilibrium ceases. The second circuit is broken by a ball traversing a frame, on which is stretched a very fine wire arranged in parallel lines very close to each other, and forming part of the circuit. This arrangement furnishes means for employing a chronoscope totally different from the former. Two pendulums, one a half-second pendulum, and the other having a little more accelerated motion, are each maintained at the extremities of their arcs of oscillation, by means of an electro-magnet. When the ball escapes from the gun, one of the pendulums is liberated, and when it breaks the wire of the frame the other pendulum is also liberated. The number of oscillations of one of the pendulums is then counted, until the motion of the two pendulums coincides; and from this fact, the time which separates the commencement of the first oscillations of the two pendulums is easily calculated.

The instruments which I really constructed had no other object than to indicate the time that had elapsed between the initial and final motion of a ball in traversing its path. M. de Konstantinoff desired an instrument measuring the times corresponding to the successive divisions of the path. Although I then thought, and still am of opinion, that it is preferable to determine them by means of successive discharges, yet I did not undertake the construction of one, because of its higher cost and its greater complexity, although it was the object of frequent conversations between us. It was in order to realise these ideas that M. de Konstantinoff, after his departure from England, and during his stay in Paris, subsequently communicated with M. Breguet, in order to profit by the well-known skill and ingenuity of that engineer. I am perfectly persuaded that M. de Konstantinoff never had the intention of attributing this invention to himself,

* Vide *Elec. Mag.*, vol. i., p. 473, which refers to the instrument seen at the United Service Museum.

and that it is entirely without his approbation, and without his knowledge, that M. Breguet has just done so.*

With regard to the instrument described by M. Breguet, I consider it as being much less exact, much more complicated, and more costly, than any of those which I have previously invented. When it is reduced to determine merely the initial and final movements of a ball, M. Breguet's instrument is furnished with five electro-magnets, each with its mechanism, whilst mine attains the same result with a single electro-magnet; and when the different divisions of a same path are to be studied, M. Breguet proposes a complementary magnet, and makes other additions to each of the partitions which the ball was to traverse. Had M. Breguet been better informed on the means by which I would obtain a series of successive measurements corresponding to a same path, he would have found that what he proposes to obtain, even with a dozen electro-magnets, would have been obtained in a much more efficacious manner by means of one alone. The following was my plan: –

A cylinder executes a rotary motion round a screw, so as to advance a quarter of an inch per revolution; to one of the extremities of the cylinder is adapted a toothed wheel of a diameter a little greater than that of the cylinder, and which communicates with a pinion whose length is equal to the total portion of the axis which the cylinder must pass over in its successive revolutions; this pinion communicates with a wheel work, put in motion by a weight suspended at the extremity of a wire winding around a cylinder, and the wheel work is furnished with a regulator which equalizes its motion; a pencil, adapted to the extremity of a small electro-magnet, is brought into contact with the cylinder, and traces upon it a helix, which is interrupted every time that the current ceases. I borrowed the idea of the chronoscopic part of this apparatus from an instrument intended for measuring small intervals of time, invented by the late Dr. Young, and which is described and drawn in his *Course on Natural Philosophy*. It may be easily comprehended, from what I have already stated, in what manner the commencement and the end of the motion of a projectile are indicated by this instrument. The intermediate processes are registered in the following manner. At any given points on the line of the passage of a projectile are erected frames closed by wire net-work; the projectile breaks the wires on passing through the frames; as many voltaic batteries are employed as there are pairs of frames, the wires of which pairs of frames communicate with the poles of these voltaic batteries, and with the wire of the electro-magnet, in such a manner that the electric current traverses the wire helix, or ceases to traverse it, according as the equilibrium is alternately destroyed or established by the successive rupture of the wires of the frames. In

---

* I here give an extract from a writing given me by M. de Konstantinoff, before quitting London: –

"M. Wheatstone having had the kindness to make for me a complete apparatus of his invention to measure the fall of bodies, and the initial velocities of projectiles I undertake," &c.

order to obtain this result, it is necessary that the resistance of the different wires be suitably proportioned.

In conclusion, I may add that the application of my electro-magnetic telegraph with a view of registering at a distance the number of the revolutions of a machine, or of all other periodic movements, has been executed by me under very various forms for several years. An apparatus with this object in view, registering up to ten thousand, may have been seen in the Museum of Natural Philosophy at King's College, since 1840; and was shown to M. de Konstantinoff during his stay in London.

3.5. Brewster: "Account of a binocular camera, and of a method of obtaining drawings of full length and colossal statues, and of living bodies, which can be exhibited as solids by the stereoscope". *Transactions of the Royal Scottish Society of Arts*, 1851, 3, 259–264.

In explaining the construction and use of the lenticular and other stereoscopes, I have referred only to the duplication and union of the dissimilar drawings on a plane, of geometrical and symmetrical solids. The most interesting application, however, of these instruments, is to the dissimilar representations of statues and living bodies of all sizes and forms, and also to natural scenery, and the objects which enter into its composition. Professor Wheatstone had previously applied his stereoscope to the union of dissimilar drawings of small statues, taken by the Daguerrotype and Talbotype processes; and in an essay on Photography, lately published,[*] I have mentioned its application to statues of all sizes, and even to living figures, by means of a binocular camera. The object of the present paper is to describe the binocular camera, and to explain the principles and methods by which this application of the stereoscope is to be carried into effect.

The vision of bodies of three dimensions, or of groups of such bodies combined, has never been sufficiently studied, either by artists or philosophers. Leonardo da Vinci, who united, in a remarkable degree, a knowledge of art and science, has, in a passage of his *Trattato della Pittura*, quoted by Dr Smith of Cambridge,[†] made a brief reference to it, in so far as binocular vision is concerned; but till the publication of Professor Wheatstone's interesting Memoir, *On some Remarkable and hitherto Unobserved Phenomena of Binocular Vision*,[‡] the subject had excited no attention.

In order to understand the subject, we shall first consider the vision with *one eye* of objects of three dimensions, when of different magnitudes, and placed at

---

[*] *North British Review*, vol. vii., p. 502, August 1847.

[†] *Complete System of Optics*, vol. ii., Remarks, p. 41, § 244.

[‡] *Phil. Trans.*, 838, p. 371; See also *Edinburgh Transactions*, vol. v. pp. 349 and 663.

different distances. When we thus view a building or a full-length or colossal statue, at a short distance, a picture of all its visible parts is formed on the retina. If we view it a greater distance, certain parts cease to be seen, and other parts come into view; and this change on the picture will go on, but will become less and less perceptible, as we retire from the original. If we now look at the building or statue from a distance through a telescope, so as to present it to us with the same distinctness, and of the same apparent magnitude, as we saw it at our first position, the two pictures will be essentially different; all the parts which ceased to be visible as we retired, will still be invisible, and all the parts which were not seen at our first position, but became visible by retiring, will be seen in the telescopic picture. Hence, the parts seen by the near eye, and not by the distant telescope, will be those towards the middle of the building or statue, whose surfaces converge, as it were, towards the eye, while those seen by the telescope, and not by the eye, will be the external parts of the object whose surfaces converge less, or approach to parallelism. It will depend on the nature of the building or the statue, which of these pictures gives us the most favourable representation of it.

If we now suppose the building or statue to be reduced in the most perfect manner, – to half its size, for example, – then it is obvious that these two perfectly similar solids will afford a different picture, whether viewed by the eye or by the telescope. In the reduced copy, the inner surfaces visible in the original will disappear, and the outer surfaces become visible; and, as formerly, it will depend on the nature of the building or the statue, whether the reduced or the original copy, gives the best picture.

If we repeat the preceding experiments with *two eyes* in place of *one*, the building or statue will have a different appearance. Surfaces and parts, formerly invisible, will become visible, and the body will be better seen because we see more of it; but then, the parts thus brought into view, being seen, generally speaking, with one eye, will have only one-half the illumination of the rest of the picture. But, though we see more of the body in binocular vision, it is only parts of vertical surfaces perpendicular to the line joining the eyes that are thus brought into view, the parts of similar horizontal surfaces remaining invisible as with one eye. It would require a pair of eyes placed vertically, that is, with the line joining them in a vertical direction, to enable us to see the horizontal as well as the vertical surfaces, and it would require a pair of eyes inclined at all possible angles, that is, a ring of eyes 2½ inches in diameter, to enable us to have a perfectly symmetrical view of the statue.

These observations will enable us to answer the question, whether or not a reduced copy of a statue, of precisely the same form in all its parts, will give us, either by monocular or binocular vision, a better view of it as a work of art. As it is the outer parts or surfaces of a large statue that are invisible, its great outline and largest parts must be best seen in the reduced copy; and, consequently, its relief, or third dimension in space, must be much greater in the reduced copy. This will be better understood if we suppose a *sphere* to be substituted for the statue. If the sphere exceeds, in diameter, the distance between the pupils of the right and left eye, or 2½ inches, we shall not see a complete hemisphere unless from an infinite distance. If the sphere is larger, we shall see only a segment, whose relief, in place of being equal to the radius of the sphere, is equal only to the versed sine of half the visible segment. Hence, it is obvious that a reduced copy of a statue is not only better seen from more of its parts being visible, but is also seen in stronger relief.

With these observations, we shall be able to determine the best method of obtaining dissimilar plane drawings of full-length and colossal statues, &c., &c., in order to reproduce them in three dimensions by means of the stereoscope. Were a painter called upon to take drawings of a statue, as seen by each eye, he would fix, at the height of his eyes, a metallic plate with two small holes in it, whose distance is equal to that of his eyes, and he would then draw the statue as seen through the holes by each eye. These pictures, however, whatever be his skill, would not be such as to reproduce the statue by their union. An accuracy, almost mathematical, is necessary for this purpose, and this can only be obtained from pictures executed by the processes of the Daguerreotype and Talbotype. In order to do this with the requisite nicety, we must construct a binocular camera which will take the pictures simultaneously, and of the same size; that is, a camera with two lenses of the same aperture and focal length, placed at the same distance as the two eyes. As it is impossible to grind and polish two lenses, whether single or achromatic, of exactly the same focal lengths, even if we had the very same glass for each, I propose to bisect the lenses, and construct the instrument with semilenses, which will give us pictures of precisely the same size and definition. These lenses should be placed with their diameters of bisection parallel to one another, and at the distance of 2½ inches, which is the average distance of the eyes in man; and, when fixed in a box of sufficient size, will form a binocular camera, which will give us, at the same instant, with the same lights and shadows, and of the same size, such dissimilar pictures of statues, buildings, landscapes, and living objects, as will reproduce them in relief in the stereoscope.

It is obvious, however, from observations previously made, that even this camera will only be applicable to statues of small dimensions, which have a high enough relief, from the eyes seeing, as it were, well around them, to give sufficiently dissimilar pictures for the stereoscope. As we cannot increase the distance between our eyes, and thus obtain a higher degree of relief for bodies of large dimensions, how are we to proceed in order to obtain drawings of such bodies of the requisite relief?

Let us suppose the statue to be colossal, and *ten* feet wide, and that dissimilar drawings of it about *three* inches high are required for the stereoscope. These drawings are *forty* times narrower than the statue, and must be taken at such a distance that, with a binocular camera having its semilenses 2½ inches distant, the relief would be almost evanescent. We must therefore, suppose the statue to be reduced n times, and place the semilenses of the binocular camera at the distance $n \times 2\frac{1}{2}$ inches. If $n = 10$, the statue will be reduced to $^{10}/_{10}$ or to 1 foot, and $n \times 2\frac{1}{2}$, or the distance of the semilenses will be 25 inches. If the semilenses are placed at this distance, and dissimilar pictures of the colossal statue taken, they will reproduce by their union a statue *one* foot high, which will have exactly the same appearance and relief as if we had viewed the colossal statue with eyes 25 inches distant. But the reproduced statue will have also the same appearance and relief as a statue a foot high, reduced from the colossal one with mathematical precision, and therefore it will be a better and a more relieved representation of the work of art than if we had viewed the colossal original with our own eyes, either under a greater, an equal, or a less angle of apparent magnitude.

We have supposed that a statue *a foot broad* will be seen in proper relief by binocular vision; but it remains to be decided whether or not it would be more advantageously seen, if reduced with mathematical precision to a breadth of $2\frac{1}{2}$ inches, the width of the eyes, which gives the vision of a hemisphere $2\frac{1}{2}$ inches in diameter, with the most perfect relief. If we adopt this principle, and call B the breadth of the state of which we require dissimilar pictures, we must make

$$n = \frac{B}{2\frac{1}{2}},$$ and $n \times 2\frac{1}{2} = B$, that is, the distance of the semilenses in the binocular camera, or of the semilenses in two cameras, if two are necessary, must be made equal to the breadth of the statue.

In the same manner we may obtain dissimilar pictures of living bodies, buildings, natural scenery, machines, and objects of all kinds, of three dimensions, and reproduce them by the stereoscope, so as to give the most accurate idea of them to those who could not understand them in drawings of the greatest accuracy.

The art which we have now described cannot fail to be regarded as of inestimable value to the sculptor, the painter, and the mechanist, whatever be the nature of his production in three dimensions. Lay figures will no longer mock the eye of the painter. He may delineate at leisure on his canvas, the forms of life and beauty, stereotyped by the solar ray and reconverted into the substantial objects from which they were obtained, brilliant with the same lights, and chastened with the same shadows as the originals. The sculptor will work with similar advantages. Superficial forms will stand before him in three dimensions, and while he summons into view the living realities from which they were taken, he may avail himself of the labours of all his predecessors, of Pericles as well as of Canova; and he may virtually carry in his portfolio the mighty lions and bulls of Nineveh, – the gigantic sphinxes of Egypt, – the Apollos and Venuses of Grecian art, – and all the statuary and sculpture which adorn the galleries and museums of civilised nations.

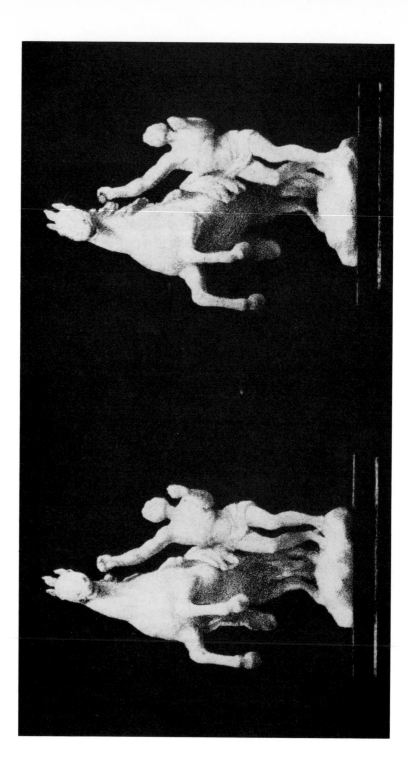

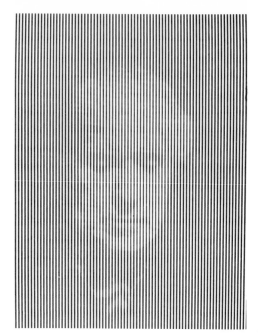

Brewster's face embedded in a geometrically periodic pattern like that in which he observed subjective colours and spatial distortions.

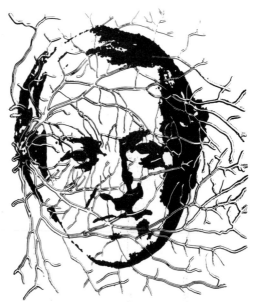

Wheatstone and the ramifications of the retinal blood vessels that he described in great detail.

4. Subjective Visual Phenomena

4.1. Introduction

The first article reprinted in this chapter is by Brewster on accidental colours (4.2). These would now be called complementary after-images, although they have also been referred to as phantasms and ocular spectra. The article is taken from the *Edinburgh Encyclopaedia* (sometimes cited as the *Encyclopaedia Edinburghiensis*), which was "conducted by David Brewster". The Encyclopaedia represented Brewster's most ambitious publishing enterprise. The first volume was published in 1808 and the eighteenth, and final, one in 1830. The complete Encyclopaedia was reprinted in 1830, together with two supplementary volumes encompassing the advances made during the preceding 22 years. Not only did Brewster contribute an astonishing number of entries to the Encyclopaedia, but it provided a continuing source of irritation to him because of the numerous problems and delays that arose throughout its production.*

Brewster commenced his discussion of accidental colours by describing the colour circle and the rules of colour mixing. However, he assumed, incorrectly, that mixing pigments yielded the same outcome as combining the same colours on a whirling disc. The combinations of colours on a rotating disc, when one was omitted, were determined from the position of the "centre of gravity" of those remaining.† Thus, if red was omitted from the circle of colours, the disc would appear bluish-green on rotation. The same interpretation was applied to accidental colours, the only difference being that, instead of omitting a colour from white light, the retina is rendered insensitive to it by the prior intense stimulation. Other than in making recourse to the colour circle, Brewster's interpretation

* Brewster's bitterness at the delays was but thinly veiled in his Preface to the reprinted edition. He attributed the delays in large measure to the indolence of the contributors. Financial considerations were also an issue: his own remuneration was contingent upon the appearance of successive volumes and it "was retarded and diminished by any stoppage in the publication" (Brewster, 1830, Vol. 1, p. vi). The publishers, Blackwoods, saw it quite otherwise, placing most of the responsibility for the delays on the Editor (see Oliphant, 1907).

† More precise and systematic experiments with the colour top were to be initiated by James Forbes, and extended by his student James Clerk Maxwell (see Maxwell, 1890).

added little to the extant theories of after-images, as advanced, for example, by Robert Darwin (1786). Brewster did make the astute observation that the fringes of accidental colours that partially surround fixated targets were due to the unsteadiness of the eye during fixation.

Brewster examined the interocular transfer of an intense after-image formed following observation of the sun's reflected image. He appeared, at that time, to be unaware of Newton's similar experiment, although he made a point of publishing the latter, which was contained in a letter to John Locke, some years later (see Brewster, 1831b). The notion of vision residing anywhere other than in the eye was so inimical to Brewster that he interpreted his observations in the following manner: "the impression of the solar image was conveyed by the optic nerve from the left to the right eye." Following these experiments Brewster suffered some "debility of the eyes" and was reluctant to conduct any more observations. Thus, Brewster can be placed alongside the foremost nineteenth-century investigators of after-images – Plateau and Fechner; all suffered long-lasting insult to their eyes as a consequence of observing the sun. Brewster's debility was, most probably, less severe than Plateau's and Fechner's, as he noted that it later disappeared.*

In concluding the article Brewster predicted that a knowledge of the theory of accidental colours would prove essential for the fabric manufacturer. At that time the distinction between simultaneous and successive contrast had not been made, but it was within the related area of simultaneous colour contrast that Chevreul, dyemaster of the Gobelin tapestry in Paris, formulated principles of colour combination that influenced both science and art (see Chevreul, 1839; Rood, 1879).

The second article by Brewster (4.3) is concerned with indirect (peripheral) vision. He commenced by discussing the occasional disappearances of objects in the periphery of vision when the eyes remained relatively steady. This phenomenon had been the topic of an earlier paper, delivered to the Royal Society of Edinburgh, but only an abstract of it was then published (Brewster, 1818). Brewster could not have known that the phenomenon had been described at the turn of the century by Troxler (1804), and it is now frequently referred to as Troxler's effect. Although Brewster stated that the effect occurred with one or two viewing eyes, he later reported, in his *Letters on Natural Magic* (1832), that it took longer for indirectly viewed patterns to disappear binocularly. The successive disappearances of directly viewed spectral colours and dimly illuminated objects were also discussed. These latter phenomena were related to the methods used by astronomers to see very faint stars, as had been reported by Herschel and South. Brewster's interpretation was, however, at variance with Herschel's suggestion that the periphery of the retina has greater sensitivity than

* This is evident from a marginal note in Brewster's handwriting by this section of the article in the Scottish National Library's copy of the 1830 Encyclopaedia.

the central parts. In its stead, Brewster proposed an optical explanation, namely that light falling peripherally on the eye is both out of focus and magnified, neither of which states obtained during direct vision. In support of this he argued that disappearances of directly viewed images could be terminated by defocussing the eye.

In this same context, but with little direct relevance, Brewster made a brief statement concerning the distortions produced by prolonged observations of a single bright line or a set of parallel lines. The lines became wavy and appeared separated by tinted colours. This represents one of the original reports of spatial distortions produced when viewing regular geometrical patterns, and probably the first report of subjective colours induced by black and white patterns (see Wade, 1977a, b).

Observations of after-images, spatial distortions, direct and indirect vision were also being reported at around the same time by the Czech physiologist, Purkinje.* Purkinje's first observations and experiments were published as his doctoral dissertation in 1819, but they were made more widely available on their republication in 1823. A series of new observations and experiments was published in 1825. Purkinje's studies were more systematic and wide-ranging than Brewster's, and it is to the perceptual effects Purkinje described that the term subjective visual phenomena is generally applied. The significance of these observations was clear to Wheatstone because, in the first of two anonymous articles published in the short-lived *Journal of the Royal Institution*, he provided a translated summary of Purkinje's first book (4.4). Moreover, it is evident that Wheatstone believed that students of vision in Britain were unaware of much important research that had been published on the European continent, and that this could be rectified, in part, by the application of his considerable linguistic skills.

Wheatstone began his selective translation by taking issue with Purkinje's use of the term subjective, but he retained it for convenience. The same reservations and uses of the "subjective" qualifier for certain visual phenomena still remain with us. The first class of phenomena described were the impressions generated by alternating light and shade. These are now referred to as stroboscopic patterns (see Smythies, 1957), although Purkinje observed them before the invention of the stroboscope! Next, the pressure figures were described and illustrated, that

---

* Jan Evangelista Purkinje (1787–1869) spent most of his active research life in Germany. His early observations on subjective visual phenomena were undertaken, in part, because of the lack of any equipment to examine other physiological processes. He was encouraged in his endeavours by Johann Goethe, to whom he dedicated his second volume of observations, because of his use of the phenomenological method (which he applied with greater success than did Goethe, himself). However, unlike Goethe, he considered that all subjective phenomena have objective physiological correlates. When Purkinje gained access to one of the new achromatic microscopes in 1832 he put his observational skills to good use, as is attested by the Purkinje cells in the cerebellum and the Purkinje fibres in the heart.

is, the geometrical patterns produced by applying pressure to the eyeball. The third class of subjective phenomena concerned those consequent upon electrical stimulation around the eye. Fourthly, the diffusely striped figures seen with the eyes closed and in darkness were described. The fifth group were the small luminous dots fleetingly seen when viewing large, uniformly illuminated surfaces. The blind-spot and peripheral target disappearances were next mentioned. Purkinje, like Brewster, did not cite Troxler's earlier reports on the disappearances of objects during prolonged viewing.

The most important section, from Wheatstone's point, was that concerning the visibility of the retinal blood vessels. Purkinje observed them by moving a candle before the open eye in a darkened room. In a long footnote (followed by the initials C. W.) Wheatstone not only described an improved method for rendering the vessels but he also gave an interpretation of their occurrence – as shadows of the vessels. Moreover, by a number of simple and elegant demonstrations he showed that no vessels were visible around the fovea (at the centre of the *foramen centrale*), and that this part of the retina was slightly concave with respect to the neghbouring regions.

Accounts were also given of Purkinje's experiments with after-images, both positive and negative, and mental images. These last were the topic of Johannes Müller's interest several years after Purkinje (see Müller, 1826b). Throughout the eighteenth and nineteenth centuries a phenomenon of recurrent interest was that of the "mouche volantes", "muscae volitantes", "fliegende Mücken", "flying gnats" and other graphic appellations – the visibility of small inclusions in the ocular media. Purkinje's contribution to their study was presented in section 10 of Wheatstone's translation.

Wheatstone concluded his survey of Purkinje's observations by suggesting that frequent repetitions of the experiments could be injurious to the eyes and he cautioned against this. He also raised the question of the generality of the various phenomena, which could have been peculiar to Purkinje's particular eyesight. This issue is made later, and more pointedly, by Helmholtz: "even now there are many of the phenomena described by Purkinje which have never been seen by anyone else" (1873, p. 226).

The topics selected by Wheatstone were but a portion, albeit the most important, of Purkinje's first book. Amongst those aspects omitted was, surprisingly, Purkinje's brief section on singleness and doubleness of vision; others were eye movements and the spatial distortions consequent upon prolonged observation of geometrical patterns like parallel lines. Purkinje returned to many of these phenomena in his second volume (1825), as well as discussing aspects of near and far sightedness, voluntary squinting and the action of drugs (belladonna) on vision. It was from a passing reference in the second volume to the changing appearance of colours in twilight – the colour shift with which he is eponymously linked – that Purkinje is best remembered in visual science.

Wheatstone concluded the article by referring to future papers which would supply these omissions, but this was not to be. Nor, alas, did the public receive the benefits of his proposed translations of Goethe, Mile, Müller and Plateau. It seems unlikely that this was for want of a journal in which to publish them (the *Journal of the Royal Institution* ran for only two volumes). Rather, he appears to have been deflected from translating the labours of others by his own research endeavours in electricity, telegraphy and binocular vision. Instead of communicating the discoveries of continental Europeans to an English-speaking audience, he was to convey to them his own "Contributions to the physiology of vision". These latter were to have a more profound influence "towards forming a more complete theory of vision" than any of the former.

There was, however, a second article in this projected series, written over the initials C. W. (4.5). The article was not a translated summary of one of the major European writers, but referred to an aspect of Purkinje's work on the disappearance of dimly illuminated objects. In the course of the discussion a translation of a short note by Benedict Prévost was given. Prévost found that colours could be seen by intercepting a beam of sunlight entering a dark room. The colours were attributed to the difference in the time required for each colour to act on the retina. Wheatstone preferred a physical interpretation in terms of the diffraction of light at the edge of the card interrupting the light.

Wheatstone proceeded to describe a novel means of producing the impression of colours from black and white patterns, by placing one on the end of an oscillating kaleidophone rod. This method is the precursor of those used by Brewster, Fechner and others, whereby rotating black and white patterns generate subjective colours.*

In assessing "all the known facts" regarding the constant stimulation of the same part of the retina Wheatstone reached the following synthesis: continuous visibility is possible either by means of retinal movement or by intermittent stimulation. Essentially the same conclusions have recently been reached using all the cumbrous impedimenta of retinal image stablization.

This same topic was the subject of the next paper (4.6), delivered by Brewster to the first formal scientific meeting of the British Association for the Advancement of Science held in Oxford in 1832. Brewster, being a prime mover in the formation of the B.A., not only delivered the review of the state of optics (Brewster, 1832c), but he also presented a number of papers in the Optics

---

* In their history of research on subjective colours Cohen and Gordon (1949) bestowed on Prévost the honour of first demonstrating them. Wheatsone argued that Prévost's results were a consequence of diffraction rather than processes underlying the perception of colours from black and white patterns. It has also been suggested that the Prévost colours bear a close resemblance to the "flight of colours" in a brief after-image (see Wade, 1977a). Wheatstone's method seems to be the first report of inducing colours with moving black and white patterns, whereas Brewster (Article 4.3) reported them earlier when viewing stationary, geometrically periodic, patterns. Because Wheatstone did not mention Brewster's demonstration of subjective colours it may well have been unknown to him.

Section, of which 4.6 was one. Brewster's initial concern was with the effects produced by viewing one or many narrow slits, and the moiré fringes generated by crossing two systems of parallel lines. He then returned to the issue of the distortions seen in regular gratings – the apparent waviness of the lines and the subjective colours. It was also maintained that the effects transferred to the closed eye. The various phenomena were attributed to movements of the pattern or of the eye. Brewster then described the radiations visible when viewing intense light sources through very small apertures, and concluded by addressing Purkinje's demonstration of the visibility of the retinal blood vessels. The latter phenomenon was interpreted in terms of differences in the sensitivity of those parts of the retina in contact with the blood vessels to incident and reflected light. The term *foramen centrale* was used frequently by Brewster, and it referred to the area at the centre of the visual axis, approximating the dimensions of the yellow spot. In this report, however, it is said that there is no retina across the *foramen centrale*, because it appeared as a dark spot.

Following Brewster's presentation the relatively unknown Wheatstone* rose to elaborate upon the conditions for seeing the blood vessels and to present an interpretation at variance with Brewster's. Wheatstone extended the views developed in his second "Contributions" article and made an elegant and succinct generalization (shown in italics) of the consequences of retinal image stabilization and the means of maintaining continuous visibility (see Wade, 1978b). He also repeated his description of the improved method for rendering the vessels visible (see Article 4.4) and demonstrated it to the meeting.

It is clear from the alacrity with which Brewster returned to this topic (see Article 4.7) that he was impressed more by Wheatstone's apparatus than by his interpretation. Indeed, Brewster borrowed the simple instrument, made of a metal disc with a central aperture and ground glass, at the Oxford meeting, and with it first observed the phenomenon. He denied that it represented the retinal blood vessels, however, and he retained his earlier interpretation (although the publication cited in 4.7 was the same article as 4.6, but reprinted in the *Philosophical Magazine*, of which he had just become an editor). That is, Brewster considered that the patterns seen were a consequence of the direction of movement of the circular aperture – similar patterns were seen with moving slits rather than circles. Furthermore, Brewster was correct in stating that Wheatstone's interpretation could only be sustained if the blood vessels were in front of the retina – he was wrong in believing that no such separations between the vessels and receptors existed. Brewster concluded by giving a brief description of yet another method for making the vessels in the retina visible: if a large convex lens of short focal length is placed close to the eye, and moved back and forth the

---

* Wheatstone did deliver a paper to the acoustics section at the Oxford meeting, and he was at that time known for his research on sound. However, his two articles on vision had been published anonymously and he was not regarded as an authority on vision.

vessels can be clearly seen, but not around the visual axis. Helmholtz (1924) recommended this technique.

Article 4.8 is taken from the *Philosophical Magazine* of 1832, Brewster's first year as one of the three editors. The title of 4.8 is the same as that for the paper presented to the B.A. directly after the "Undulations" article, but this version is expanded somewhat. Reference was made initially to Newton's "pressure figures" (which were not cited by Purkinje) and also to his observations on the persistence of vision. Various aspects of Newton's description, which was given in its entirety, were disputed by Brewster: the "circle of light" was considered to remain as long as pressure was maintained, and it did not appear coloured to Brewster. The range of effects observed were related to the degree of pressure applied to the eye. The influence of pressure on the visibility of an after-image was described – the colour was changed by gentle pressure. The effects were related generally to a disease of the eye called *Amaurosis*, although this was a form of blindness attributed at the time to malfunction of the visual nervous system.

Brewster returned to the issue of subjective patterns in the next article (4.9) – those produced by intermittent stimulation. First, he described the action of bright sunlight interrupted when passing railings. The patterns described are similar to Purkinje's checkerboard figures, but in Brewster's case they were coloured – like the "brightest tartan". The same phenomena could be seen using Purkinje's distended finger method, though Brewster did not refer to Purkinje's work. The phenomenon could be seen more conveniently using the phenakistoscope, so that the apertures in the revolving disc produced regular and successive stimulation. Again colours were visible, and the network pattern described were in many ways similar to Purkinje's figures (see Article 4.4). These various coloured effects were interpreted in terms of the time course of persisting images and after-images, and the optical conditions for eliciting them were formulated.

Following the flurry of publications on vision that coincided with shouldering the Edinburgh editorial mantle of the *London and Edinburgh Philosophical Magazine and Journal of Science*, to give its full title, Brewster had a fallow period for research. His energies were directed elsewhere. In 1838 he assumed the Principalship of St. Andrews University and he sought to change the course of that venerable institution by introducing a greater scientific content. This was not a happy time for Brewster, as his visions of the University's future were not shared by the Professoriate. The dispute reached such a pitch that a Royal Commission was appointed to investigate the running of the University. Although the Commission did not support the removal of Brewster from office, he was severely censured in their report for his style of administration (see Anderson, 1983).

By contrast, this was a very productive period for Wheatstone. He was appointed to the Chair of Experimental Philosophy at King's College, London in

1834. He published his measures on the velocity of electricity, his description of the stereoscope and patented the electric telegraph. Wheatstone's connections with King's College seem to have been more congenial than were Brewster's with St. Andrews. On the other hand, Brewster appeared to have closer contacts with students than did Wheatstone. Brewster gave frequent lectures to interested students, and one of his popular courses was on "The Philosophy of the Senses".* This willingness to lecture contrasts with his earlier reticence for giving sermons, as they so debilitated him. Indeed this was one of the reasons he decided against entering the Kirk. Wheatstone does not seem to have overcome his shyness. It is uncertain whether he actually delivered any lectures to his students, following his first professorial series in 1835 (see Bowers, 1975). His papers to to the Royal Institution and to the Royal Society were almost always delivered by Michael Faraday. On one occasion, in April, 1846, Wheatstone steeled himself to give his own Friday evening lecture at the Royal Institution. He approached the open door of the lecture theatre, accompanied by Faraday, but fled before entering.† Wheatstone thus initiated a tradition at the Royal Institution whereby the Director always stands behind the lecturer to discourage any such hasty departure (see Williams, 1965).

When Brewster returned to his visual researches it was to the topic of Wheatstone's stereoscopic phenomena that he addressed himself (see Articles 2.5–2.7). These three articles were punctuated by another, also in the Edinburgh Transactions, on *muscae volitantes* (4.10), because he had encountered a particularly good example of the phenomenon in one of his eyes. Accordingly, he was able to illustrate the form they took, and he calculated their location within the eye from the separation of double images produced by two light sources.

Both Brewster and Wheatstone attended the York meeting of the British Association in 1844, and both presented papers to the Optics section. Brewster's first paper (4.11) was concerned with communicating an account of a phenomenon described to him by a Rev. Selwyn. This was the appearance of white spots at the intersections of black lines, crossing at right angles in the form of a grid. It is now referred to as the Hering grid, and the complementary configuration, with white intersecting lines on a black background, is called the Hermann grid. Hermann (1870) first noticed the effect when reading a German translation of Tyndall's lectures on *Sound* which were delivered at the Royal Institution in 1867. One of the illustrations consisted of a matrix of Chladni figures, each drawn in a separate black square on a white ground. Fortuitously, the separation of the regular black

---

* No records of these lectures have been kept, and, because Brewster's papers were destroyed by fire at the family home near Kingussie early in this century, their contents are likely to remain a mystery. A book with the same title is dedicated to Sir David Brewster, but the author did not attend the lectures (see Wyld, 1852).

† Faraday gave an extemporized talk entitled "Thoughts on ray vibrations". This is taken as one of the first hints of an electromagnetic theory of light.

squares was suitable for generating the dark dots at the white intersections. Hermann published a brief note describing the effect and attributing it to simultaneous contrast. Several years later Hering described the alternative figure of black intersecting lines yielding white dots. Perhaps the reason why Brewster's earlier account has been neglected is that there is little in the title to suggest the nature of the optical phenomenon that the Rev. Selwyn had observed. Retrospective justice might be served by renaming it the Selwyn grid!

Sandwiched between the seven papers (mainly concerned with physical optics) presented by Brewster to the Optics Section at the York meeting was a brief note by Wheatstone (4.12), with a singularly enigmatic title. It described the apparent motion seen in patterns of red and green when viewed in dim light. It is clear from the following paper by Brewster (4.13) that they had discussed the phenomenon privately, and that both had intended talking of it at the formal sessions. Moreover, it would seem from Brewster's account that it had been known informally for some time, and it had been called the "fluttering hearts", because the colours, red or blue, had been represented in the shape of hearts on the other coloured background. This descriptive origin of the term "fluttering hearts" seems to have been lost: it was referred to subsequently, particularly in the German literature, as the "so-called fluttering hearts". Here is another instance in which the title of the paper, "On the same subject", would have provided little to assist the researcher in divining its contents.

The following meeting of the British Association, in Cambridge, was attended by Brewster. Amongst his usual crop of optical papers was a very short abstract (4.14) which described a motion after-effect he had observed whilst travelling by rail. After viewing the laterally moving stones by the side of the railway track and closing the eyes he perceived motion in the direction perpendicular to that of the stones. This after-effect is closely related to one described by Purkinje (1823): following observations of a stationary pattern of parallel lines there was apparent motion in the direction perpendicular to the lines. As with many of the closely related phenomena examined both by Purkinje and by Brewster, the latter rarely referred to the observations of the former. Where such reference was made, as in the case of the visibility of retinal blood vessels, it was a consequence of others, like Wheatstone, having first drawn attention to them. It is likely, therefore, that Brewster did not have first-hand knowledge of Purkinje's books on subjective visual phenomena.

In the 1850s Brewster published his treatise on *The Stereoscope* (1856) and revised that on *The Kaleidoscope* (1858), in addition to opening his debate with Wheatsone on the priority of invention of the stereoscope. Relatively little original work was published in the area of vision by Brewster during this period, and when he did present two papers (4.15 and 4.16) to the Manchester meeting of the British Association, in 1861, they amplified observations and interpretations he had made previously.

It is a fascinating coincidence that these two students of vision, who had examined many related phenomena, should also have suffered from similar forms of ophthalmic migraine attacks – for so it would appear from the last of Brewster's papers, and from a reference to Wheatstone in Airy's (1870) classical article on "transient hemiopsia". In his first discussion of "hemiopsy" (4.17) Brewster described some earlier accounts on the phenomenon and related his own afflictions. His interpretation of this effect, as with so many other phenomena, was retinal. Pressure on the retina was considered to be the cause, because the appearance was similar to that from the application of external pressure to the eyeball; furthermore, the affected part of the field still appeared luminous in a dark room. Brewster discussed the views of Wollaston and others on hemiopsy, and in so doing he surveyed the tangled state of knowledge concerning the nervous pathways from the eyes to the brain. Brewster, himself, had considerable difficulty in reconciling the visibility of the disturbance by either eye with his belief in the retinal origins of the effects.

Brewster's second article on hemiopsy (4.18) commenced with a reference to his old adversary, George Biddell Airy,* who was similarly afflicted by occasional attacks of hemiopsy. It was the Astronomer Royal's son, Hubert Airy, who produced the most complete survey of "transient hemiopsia" available at that time, together with detailed and coloured representations of the "fortification" effects. In the course of his survey, Airy reproduced an account of one of Wheatstone's attacks (4.19), which had first occurred in 1849. Wheatstone endorsed Airy's use of the report. The description represents a classical ophthalmic migraine attack (see Richards, 1970), and the reference to the "motion of a luminous liquid" is particularly apposite.

In both Brewster's and Wheatstone's cases it appears that the attacks were induced by reading. It seems only fitting that this collection should end with reports by both visual scientists on the same phenomenon, because their earlier interests in vision overlapped so closely. It is equally appropriate to find them describing it in different terms!

---

* George Biddell Airy (1801–1892) was Astronomer Royal from 1835–1881. As Professor of Astronomy at Cambridge University he, together with Whewell and Herschel, promoted the wave theory of light and attacked those, like Brewster, who were not convinced by it (see Cantor, 1978; Morrell and Thackray, 1981). Airy (1847) was also a major critic of Brewster's theory of the triple spectrum.

4.2. Brewster: "Accidental colours". In *Edinburgh Encyclopaedia*, 1830, Vol. I, pp. 88–93.

Accidental Colours, a name given by Buffon to those colours which arise from the continued action of light upon the retina, in order to distinguish them from those which are produced by the decomposition of white light.

A few of the phenomena of accidental colours were first observed by De la Hire, and our countryman Dr Jurin; but we are indebted to Buffon, Professor Scherffer, and Æpinus, for a complete series of experiments, by which the nature and cause of these colours have been almost completely unfolded. The limits of our work will not permit us to give a detailed view of the various experiments by which this subject has been illustrated; but by directing the attention of the reader to the most important facts, and to the theory by which they may be explained, he will be enabled to account for the various optical illusions which are referable to the same cause.

When we look steadily, and for a considerable time, at a small square of red paper placed upon a white ground, we perceive a light green border surrounding the red square: by removing the eye from the red square, and directing it to another part of the white ground, we perceive very distinctly a square of light-green approaching a little to blue, and of the same size as the real red square. This imaginary *green* is the *accidental colour of red*, and continues to be visible till the impression made upon the retina by the red square has been effaced by other images. By making the same experiment with squares of different colours, it will be found that

Black is the accidental colour of	White.
White that of	Black.
Red	Blue.
Purple	Green.
Blue	Yellow.
Green	Red.

In these experiments of Buffon, the ground on which the squares of natural colours were viewed, was white, except in the case of the white square, which was placed upon a black ground. Professor Scherffer has found, that the accidental colours will be much more vivid, and their outlines more distinct, if the natural colours are viewed upon a black ground, and the eye transferred to a white ground. The most convenient way of making the experiments, is to use coloured wafers, fixed either upon a piece of white or black paper.

In order to explain these phenomena, we must recollect, that white light is composed of seven different colours, in the following proportions; the colours being supposed to be arranged in the circumference of a circle.

Violet	$2/9$ or 80°
Indigo	$1/9$ or 40
Blue	$1/6$ or 60
Green	$1/6$ or 60
Yellow	$2/15$ or 48
Orange	$3/40$ or 27
Red	$1/8$ or 45

Hence, if we take seven powders of the same colour as the seven prismatic colours, and proportion the quantities of each to the numbers in the preceding Table, the mixture of all these powders will be of a white colour; but if the red powder, or any of the others, be withdrawn, the mixture of the remaining colours will not be white, as before. To illustrate this in a more simple manner, let us suppose, that a circular wheel has its circumference divided into sectors, whose arches are in the same proportion as the preceding numbers, and that each sector is painted of its proper colour, viz. the sector of 80° violet, that of 40° indigo, and so on with the rest, as is represented in Fig. 4; then if this wheel be whirled briskly

ACCIDENTAL COLOURS

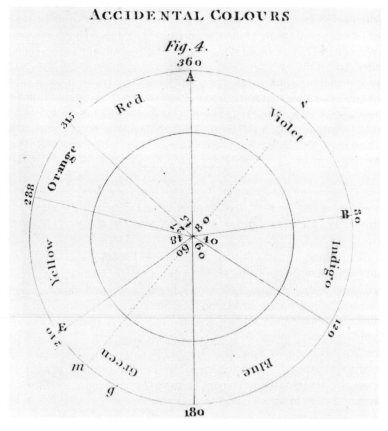

Fig. 4.

round its axis, its colour will be white. But if the red sector is taken out, or painted black, and the wheel again put in motion, the colour of the wheel will then be green; and, by leaving out the other colours successively, the following results will be obtained:

Colours omitted.	Colour of the wheel in motion.
Red	Green.
Yellow	Blue.
Green	Purple.
Blue	Red

As this experimental method of determining the colour which arises from mixing any number of the prismatic colours is too circuitous to be used in practice, we shall proceed to point out a method by which the resulting colour may be determined by a very simple calculation.

Let the seven prismatic colours be arranged in a circle, as in Fig. 4, where each colour occupies its proper arch of the circumference; and let us suppose each colour concentrated in the centre of gravity of its arch; then, if we omit any of the colours, it has been found, that the colour resulting from the mixture of all the remaining colours, is that which is nearest to the centre of gravity of the remaining arch. Thus, if we omit violet, the remaining arch will be AEB, whose centre of gravity is the point m, which falls in the green arch: but as the point m does not coincide with g, the centre of gravity of the green arch, the colour arising from a mixture of all the colours, except violet, will not be exactly green, but green mixed with a yellow, as the point m lies between the centres of gravity of the green and yellow arches. Since v is in the centre of the arch AB, and m the centre of AEB, it is evident, that the point m will always be directly opposite to the centre of gravity v of the violet, or omitted colour; hence we have only to draw a diameter from the centre of gravity of the omitted colour, and the extremity of that diameter will point out the colour which results from the combination of the rest.

If we suppose the divisions of the circle to commence from A, the boundary of the red and violet, we shall have the following Table, which will enable us to determine the resulting colour without the aid of a diagram.

Colours.	Position of the centre of gravity of each coloured arch.	Position of the point m, or the point opposite the centre of gravity of each coloured arch.	Limits of each coloured arch.	
Violet,	40th deg.	220th deg.	From 0° to 80	
Indigo,	100th	280th	80	120
Blue,	150th	330th	120	180
Green,	210th	30th	180	240
Yellow,	264th	84th	240	288
Orange,	301st ½	121st ½	288	315
Red,	337th ½	157th ½	315	360

As the construction of the preceding Table is very obvious, from the inspection of Fig. 4, a single example will be sufficient to explain its use. Let it be required, therefore, to determine the colour which results from a mixture of all the colours, except *blue*. In the third column, we find, that the point *m*, opposite to the centre of gravity of the blue arch, is in the 330th degree of the circle, which appears, from the fourth column, to lie between the limits of the *red* arch, viz. 315 to 360: therefore the resulting colour will be red, but with a small mixture of orange, as the 330th degree, or the point *m*, is between the centres of gravity of the red and that of the orange arches, being 7° from the former, and 28½° from the latter.

With the aid of these preliminary observations, we are in a state of preparation for explaining the phenomena of accidental colours. When the eye is fixed for some time upon a red square, the part of the retina, which receives the image of the square, is strongly excited by the continued action of the red rays. The sensibility of that relaxed portion of the retina to red light, must therefore be diminished, in the same way as the palate, when accustomed to a particular taste, ceases to feel its impression. But if the red rays, which afterwards fall upon the relaxed part of the retina, are feeble compared with those which issued from the red square, and produced the relaxation; or if the taste, which is afterwards presented to the palate, is much weaker than that which first diminished its sensibility, then it is still more obvious, that the debilitated portion of the respective organs will not be susceptible of these feebler excitements.

When the eye, therefore, is turned from the red square to the white paper, the enfeebled portion of the retina is excited by the white light which flows from the paper, but is not sensible to the impression of the red rays which enter into the composition of this white light. The debilitated part of the retina, therefore, is excited by all the component colours of white light, except the red, or by the colour resulting from their combination. But it will be found, from the preceding Table, that this resulting colour is blue with a mixture of green, or bluish-green, consequently the relaxed part of the retina will be sensible only to this colour, and will perceive a bluish-green square upon the white paper, of the same size as the red square, if the white paper and red square were held at the same distance; but of a greater or less size, according as the distance of the white paper is greater or less than the distance of the red square. Hence the accidental colour of red is bluish-green, or, in general, the accidental colour of any natural colour is that which results from the mixture of all the colours of the spectrum, except the natural colour itself. When the square first viewed by the eye is black, it is obvious that the part of the retina on which its image falls, is not excited by any rays, while all the surrounding part of the membrane is excited, and enfeebled, by the image of the white paper upon which the black square is placed. If the eye, therefore, be fixed upon a white ground, the light of this ground will make the strongest impression upon the unexcited part of the retina, and, consequently, there will appear, on the white ground, a square whiter than the surrounding portion. The very reverse of this will happen, when a white square, upon a black ground, is viewed by the eye.

From this hypothesis we may now construct a table of accidental colours more accurate than that which Buffon deduced from experiment. The Table, however, which is thus formed, is founded on the supposition, that the natural colours employed are of the same kind as the prismatic ones.

Natural Colours.	Accidental Colours.
RED,	BLUE, with a small mixture of GREEN.
ORANGE,	BLUE, with nearly an equal part of INDIGO.
YELLOW,	INDIGO, with a considerable mixture of VIOLET.
GREEN,	VIOLET, with a mixture of RED.
BLUE,	RED, with a mixture of ORANGE.
INDIGO,	YELLOW, with a considerable mixture of ORANGE.
VIOLET,	GREEN, with a considerable mixture of BLUE.

There is one appearance observed by Buffon, which does not seem to have been explained, either by that philosopher, or by any succeeding author. The writer of the article "Accidental Colours", in the Suppl. to the Encyc. Brit., has attempted to account for it; but it is easy to shew, that he has ascribed the phenomenon to a wrong cause. The appearance, to which we allude, is the fringe of accidental colour, which seems to surround the coloured square, before the eye is transferred to the white ground. This fringe is ascribed, in the article now quoted, to a dilatation of the pupil, without any explanation of the process by which the fringe is generated.

We presume, however, that, in this explanation, the dilatation of the pupil is supposed to increase the image of the square upon the retina; so that the white light from the paper, immediately surrounding the real square, falls upon that part of the retina over which the increment of the image is expanded, and produces the accidental colour of the square, stretching as far beyond the real square, as the image on the retina, increased by the dilatation of the pupil, stretches beyond the image which is formed before the pupil begins to expand. Admitting the dilatation of the pupil, which, in the present case, we are disposed to call in question, the only effect of it would be to give us a larger image of the real square; or if, from any occult cause, a fringe should be produced, its colour ought to be much fainter than the accidental colour of the square; for the part of the retina, which produces the fringe, has not been so long excited as the part which produces the accidental colour. There is, however, no perceptible difference between this colour and the fringe, so that the phenomenon must be traced to a different cause.

If we examine with accuracy this coloured fringe, we shall find, that, in general, it does not completely surround the real square, but appears only on one or two sides of the square at the same time; and if a circle is used instead of a square, the fringe will be a lunula, or lucid bow, surrounding only one half of the circumference. Had this single circumstance been attended to, philosophers might have readily discovered, that the fringe arose from the unsteadiness of the observer's eye, which cannot remain fixed on the same point of the square, or circle. The smallest aberration of the eye, which begins to be unsteady in a short time, will therefore make the image of the white paper, contiguous to the square, fall upon the excited part of the retina, and thus produce the accidental coloured fringe, which will increase with the unsteadiness of the eye. If, from the unsteadiness of the head or hand of the observer, the paper, on which the square is placed, should be removed to a greater distance from the eye, than when the impression was made upon the retina, the fringe will surround the whole square; and may be made to assume any size, by increasing the distance of the paper from the eye, after the retina has been sufficiently excited. In this case, the natural-coloured square will be surrounded with a square of accidental colour, the sides of the squares forming any angle with each other, according to the position of the real square.

When the retina is highly excited by the action of the coloured light, the accidental colour appears, though with much less brilliancy, which the eye is shut. This, however, evidently arises from a small quantity of light, which is transmitted through the eye-lids. It has been maintained, (Sup. Encyc. Brit.) that the accidental colours will appear, even if we retire into a dark room; but this is physically impossible. From the duration of the impressions of light upon the retina, the square may, in this case, appear of its natural colour, and actually does so; but the presence of light is absolutely necessary to the generation of accidental colours.

In order to shew, that the same colour results from the combination of accidental colours, as from the combination of real ones, Professor Scherffer placed two small squares, in contact with each other, upon a black ground, the square on the left being yellow, and that on the right red. He then fixed his eye for a few seconds on the centre of the yellow square, and, without moving his head, he fixed it for the same time on the centre of the red square; his eye was then returned to the yellow square, and the operation of viewing each square alternately was repeated three or four times. When this part of the experiment was completed, he turned his eye to a white wall, on which there appeared three squares, in contact with each other. The square on the left was *violet,* the middle square was a mixture of *green* and *blue,* and the colour of the right hand square was a *vivid green.* When the eye is fixed on the yellow square, the image of it falls upon the centre of the retina, and produces an accidental colour of indigo-violet; but when the eye is transferred to the red square, its image falls likewise upon the centre of the retina, and produces an accidental colour of bluish-green; consequently the mixture of these accidental colours produces green and blue, which is therefore the accidental colour that appears in the middle square. But while the eye was fixed on the yellow square, the image of the red square fell upon one side of the centre of the retina, and produced the accidental colour of green, which appeared in the right hand square; and, while the eye was fixed on the red square, the image of the yellow square fell upon the other side of the centre of the retina, and produced the accidental colour of indigo-violet, which appeared in the left hand square. This, we presume, is the true explanation of the phenomena, and may be applied to the following experiments of Scherffer.

Number and order of the natural-coloured Squares.

	Yellow	Green	....	Deep Blue
	Green	Blue	....	Reddish
	Red	Green	....	Green
Green	Yellow	Red	....	Reddish
Blue	Yellow	Red	....	Pale Yellow

Number and order of Accidental Colours.

Violet with much Red			Pale Red
Orange			Pale Yellow
Dark Brown			Red
Deep purple	Deep blue	Green and blue	Green
Greenish blue	Deep green	Green and blue	Green

The preceding experiments, which were intended merely to prove the mixture of accidental colours, might have been conducted with much more simplicity. If, for example, in the case of the yellow and red squares, the one were always concealed when the eye was examining the other, then, if the eye, after an alternate examination of each square, were transferred to a white ground, instead of three squares, it would perceive only one, which will be found to be a combination of the two accidental colours, like the middle square in Scherffer's experiment. The effect of the experiment will be still more beautiful when one of the squares is larger than the other. If we make the red square largest, and examine the two squares as before, we shall have, by turning the eye to a white surface, the appearance of one square inclosed in another: the interior square will be green and blue, or the mixture of the accidental colours of the red and yellow squares, while the exterior square is the accidental colour of the red square. If the yellow square is the largest, the interior square will be the same as before, but the exterior one will be the accidental colour of yellow.

In the course of his experiments, Buffon remarked, that the figure and colour of a red square underwent several curious transformations, by looking at it steadily for a very long time. These phenomena, however, were observed after his eye had been reduced by fatigue to an extreme degree of debility; and, therefore, it would be absurd to attempt an explanation of appearances, which probably arose from the diseased state of the organ.

The subject of accidental colours has been investigated by M. Æpinus; but he has attended only to those phenomena which were produced by the impression of the solar image upon the retina. When the sun was near the horizon, and the brilliancy of his light diminished by the interposition of thin clouds or floating exhalations, M. Æpinus fixed his eye steadily on the solar disc for the space of 15 seconds. After shutting his eye, he perceived an irregular pale yellow image of the sun, verging to green like sulphur, and surrounded with a faint red border. As soon as he opened his eye, and turned it to a white ground, the image of the sun was brownish red, and its encircling border was sky-blue. When his eye was again shut, the image of the sun became green, and the border a red colour, different from the last. Upon opening his eye, and turning it to the white ground as before, the image was more red than formerly, and the border a brighter sky-blue. His eye being again shut, the image appeared green approaching to sky-blue, and the border red, still differing from the former. When his eye was opened as before, upon a white ground, the image was still red, and its border sky-blue, but the shades of these colours were different from the last. At the end of four or five minutes, when his eye was shut, the image was a fine sky-blue, and the border a brilliant red; and upon opening his eye as before, the image was a brilliant red, and the border a fine sky-blue. By considering that the colour of the sun approached to orange, and that when the eyes are shut, red light is still admitted through the eye-lids, the preceding phenomena may admit of satisfactory explanation. It was observed by Æpinus, that the image of the sun, after his eye was fixed on the white ground, frequently disappeared, returned, and disappeared again, and that it generally disappeared when he wished to examine it, but returned when the eye was not prepared for observing it.

These experiments of Æpinus were repeated under different circumstances by the Editor of this work. Instead of looking at the sun when obscured and tinged with yellow by the interposition of clouds and vapours, I took advantage of a fine summer's day, when the sun was near the meridian, and formed a very brilliant and distinct image of his disc by means of the concave mirror of a reflecting telescope. My right eye being tied up, I viewed this luminous disc with the left through a tube, which prevented any extraneous light from failing upon the retina. When the retina was highly excited by the solar image, I turned my left eye to a white ground, and perceived the following appearances by alternately opening and shutting it.

Spectra with the left eye open.	Spectra with the left eye shut.
1. Pink surrounded with green	Green
2. Orange mixed with Pink	Blue
3. Yellowish Brown	Bluish Pink
4. Yellow	
5. Pure Red	Sky Blue
6. Orange	Indigo

This series of colours is much more extensive than that observed by Ӕpinus, because the retina was more strongly excited by the sun's light.

After uncovering my right eye, a remarkable phenomenon appeared; but as I am afraid that there was some illusion attending it, I shall insert the account which I drew up at the time for a scientific friend, and request the reader to consider it, not as a scientific fact, but as a point which is to be confirmed or overthrown by subsequent experiments.

> I was surprised to find, upon uncovering my right eye, and turning it to a white ground, that it also gave a coloured spectrum exactly the reverse of the first spectrum, which was *pink* surrounded with *green*. This result was so extraordinary, that I repeated the experiment twice, in order to be secure against deception, and always with the same result. The spectrum in the left eye was uniformly invigorated by closing the eye-lids, because the images of external objects efface the impression upon the retina; and when I refreshed the spectrum in the left eye, the spectrum in the right was also strengthened. On repeating the experiment a third time, the spectrum appeared in both eyes, which seems to prove, *that the impression of the solar image was conveyed by the optic nerve from the left to the right eye*; for the right eye being shut, could not be affected by the luminous image.* After these experiments, my eyes were reduced to such a state of extreme debility, that they were unfit for any further trials. A spectrum of a darkish hue floated before the left eye for many hours, which was succeeded by the most excruciating pains, shooting through every part of the head. These pains, accompanied with a slight inflammation in both eyes, continued for several days, and prevented me from varying the experiments.

This debility of the eyes has continued for two years, and several parts of the retina in both eyes have completely lost their sensibility. I must therefore leave it to other observers to confirm or overthrow this experiment.

Dr R. Darwin has made some ingenious observations on the subject of accidental colours. The images which arise from the duration of the impression of light upon the retina, and those which are accidentally coloured, he calls spectra, some of which, as the black spectrum from a white object, arise from a defect of sensibility; and others, as the white spectrum from a black object, arise from an excess of sensibility. The spectra which have the same colour as the object that makes the impression upon the retina, such as the red spectrum of a red square, which appears after the eye is shut and all light excluded, he calls *direct spectra*, and those which have the accidental colour of the object examined, he calls *reverse spectra*. The various experiments which he relates, may be easily explained from the principles already laid down: the physiological conclusions which he has deduced from them, do not belong to this article. See *Phil. Trans.* 1786, p. 313.

It can scarcely be expected, that, in a work like the present, we can enumerate the various phenomena which may be explained by the theory of accidental

---

* Immediately before the spectrum given by the right eye vanished, the green image was surrounded to a considerable distance with total darkness, so that the corresponding part of the retina was completely insensible to light.

colours. That the reader, however, may be able to trace these phenomena to their proper source, it may be necessary to mention, that the general causes of such appearances in the open air, are to be found in the verdure of the fields, the azure colour of the sea, the blueness of the sky, the golden brilliancy of the rising and setting sun, and the ruddy hue of the morning and evening clouds. When such phenomena are seen in a room, they are generally to be traced to the colour of the walls, or the window-curtains, and sometimes to that of the carpet or the furniture, when strongly illuminated by the sun.

Dr Darwin very properly infers, from the theory of accidental colours, that in the dial-plate of a clock or watch, or in a book printed with small types, the letters or figures should be of such a colour, that their spectra or accidental colours may be of the same hue as the ground on which they are placed. When this is done, the letters will appear more distinct, because the spectra arising from the unsteadiness of the eye cannot become visible. We conceive, however, that the theory is capable of a much more extensive application, and that, at some future time, which is not far distant, a knowledge of accidental colours will be deemed absolutely necessary to the manufacturer in the fabrication of coloured stuffs. It will be uniformly found, that, in every combination of colours, those are the most pleasing to the eye, in which the prominent colour is placed upon a ground similar to its accidental colour: the general effect will not be injured by the appearance of partial or complete spectra, and the organ of sight will not be distracted by floating images alternately soliciting his attention, and escaping from his view. Whenever theory seems to come in contact with practice, the connection should be diligently traced through all its consequences; for it is frequently thus that philosophy becomes the handmaid of the arts.

Before concluding this article, we shall present the reader with a new theory of accidental colours, proposed by the celebrated La Place, and published in the 2d edition of Haüy's *Traité de Physique*. La Place supposes,

> that there exists in the eye a certain disposition, in virtue of which, the red rays comprised in the whiteness of the ground are at the moment when they arrive at that organ, in a manner attracted by those which form the predominant red colour of the circle; so that the two impressions become blended into one, and the green colour finds itself at liberty to act as though it existed alone. According to this method of conceiving things, the sensation of the red decomposes that of the whiteness, and while the homogenous actions combine together, the action of the heterogenous rays which are disengaged from the combination produces its effect separately.

This hypothesis, unauthorised by experiment, is entitled to our regard solely from the unrivalled genius of its illustrious author. In a subsequent article, in which we propose to give a new theory of accidental colours, founded on a number of experiments, we shall be able to give a direct refutation of La Place's theory.

The writer of this article is engaged in a set of experiments connected with accidental colours, by which he expects to reduce the various colours in nature to a fixed nomenclature, – to ascertain the elements of which they are composed, and the proportion in which these elements are combined; and to determine the duration of the impression of light upon the retina, when proceeding from bodies of various colours, and under different degrees of illumination. The results of these experiments may probably be communicated in some subsequent article. Those who wish to study the subject of accidental colours, are referred to the works already quoted, and to *Jurin's Essay on Distinct and Indistinct Vision*, at the end of *Smith's Optics. Observations sur la Physique, par Rozier*, &c. vol. xxvi. p. 175.273.291. *Porterfield on the Eye*, vl. i. p. 343. Buffon, *Mem. Acad. Par.* 1743. p. 215. Æpinus, *Nov. Comment. Petrop.* tom. x. p. 283. Gregory's *Translation of* Haüy's *Nat. Phil.* vol. ii. p. 424. *Addenda. Mem. Acad. Berlin*, vol. ii. for 1771.

4.3. Brewster: "On some remarkable affections of the retina, as exhibited in its insensibility to indirect impressions, and to the impressions of attenuated light". *Edinburgh Journal of Science*, 1825, 3, 288–293.*

Among the various phenomena of vision which were observed by the philosophers of the last century, those which arise from indirect impressions, and from the influence of highly attenuated light upon the retina, seem to have escaped their notice.

If we look at a narrow slip of white paper placed upon a black or a coloured ground, it will never appear to vanish, however long and attentively we view it. But if the eye is fixed steadily upon any object within two or three inches of the paper, so as to see it only *indirectly*, or by oblique vision, the slip of paper will occasionally disappear, as if it had been removed entirely from the ground, the colour of the ground extending itself over the part of the retina occupied by the image of the slip of paper.

If the object seen indirectly is a *black* stripe on a white ground, it vanishes in a similar manner; and, what is still more remarkable, the same phenomena of disappearance take place *whether the object is viewed with one or with both eyes.*

When the indirect object is luminous, like a candle, it never vanishes entirely, unless it is placed at a great distance; but it swells and contracts, and is surrounded by a halo of nebulous light, so that the excitement must extend itself to contiguous portions of the retina which are not influenced by the light itself.

If we place two candles at the distance of about eight or ten feet from the eye, and about twelve inches from each other, and view the one directly and the other

---

* This paper formed the third section of a Memoir *On the Structure and Functions of the Human Eye*, which was read before the Royal Society of Edinburgh on the 2nd December 1822.

indirectly, the indirect image will be encircled with a bright ring of *yellow* light, and the bright light within the ring will have a pale blue colour. If the candles are viewed through a prism, the red and green light of the indirect image vanish, and leave only a large mass of yellow, terminated with a portion of blue light.

While performing this experiment, and looking steadily and directly at one of the prismatic images of the candle, I was surprised to observe that the red and green rays began to disappear, leaving only *yellow* and a small portion of *blue*; and when the eye was kept immoveably fixed on the same part of the image, the yellow light became almost pure white, so that the prismatic image was converted into an elongated image of white light.

If the slip of white paper, viewed indirectly with both eyes, is placed so near as to be seen double, the rays which proceed from it no longer fall on corresponding points of the retina. In this case, the two images do not vanish simultaneously; but when the one begins to disappear, the other begins soon after it, so that they sometimes appear to be extinguished at the same time.

In order to ascertain whether or not the accidental colour of an object seen indirectly would remain after the object itself had disappeared, I placed a rectangular piece of a *red* wafer upon a white ground, and having looked steadily at an object in its vicinity, the wafer disappeared, and though the accidental colour showed itself just before the wafer had vanished, yet no trace of colour was visible afterwards.

The insensibility of the retina to *indirect impressions* has a singular counterpart in its insensibility to the *direct impressions* of attenuated light. When the eye is steadily directed to objects illuminated by a feeble gleam of light, it is thrown into a condition nearly as painful as that which arises from an excess of splendour. A sort of remission takes place in the conveyance of the impressions along the nervous membrane; the object actually disappears, and the eye is agitated by the recurrence of excitements which are too feeble for the perfomance of its functions. If the eye had, under such a twilight, been making unavailing efforts to read, or to examine a minute object, the pain which it suffers would admit of an easy explanation; but, in the present case, it is the passive recipient of attenuated light, and the uneasiness which it experiences can arise only from the recurring failures in the retina to transmit its impressions to the optic nerve.

The preceding facts respecting the affections of the retina, while they throw considerable light on the functions of that membrane, may serve to explain some of those phenomena of the evanescence and reappearance of objects, and of the change of shape of inanimate objects, which have been ascribed by the vulgar to supernatural causes, and by philosophers to the activity of the imagination. If in a dark night, for example, we unexpectedly obtain a glimpse of any object, either in motion or at rest, we are naturally anxious to ascertain what it is, and our curiosity calls forth all our powers of vision. This anxiety, however, serves only to baffle us in all our attempts. Excited only by a feeble illumination, the retina is not capable of affording a permanent vision of the object, and while we are straining our eyes to discover its nature, the object will entirely disappear, and will afterwards appear and disappear alternately.* The same phenomenon may be observed in day light by the sportsman, when he endeavours to mark, upon the monotonous heath, the particular spot where moor-game has alighted. Availing himself of the slightest difference of tint in the adjacent heath, he keeps his eye steadily fixed upon it as he advances; but whenever the contrast of illumination is feeble, he invariably loses sight of his mark, and if the retina is capable of again taking it up, it is only to lose it again.

Since the preceding paper was read, Mr Herschel and Mr South† have described a very curious fact, which has some analogy with the phenomena now described.

"A rather singular method", they remark,

> of obtaining a view, and even a rough measure of the angles of stars, *of the last degree of faintness*, has often been resorted to, viz. to *direct the eye to another part of the field*. In this way, a faint star, in the neighbourhood of a large one, will often *become very conspicuous*, so as to bear a certain illumination, which will yet *totally disappear*, as if suddenly blotted out, when the eye is turned full upon it, and so on, *appearing* and disappearing alternately, as often as you please. The lateral portions of the retina, less fatigued by strong lights, and less exhausted by perpetual attention, are probably more sensible to faint impressions than the central ones, which may serve to account for this phenomenon.‡

As it is with much diffidence that I venture to controvert any opinion entertained by Mr Herschel, I have been at some pains to investigate the subject experimentally. I was, at first, disposed to ascribe the evanescence of the faint star, solely to the same cause as the evanesence of faintly illuminated surfaces, and the reappearance of the star by indirect vision, to the circumstance of the retina recovering its tone, by contemplating another object sufficiently luminous for vision; but this opinion was not well founded.

If a given quantity of light, which is unable to afford a sustained impression when expanded over a surface, is concentrated into a luminous point, it is still less fitted for the purposes of vision. It then acts upon the retina somewhat in the same way as a sharp point does upon the skin. The luminous point will alternately

---

* An analogous phenomenon, but arising from a quite different cause, must have often been observed by persons who are very long-sighted. In a dark night, the pupil dilates to such a degree as to deprive the eye of its power of adjusting itself to moderate distances. (See this *Journal*, vol. i. p. 80.) Hence, if an object presents itself within that distance, the observer must see it with a degree of indistinctness which cannot fail to surprise him, especially as all distant objects, particularly those seen against the sky, will appear to him with their usual sharpness of outline.

† See the *Phil. Trans.* 1824, part iii, p. 15, and page 283 of this Number.

‡ If we recollect rightly, a similar fact, with regard to the satellites of Saturn, is recorded in a late number of the *Ann. de Chimie*, and a similar explanation given. It was, we think, noticed by some of the astronomers in the Royal Observatory of Paris; but we have not the Number at hand to refer to.

vanish and reappear; and if the retina is under the influence of a number of such points, it will be thrown into a state of painful agitation. The same effect is produced by a sharp line of light; the retina is, in this case, thrown into a state of undulation, so as to produce an infinite number of images parallel to the luminous line; and when this line is a narrow aperture held near the eye, a sheet of paper, to which it is directed, will appear covered with an infinity of broken serpentine lines parallel to the aperture. When the eye is stedfastly fixed, for some time, upon the parallel lines which are generally used to represent the sea in maps, the lines will all break into portions of serpentine lines, and *red, yellow, green,* and *blue* tints will appear in the interstices of them.

The evanescence of stars, therefore, of the last degree of faintness, must be ascribed, both to their deleterious action upon the retina as points of light, and to the insufficiency of their light to maintain a continued impression upon the retina.

When the same star is seen by indirect vision, it reappears with a degree of brightness which it never assumes when seen directly by the eye. When the eye is adjusted to the distinct perception of an object placed in the axis of vision, an object placed out of the axis cannot be seen with the same distinctness, both from the pencils not being accurately converged upon the retina, and from the expansion of the image, which, as we have already described, accompanies indirect vision. A luminous point, therefore, seen indirectly, swells into a disk, and thus loses its sharpness, and acts upon a greater portion of the retina.* In order to determine whether this expansion, and the image of the luminous point, was the cause of its superior visibility, I turned my eye full upon a luminous point till it ceased to be visible, and then, re-adjusting my eye, so as to swell the point into a circular disk by direct vision, I invariably found that its visibility was instantly increased. If this explanation of the phenomenon be the correct one, the practical astronomer may, with direct vision, obtain a clearer view of minute and faint stars, either by putting the telescope out of its focus, or by adjusting his eye to nearer objects.

Allerly, *September 5th* 1825.

4.4. Wheatstone: "Contributions to the physiology of vision. No. I". *Journal of the Royal Institution*, 1830, **1**, 101–117. (Published anonymously)

Under the above title it is proposed to bring forward those stores of knowledge on this subject which have been hitherto locked up in the repositories of foreign scientific literature. The physiology of vision has a peculiar claim on the attention

---

* The eye is not capable of observing the *colours* of luminous points seen indirectly. A *blue* luminous point, for example, appears nearly *white*.

of philosophers, as presenting some of those links which connect physical with mental phenomena. Metaphysicians, physiologists, natural philosophers, and artists, have equally made it an object of their study; and the names of Baptista Porta, Leonardo da Vinci, Kepler, Descartes, Newton, Berkeley, Reid, Buffon, Darwin, Wells, Brown, Young, &c., are among those who have advanced the inquiry by their investigations and discoveries. That the subject is of such equal interest to so many different classes of inquirers, is perhaps the cause that, as a whole, it is so imperfectly known. Each person who occupies himself with its study, looking at it only from his own point of view, disregards those facts which he considers as belonging to the province of others, and thus is unable to arrive at those general conclusions which can only be obtained from a complete survey of all the various phenomena and their relations. To render some assistance towards forming a more complete theory of vision, we shall successively give an account of the discoveries of Purkinje, Goethe,* Mile, Müller, Plateau, &c. The number of these interesting memoirs on this interesting branch of science, which have been entirely unnoticed in this country, might surprise us, did we not know that the same neglect extends to many other important departments of knowledge.

'*Beiträge zur Kenntniss des Sehens in subjectiver Hinsicht, etc.*' (Essay on the Subjective Phenomena of Vision, by Dr. J. Purkinje, Professor of Physiology at the University of Breslau.) Prague. 1823.

This little volume has excited considerable interest in Germany; it relates to those appearances which, independently of external objects, are perceived in the organ of sensation itself. To distinguish these phenomena from those which arise on the presence of their appropriate external objects, the author employs the term subjective, which, as denoting this class of phenomena better than any other we are acquainted with, and, to avoid circumlocution, we have purposely retained; it will, however, on consideration, be perceived, that the term is not strictly proper, as, correctly speaking, all phenomena, *as such*, are subjective, *i.e.* in the mind; and were we, without qualification, to admit the classification of phenomena into objective and subjective, we should be unable to determine, with any degree of accuracy, where the objective ends or the subjective begins. Thus, the vessels of the eye and the retina itself are subjective, considered as parts of the visual organ; yet we shall see that in some of Dr. Purkinje's experiments they become real objects, and are perceived as such. But we shall not further discuss this question; what we have said will be sufficient to explain the term subjective as employed by Dr. Purkinje and by ourselves in the following extracts. We now proceed to an abridged description of the most interesting of Dr. Purkinje's experiments.

---

* An account of the 'Farbenlehre,' or theory of colours, of this illustrious poet and philosopher, will form one of the subsequent papers of this series.

I. *Luminous Figures produced by rapid alternations of Light and Shade.* – These figures are most distinctly seen in the following manner: the eye-lids being closed and the eyes directed towards the sun, the observer quickly moves his hand with the fingers spread, from one side to the other, so that the luminous rays are alternately intercepted and admitted; at the beginning of the experiment a yellowish-red glare is perceived which is afterwards replaced by a beautiful and regular figure, which it is, however, impossible to fix or determine, unless the experiment be continued for some length of time. Figs. 1, 2, 3 and 4 represent the phenomena as observed by Dr. Purkinje in his right eye.

Fig. 1 consists of small squares, chequered as in a chess board, and alternately bright and dark; this entire figure is bounded by zigzag lines, which are continually varying in direction, length, and brightness, and which appear rather more illuminated than the squares; at the centre of the square field is a dark point, with a luminous area, surrounded by rapidly moving semicircular lines, which nearly resemble rose-leaves in form; these are around and principally below the luminous area; below these semicircular lines is a field of hexagons, the circumferences of which are gray, and the centres white. This figure, Dr. Purkinje says, may be obtained very distinctly, and without any admixture of the other figures, if the experiment be modified so that the eye, being open, is directed towards an equally illuminated white wall, and the spread fingers are moved before it; if the experiment be made as before described, the secondary figures rather predominate. The appearances also take place under various other circumstances and modifications; for instance, the semicircular lines at the centre of the figure are particularly visible when the eyes are directed as near as possible to the flickering flame of a candle. The square field is also seen by looking at Newton's circle of colours, when it is in rapid motion; in this case it is not necessary that the colours be distributed in any particular manner, for the experiments will succeed, if the segments of the disc be merely alternately light and dark; the nearer the segments are to each other, the less rapid the motion of the circle is required to be, but bright sunshine is indispensable to the experiment. Lastly, the figure is seen when a wheel rapidly revolves between the eye and the sun, or a strong light; and it appears accordingly that the general condition of the phenomenon is a rapid alternation from light to shade.

The secondary figures, as Dr. Purkinje calls them, are indistinct when the experiment is made whilst the eyes are open; they appear under two modifications, the rectangular spiral, and the star with eight rays: at the commencement of the experiment, whilst the eyes are not over excited, both figures appear, as it were, mingling with each other, the radiated figure evidently predominating (Fig. 2); but as the experiment continues, the rectangular spiral (Fig. 3) becomes more visible, and the star gradually disappears: the central line of the spiral is the smallest and darkest, as will be seen by the figure, and has an oblique direction to the right and below; the line itself consists of a darker axis and a bright margin, and is divided, as it were, into joints; towards the periphery of the figure the axis becomes enlarged, and fades to a greyish tint; the lateral margin also loses its brightness, and at the termination of the spiral line the illumination seems even to be inverted – that is, the centre appears light, and the circumference dark: it is, however, impossible to determine with great accuracy the external parts of the figure; the intervals between the coils of the spiral are occupied by a faint gleam of the squares of Fig. 1.

In the two oblique lines of the star (Fig. 4), the light axes are brighter than in the other two lines; in the latter, on the contrary, the dark borders are of a deeper black. The spiral and radiated figures are in continual motion and fluctuation: sometimes the rectangular spiral changes into a triangular one; at other times the centre of the star dissolves, and the rays intersect each other at various points, or become parallel, or form squares, triangles, &c. The four figures above described are, however, whose which most frequently occur; and though, as Dr. Purkinje judiciously remarks, these subjective phenomena might appear to other eyes different from what he observed, yet the experiments made by others at his request seem to confirm his own observations: we may therefore, perhaps, be justified in concluding that the above phenomena do not depend on a morbid or individual condition, but physiologically result from the very organization of the human eye.

The figures in Dr. Purkinje's left eye, the sight of which was very weak, were very indistinct, but did not in any other respect appear different from those perceived by the right eye: the squares were more like network formed by curved lines; the secondary figures were apparently the same as before, but, as might be supposed, were in the opposite direction.

II. *Figures produced by pressure on the eyeball.* – If gentle pressure be exerted on the middle of the eye, a large luminous ring is seen, which, on close attention, will be found to resemble Fig. 5. It consists of numerous small oblong rectangles, obliquely arranged, and more or less bright and obscure; the sides of the figure have an oblique position, and its form is that of a rhombus with obtuse angles; the centre, as well as the space round the rhombus, is dark, but gradually becomes traversed by a luminous star (Fig. 6). The rectangles become more intensely illuminated, and after some time one of the angles is filled by a yellowish-white spot with distinct edges (Fig. 7), which progressively enlarges, and ultimately occupies the entire rhombus. In this luminous space, which is now of a bluish colour, very small circular lines are observed, which are either concentric or variously intersect each other, and seem to be in a continual glimmering fluctuation (Fig. 8): at the circumference of the rhombus there is a very narrow orange-coloured ring, and round this is occasionally seen beyond a dark interstice a larger ring of the same colour. On discontinuing the pressure, the figure successively repasses through all the metamorphoses in an inverse manner to that in which they have taken place.

When a strong pressure is made on the eye, the Fig. 9 is seen. The serpentine rays seem to proceed from the centre, and are in continual fluctuation from brightness to obscurity; after some time the black intervals between them become filled with squares (Fig. 10); the radiated figure then gradually disappears, and the square field itself terminates at last in the luminous rhombus. The pressure being still increased, the appearance represented in Fig. 11 is perceived; the luminous spots alternately appear and disappear, and during their disappearance are replaced by black spots, which again give place to the luminous ones; the larger spots, which are of a bluish tint, appear and disappear more slowly than the smaller ones, which occur nearer the centre. On continuing the pressure, the small luminous spots gradually fade away, while the larger spots near the circumference remain much longer, but they ultimately also disappear in succession: in the mean while a vague and continually fluctuating gleam has been dawning, which now develops itself into various groups of spots, rings, and squares, which after some time arrange themselves into small squares and larger hexagons (Fig. 12). To see this figure distinctly the pressure must be equal, and the eye be kept steady, for on the least motion of the eyeball a general fluctuation prevails, and no defined figure can be distinguished: sometimes curved lines are seen, which rapidly move round a centre in alternate directions. If the pressure be discontinued, luminous ramifications, the fragments of a figure which will be hereafter described, appear (Fig. 13): the appearance subsequently terminates in the luminous rhombus, &c.

When the luminous rhombus has been produced by gentle pressure, if the eye be opened and directed towards an unclouded sky, numerous parallel and converging grey semitransparent lines will be perceived, which evidently correspond to the bright oblong rectangles, and on closing the eye they again become luminous. On opening the eye during the appearance of Figs. 9 and 10, the daylight is at the first moment invisible: suddenly the figure bursts, as it were, at the centre, rapidly opens towards the circumference, and at last entirely disappears. If the eye be opened when Fig. 12 has been produced by strong pressure, twenty seconds sometimes elapse before the daylight can be seen, and even then it is obscured for a considerable time by opaque lines and spots.

Similar figures to those produced from pressure, particularly the rectangles, are produced by impeded circulation through the brain, violent exertions, and the use of narcotics; they appear also during fainting fits, strong mental emotions, &c.

Dr. Purkinje institutes a comparison between the above and acoustic figures, and concludes that both phenomena are objectively identical: the primary rectangular, &c., figures he considers to be analogous to the small reticulated undulations communicated from a sounding plate to the surface of a liquid; the secondary ones to those which are caused by the intersection of the undulations.

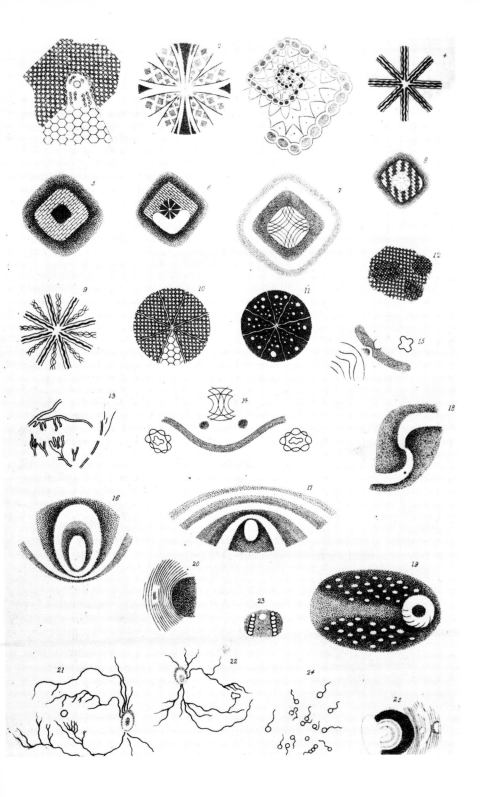

He does not, however, state where he conceives this undulatory motion to be: probably they arise in the humours of the eye, and are thence communicated to the retina; but he speaks only of a contraction of the eyeball as its immediate cause. The luminous rhombus he considers to be caused by the lens; the Fig. 13 by the central vessels of the eye, &c.

III. We come now to some most interesting experiments, viz., those concerning the *luminous figures produced by galvanism.* These experiments were made with a pile of twenty pairs of copper and zinc plates, and layers of cloth dipped in a solution of muriate of ammonia. The pile was constructed in the following manner: zinc, copper, moistened cloth, zinc, copper, &c.; zinc being the undermost. When the eyes were shut, whilst the positive conductor was placed in the mouth, and the negative wire made to touch the middle of the forehead, Fig. 14 was perceived: it consisted of a dark arch, traversing the centre of the common field of vision, with its concavity upwards, and the extremities losing themselves imperceptibly in a lateral direction. Above the arch there was a bright violet gleam, the greatest intensity of which was towards the middle of the arch; laterally from this gleam there were two distinct dark spots, which apparently correspond with the insertions of the optic nerves: the space below the arch was also filled with a bright violet gleam, but so that the greatest intensity was seen externally, in the form of luminous roses. When, during the experiment, the right eye only was kept shut, one half only of the figure was seen, but with this difference, that the brightest point of the upper light was seen in the visual axis. When the galvanic poles were changed, the contours of the figure remained the same, but the violet light was changed into a faint yellow glare, the intensities of which were also distributed in an inverse manner, viz., the middle of the field of vision above the arch, and the lateral points below it, being darkest, and the dark points which correspond with the insertions of the optic nerves appearing as distinct bright violet-coloured spots. The direction of the transverse arch was further observed to change in a remarkable manner, according to the different places which the conductors were made to touch during the experiment. When the wire was transferred from the middle of the forehead to the bridge of the nose, the centre of the arch became depressed, and its extremities were raised; when it was carried along the lower eyelid from the inner towards the outer angle, the arch gradually became indistinct, and ultimately seemed to be divided. At the outer angle the appearance was similar to Fig. 15: the oblique and almost perpendicular direction of the arch was of course gradually changed into the former horizontal one, when the wire was carried back to its former place. During a quick repetition of shocks, there appeared, in the light places above and below the arch, parallel curved lines, alternately light and dark, which intersected each other and formed squares, but of much larger size than were observed in any of the former experiments: these squares were also, and still more distinctly, seen when the lower conductor was brought into contact with that near the eye. When, during the galvanic experiment, the eye was pressed, the luminous rhombus, &c., appeared, and nothing could be seen of the galvanic figure; when strong pressure was exerted, Figs. 21 and 22 were perceived, and on every shock the ramifications proceeded from the dark centre with a most beautiful violet-coloured light.

IV. *Nebulous striæ.* – If the eyes are well protected against external light, and the observer fixes his attention to the darkness before them, nebulous figures and glares are soon seen to arise, which at first are extremely vague and almost formless, but gradually acquire a more distinct and perceptible shape; they consist of luminous streaks with dark intervals, and move in a centripetal, transverse, or circular direction (Figs. 16, 17, 18). Their motion is rather slow, and, in Dr. Purkinje's eye, about eight seconds elapsed between the rising and disappearing of one of the transverse streaks. When the experiment was continued for a few minutes, Dr. Purkinje distinguished the following figures: –

1. A feeble glare in the middle, surrounded by dark concentric rings, and the intervals between them filled with a faint light, which gradually loses itself in the darkness of the rings; the whole figure is in continual centripetal motion, the gleam of light in the middle gradually fades and makes room for the shade of the next ring, which, having now become a dark spot, also disappears, &c.
2. At other times the light comes from above as a large horizontal luminous streak (Fig. 17); it slowly moves downwards, and, on approaching towards the middle, its lateral ends bend until they unite and form a luminous ring, which is then dissolved into darkness, as in the preceding case.
3. The luminous streak comes from below and moves upwards. Sometimes the streaks move in rather an oblique direction.
4. The appearance is as in Fig. 18, and the nebulous streak moves in a circular direction, like the sails of a windmill.

When the experiment has been continued some time, and the attention becomes exhausted, all regular appearances dissolve themselves into a fluctuation between light and obscurity, which ultimately terminates in a feeble gleam covered as it were by a veil.

V. The following is another instance of subjective vision. When the eyes are fixed on a large illuminated surface (a white wall, a regularly clouded sky, &c.), the observer sees, after a few seconds, bright points suddenly starting up in the midst of the field of vision; they rapidly disappear, making room for black spots, which also quickly dissolve. If, after the appearance of the bright points, the eyes are shut or directed to a dark surface, the phenomenon continues; but in a milder light the bright appearances are changed into a feeble glimmer. The bright points are also seen when the eyes are shut before they have appeared.

VI. *Place of insertion of the optic nerve.* – It was first shewn experimentally by Mariotte, and was afterwards mathematically ascertained by Euler and Bernoulli, that the image of an object disappears in that point of the field of vision which corresponds with the insertion of the optic nerve. Besides this, there are some other circumstances under which objects within the field of vision will disappear. If a number of black dots are made on an equally illuminated surface, with one of them in the middle, and the eye is fixed to the central dot, an indistinct nebulous floating begins, and some of the dots, sometimes all of them, alternately disappear and reappear, whilst the light ground on which they are marked remains unaltered.

That the place of insertion of the optic nerve is not entirely insensible to light, as has been sometimes stated, appears from the following simple experiment: If a small flame be placed in the projection of that part of the field of vision which corresponds to the insertion of the optic nerve, it will directly disappear, but in its stead a beautiful red nimbus is seen; if the flame is slightly moved in a lateral direction, upwards, or downwards, there appears in the opposite side of the nimbus a dark gap, which spreads parabolically downwards or upwards, and the margin of which is coloured with the light of the flame. If the flame is moved in a small circle, the shade also shews a circular motion, being always opposite to that of the flame.

VII. If the eye, being well covered, is quickly turned outwards, a large luminous ring (Fig. 19) will be seen, the light of which is in a constant glimmering fluctuation: this phenomenon is particularly striking in the morning, immediately after awaking, and then, besides the luminous orb, the entire field of vision, but particularly the upper and lower parts of it, is filled with large equidistant sparks. The central area of the orb appears of a grey colour if, during the experiment, the eyes are open and directed towards a white surface; and of a deep-blue colour if they are shut and directed towards the sun. If, during the experiment, the eye is directed to any other colour, the inner surface of the ring is not of the complementary, but of the same colour, though rather deeper. Round the luminous orb, towards the centre of the field of vision, there are concentric bright streaks with dark intervals (Fig. 20). It appears that the luminous orb is produced by the nerve being forcibly stretched by the rapid lateral motions of the eye.

VIII. Another very interesting experiment is the following. If a flame, at about two or three inches distance, is slowly moved before the right eye in various directions, Fig. 21 appears painted as it were in the luminous area round the flame. The vessels, for such they evidently appear to be, seem to proceed from the insertion of the optic nerve, and consist of two upper and two lower principal branches, which are variously ramified towards the middle of the field of vision, where a dark point is seen, which sometimes appears concave. A similar, but inverted figure is perceived in the left eye; but to Dr. Purkinje, who is weak-sighted in this eye, it appeared rather irregular and incomplete (Fig. 22). The origin of the vessels is a dark oval spot, with a light areola; the figure itself, or rather fragments of it, are seen under various other circumstances. As was observed above, there can be no doubt that the figure is formed by the central vessels of the retina.*

* This is an easy experiment to repeat, and is certainly a singularly beautiful one; the blood-vessels of the retina, with all their ramifications, are distinctly seen projected, as it were, on a plane without the eye, and greatly magnified. I have found the experiment to succeed more perfectly when, the eye being stedfastly directed forwards, the light is made to move right and left below the eye, or upwards and downwards at the side of the eye; for when the flame is in the field of view the image is indistinct; the eyelids of the unemployed eye should not be closed, but the light should be obstructed by the hand or any other covering. It is indispensable that the light be in motion, for directly it becomes stationary the image breaks into fragments and disappears: during the motion of the light the image also moves, and in a contrary direction to that of the light. No image arises when the light moves to and from the eye, nor when it is alternately shaded and uncovered; the effect, therefore, cannot be attributed to variations of intensity in the light. One of the most remarkable circumstances of this phenomenon is that at the point corresponding to the projection of the foramen centrale, a crescent-formed image is occasionally observed; its appearance depends on the position of the light with respect to the axis of the eye: for instance, when the light is placed below the eye, the image appears on looking downwards, and becomes obliterated on looking upwards, and in general it appears on looking towards the light, and disappears on looking from it: the mark always appears concave in the direction opposite to the light. That the variable mark just mentioned is in the centre of distinct vision I ascertained by the following experiment: I impressed on my eye the spectrum of a coloured wafer, by looking intently on a black dot at its centre; on causing then the vascular image to appear, I saw the centre of the spectrum coincide with that of the mark. Dr. Purkinje has given no explanation of this phenomenon; the following is an endeavour to supply the omission. Were the blood-vessels which are spread on the anterior surface of the retina entirely opaque, they would prevent the transmission of light to the nervous matter beneath them, and their distribution would be constantly visible; but they are transparent, and in ordinary cases the intensity of the light which passes through them does not materially differ from that which falls directly on the retina. When, however, the retina is fatigued by a strong light, the veins become visible, because the retina is rendered insusceptible to a portion of the light they transmit; but this effect is only momentary, for those parts which are thus shaded from the more intense light promptly recover their usual susceptibility, and the images vanish: but they may again be made perceptible by displacing them on the retina; and by making them constantly change their places the images may be rendered permanent. The momentary appearance of these images may be frequently observed on looking at a strong light immediately after waking in the morning, and may be reproduced several times by successively shutting and opening the eyes. The mark in the middle of the field of vision is most probably a shadow, occasioned by a slight convexity or concavity in the retina at that point.

The more minute vessels of the retina may be rendered visible in the following manner: place as near to the eye as possible a plate of ground glass, and upon its external surface lay a card, in which a large pinhole has been made; adjust this aperture so that it shall be in a right line drawn from the eye to the flame of a candle. When the card is kept in motion so as to displace continually the image of the light in a small degree (*vide* Scheiner's experiments), the veins will be seen distributed as above, but they will now appear brighter than before, and the spaces between the ramifications will be seen filled with innumerable minute tortuous vessels, which were in the former experiment invisible: in the very centre of the field of vision there is a small circle, in which no traces of them appear, and in the centre of this circle is seen a darker point. The same appearance will be seen by moving a pinhole close to the eye when looking at a ground-glass window-pane, an illuminated white wall, or a sheet of paper. The absence of vessels at the centre of the retina will probably account for the greater distinctness with

VIII. Dr. Purkinje has made numerous experiments on what are generally called ocular spectra, *viz.*, the images which remain after objects have been regarded for some time; he gives a more detailed account of them than we believe is elsewhere to be found, and the following extract will, we trust, be read with interest.

1. Looking stedfastly for a very short time at the flame of a candle, then quickly covering the eye, the bright image of the flame remains, but instantly disappears from the circumference towards the centre, leaving red shining flame, which becomes invisible in the same manner, and is replaced by a white image; this also, though rather slowly, fades away, and after having completely disappeared, leaves a dark coloured contour of the flame with a greyish nimbus, which ultimately enlarges towards the centre, and thus terminates the whole appearance. If, at the beginning of the experiment, the eye, instead of being covered, is directed towards a white surface, the first two images of the flame are the same, but the former white spectrum is now of a dark grey colour with a white margin. The same appearances are obtained when the flame has been regarded for a longer time, except that the metamorphoses take place more slowly, and the proportion between the time during which the flame has been looked at, and the duration of the spectrum remains always the same, *viz.*, about 1 : 20.

2. When the flame has been stedfastly looked at for a much longer time (from twelve seconds to a minute) the succession of the images is nearly the same as in the first experiment, except that the bright and coloured ones rather predominate. First the bright image of the flame is seen, then the yellow, red, blue, white, and black images follow, and the whole appearance is ultimately covered by the grey gleam, as in the above case. All the images disappear in a

---

which small objects are there seen, and also for the difference of colour observed by anatomists in that part of the nervous expansion.

The following experiment, as well as the preceding, is original, both having been observed by myself in attempting to verify the discoveries of Purkinje. In the ordinary circumstances of vision, particles floating in the humours of the eye, or specks in the cornea or crystalline lens, are invisible, because their shadows are projected by different rays of light on every part of the retina, thus permitting no distinct image of them to be formed; but they may be rendered visible by allowing only a single ray of light to fall on the eye through a hole made in a card by a very fine needle, and placing the light and aperture so that the object within the eye may be in a right line with them and the centre of the retina: they may be projected on any part of the retina, but they will be most distinctly seen at this point of most perfect vision. I have thus observed, in my own eye, collections of transparent globules which, from their free motions, evidently exist in the humours; and one remarkable spot (in my left eye), which, from its permanence, must be either in the cornea or the lens; after winking, the secretion from the lacrymal ducts is also very obvious.

These experiments may probably afford to the oculist a means of ascertaining, from the direct observation of his patient, various morbid changes in the retina and lenticular apparatus of the eye. – C. W.

centripetal direction, the first much more rapidly than the others, the black remaining visible for the longest time. During the experiment, fragments of the vascular figure are frequently observed; they are of the same colour as the image in which they are perceived.

3. If the sun or the focus of a lens has been stedfastly regarded for a short time, a bright white image remains, and lasts for a considerable time; the coloured spectra then appear, and follow each other in rapid succession.

4. If the windows be regarded on a cloudy day for about twenty seconds, and the eyes be then quickly covered, at first the panes are seen white and the frame black, but the former rapidly change into black and the latter into white; and after a repetition of these changes four or five times, the whole appearance is dissolved in a grey gleam.

IX. Very different from the ocular spectra are what might perhaps be called the mental spectra, viz., the images of objects before the internal eye, (if the expression may be allowed,) after they are inaccessible to the external sense, as for instance, during winking, or whilst shutting the eyes during meditation. They seem to depend entirely on the observer's will and attention, and may even be recalled after having completely disappeared: this is, in fact, a memory peculiar to one particular sense, and thus far, perhaps, the purest instance of *subjective* vision. The ocular spectrum goes through its regular metamorphoses; and so far from its distinctness being proportionate to the observer's attention, it is most prominent if his look only is fixed to the object – his thoughts being otherwise engaged. The ocular spectrum further follows the rotation of the eye, whilst in the mental spectrum the objects maintain their real position, independent of the motions of the eye and the body. Narcotic and spirituous substances, an excited state of mind, some febrile diseases, congestions towards the brain, &c., appear to augment the permanence and clearness of the mental spectra; that of the ocular spectra is increased during a nervous asthenic state, &c.

X. Dr. Purkinje says, 'I am standing before a white surface, and direct my eyes as if I were looking at a very near object. I perceive in the midst of the field of vision a white transparent circle, with a brownish, semitransparent area, and an indistinct border. If I now discontinue the effort, the brownish area disappears, and the white surface is at its circumference brighter than anywhere else. If, whilst the effort continues, a slight lateral pressure is made on the eyes, the area becomes opaque, of a dark-brown colour, and lined at its outer side with a light violet semitransparent border; the white circle in the midst continues, but on increased pressure a brown central point is seen in it. If the eye is closed, and well secured against external light, the circle in the middle appears dark, and the brown colour of the area is changed into a feeble gleam.'

During this experiment the brownish area sometimes presents a peculiar phenomenon, which, according to Dr. Purkinje, is the circulation of the eye becoming visible, in the shape of a series of globules (Fig. 23) on each side of the white circle, ascending on the left and descending on the right side. The 'mouches volantes,' Dr. Purkinje is inclined to consider as depending on the same cause: they are best seen if, after violent exertion, the eyes are steadily directed towards a white equally illuminated surface, as the clouded sky, or a snow-field; a large quantity of bright points (Fig. 24) are then seen, which, like shooting stars, suddenly arise and disappear after a rapid motion, in various straight and curved lines. On close attention, it will be found that every light point is accompanied by a shade at the opposite side of the field of vision, and that also between the small, larger but less bright points are slowly moving. These larger points are very distinctly seen after violent exertion, particularly after lifting a weight: they move from the extreme margin of the field of vision towards the middle, and are in a straight or bent direction, always accompanied by a shade at the opposite side; the nearer they come to the middle, the less distinct and shining do they appear, and the less dark are their shadows. As they are visible only as long as the eyes are held open, and as they require a strong and equal light, in order to be seen, they must be considered as differing from the bright points described above, as far as these evidently depend on the different state of the various points of the retina, whilst phenomenon in question is caused by external bodies, with reference to the retina, viz., according to Dr. Purkinje's opinion, by free blood-globules in the aqueous humour; which, according to their different distances from the crystalline lens, are seen of different size and distinctness.

XI. *Luminous Rings.* This phenomenon, which is sufficiently known to be caused by lateral pressure on the eye, has been carefully examined by Dr. Purkinje: the following are the results of his experiments: –

1. If the observer makes an effort, as if to look at something very near, the slightest pressure produces the luminous ring; whilst, on looking at a distance, the pressure must be considerably increased.

2. The rings, as well as the places of insertion of the optic nerves, are most vivid in the morning, and the proximate cause of both phenomena appears to be identical, viz.; pressure on the retina.

3. If a piece of white paper is held in the inner angle, and whilst the eye is as much as possible directed towards it, the observer presses, with a small conical piece of wood, on the external side of the globe, near the orbit, a great number of concentric white and black lines are seen (Fig. 25), similar to the appearance of Fig. 20; they extend over the spot in the middle of the visual field (Fig. 20),

and are always parallel wherever the pressure may be exerted. On the paper there appears, at the same time, a large black circular spot, the centre of which is of a dark bluish green, or deep violet, similar to the eye of a peacock's tail, sometimes with fragments of the vascular figure (Fig. 13). That side of the spot which is directed towards the middle of the field of vision, touches at the above-mentioned parallel lines; the opposite side is bordered by a yellowish-white gleam, which, on increased pressure, reached as far as the middle of the black spot.

4. If by placing the piece of wood between the orbit and eye-lid, the pressure is exerted on the posterior point of the globe, the parallel lines are seen extending towards the middle of the field of vision, and terminating in a white semilunar streak, which, in its concavity, contains a small bright circle, and at the convex portion of which there is a brownish semilunar spot; both spots follow all the motions of the coloured eye, and turn round the centre of the field of vision as on an axis. If the pressure is increased, the coloured eye advances towards the white semilunar streak, so as to cover it entirely with the exterior of its middle portion, which remains as a white circular spot in the middle; the brown semilunar spot also disappears.

5. If the pressure on the globe is suddenly discontinued, the white circular spot as suddenly moves outwards, and in its stead a light-brown violet cloud remains, which is divided by a white streak into two parts, the upper of which is larger and darker; this cloud, especially the middle portion of it, generally remains for a considerable time, and greatly impedes clear vision.

6. The experiment in question shews also the coincidence of the two fields of vision; for if each eye is pressed at the corresponding place, the luminous rings are always seen to coincide.

7. If the eye is well covered during the experiment, the colours in the middle of the circular spot, as well as the margin round the periphery, are luminous; the concentric lines are very indistinct, and of a faint gleam, and the yellowish-white glare at the outer side of the circular spot is black. On suddenly discontinuing the pressure, a bright luminous streak flashes from the inner towards the outer side.

Dr. Purkinje has evidently bestowed much time upon these experiments. It appears from some passages in his work, that he began, even in his boyhood, to amuse himself with some of the luminous appearances therein described. The study of physiology afterwards led him to an accurate and scientific inquiry, which he even pursued at the risk of health; for, although he in one passage of his work states that his experiments had not been injurious to his sight, the circumstance of his right eye being myopic, and the left near-sighted (amblyopic,) seems almost to contradict this assertion; we ourselves cannot, after a great number of experiments which we made before and since our perusal of Dr. Purkinje's work, withhold our conviction, that their frequent repetition may be attended with dangerous effects on the eyes. On the other side, it is indispensable that the experiments should be frequently repeated and varied; for at the commencement of the inquiry the observer must be quite unaccustomed to this new field of experiment. The condition of Dr. Purkinje's sight might further raise some doubts whether some of his experiments be not the effects of a morbid state, rather than depending on the organization of the human eye.

We have not yet exhausted the experiments which this interesting pamphlet contains; some of those which are now omitted we shall have occasion to refer to in our suceeding papers.*

4.5. Wheatstone: "Contributions to the physiology of vision. No. II". *Journal of the Royal Institution*, 1831, **1**, 534–537. (Published anonymously)

On the Insensibility of the Retina to feebly-illuminated Objects, when continuously presented. – In accounting for the beautiful and extraordinary phenomenon described at page 111 of this volume, I have admitted as an established fact, that weak impressions on the retina become obliterated when rendered continuous. To confirm the explanation there offered, it will be satisfactory to adduce a few instances equally illustrative of the rule, which is only one case of a more general law, confirmed by numerous observations, viz., that *all* luminous objects, when continuously presented to the same points of the retina, become invisible; and that the rapidity of their disappearance is in proportion to the feebleness of the light emitted by or reflected from the object. Astronomers are well aware that, on looking intently at a star through a telescope, it will sometimes completely disappear, and again become visible on changing the position of the eye, so that its image may fall on another part of the retina; stars also, which, from the feebleness of the light they emit, are ordinarily invisible, may be made apparent by the same means; and if the statement of Majendie and Desmoulins be correct, stars may be thus made to appear in full daylight.†

---

* Since the preceding pages were printed, we have ascertained that the interesting experiment of § VIII, was first described by Steinbuch, in his *Physiologie der Sinne*, 1811.

† During day-time, in an unclouded sky, the light of the stars, which is but one sixty-fourth of the luminous splendour of the atmosphere, is insensible to our eyes. In general, any body projected and immoveable on a plane with which it has this same degree of luminous intensity, is invisible. But if by a displacement, either of the body upon this plane, or of the image of a star in a telescope, it is made to pass over a certain arch, repeated on the retina by the displacement of the focus of its rays, this body or the image of the star becomes visible. – (Majendie et Desmoulins, Anatomie des Systêmes Nerveux des Animaux à vertèbres. Tom, ii. p. 670.)

Dr. Brewster has described several analogous cases of the disappearance of visible objects;* and the following experiments of the late Benedict Prévost of Geneva (published posthumously in the 'Mem. de la Soc. de Phys. et d'Hist. Nat.,' t. iii. 2d part) will afford an additional instance, and will at the same time prove to us that the employment of very simple means may greatly assist our powers of observation with regard to a variety of optical phenomena, in which the feebleness of the objects might otherwise be deemed an obstacle to successful inquiry.

On an appearance of Decomposition of White Light, by the Motion of the Body which reflects it. – In a chamber sufficiently dark, into which a ray of the sun penetrates, move a rectangular piece of white card, about two inches in breadth, backwards and forwards, as if you would cut this ray nearly perpendicularly to its axis.

At the moment the white card traverses this axis, the eye which regards it evidently receives from this object a white light, as if the card remained stationary at this place. But it happens, however, that the disc, illuminated by the ray, the section of which it represents, appears coloured; it is white only in the centre. The very small white space which surrounds the centre, changes to violet, deepening as it recedes. The violet spot is surrounded by a zone of a deep indigo colour, very distinct and well defined, and exactly resembling the colour of the heart's-ease (*viola tricolor*). Around this indigo zone is a zone of greenish-yellow, equally well defined; then, surrounding it externally, a red tint. If the observer be very attentive, and seize the most favourable moments and situations, it will be seen that the white ray reflected by the disc has been decomposed, as it would have been by the prism, into seven principal colours, arranged nearly in the same order.

If a red or pink card be susbstituted for the white card, the decomposition of the ray appears still more distinctly.

If, on the contrary, a blue tinted card be employed, this decomposition is less distinct than with the white.

Besides, all these colours are subject to vary according to different circumstances, such as the velocity of the motion, the obliquity of the axis to the card which cuts it, the distance from the section to the origin, or to the base of the luminous ray, the different shades or tints of the card, the intensity of the light, &c. But there is always an apparent decomposition.

With a yellow card, a circular areola, of a more brilliant yellow than that of the card itself, is seen externally, when there is no motion.

With a black card there is no coloration, unless a nebulous shade in the centre may be so considered. Besides, it is probable that this shade arises from the black of the card being far from perfect. A card covered with black velvet did not present the slightest appearance of decomposition.

The phenomenon is observed if the card passes the ray but once; this proves that it is independent of the fatigue of the eye.

Neither does it depend immediately on the agitation or motion of the card, but doubtlessly only on some effect of this motion, most probably because the illuminated space strikes the eye during a short time only: for if the card be so large that the illuminated space always remains upon it, and that, notwithstanding the motion, the eye continues always to see it, it appears white, as if it were at rest, and there is no appearance of the decomposition of the light.

* Edinburgh Journal of Science, No. IV.

In the preceding experiments the coloured rings evidently result from the diffraction of the light at the edges of the aperture which admits the ray; the colours thus produced, being of very feeble intensity, become almost immediately invisible when constantly presented to the same part of the retina; but the intermittent action of the luminous object produces an analogous effect to the shifting of its place on the retina in the previously mentioned experiments. The explanation of these phenomena given by Prévost himself, is founded on Cuvier's theory, which supposes that the visual sensation is occasioned by the chemical action of material light on the nervous substance of the retina; and that each colour, having a different affinity for this substance, requires a different time to exert its energy upon it; but admitting for a moment this totally unsupported hypothesis, the attempted explanation does not accord with the facts of the case.

There is another case of coloration which, I believe, has not yet been noticed, and which admits of a similar explanation. If a sheet of paper, with black characters, either printed or written, be moved rapidly backwards and forwards at the ordinary distance of distinct vision, the lines described by the motion will appear accompanied by very evident colours, the green and red obviously pre-dominating. The experiment succeeds better if the lines are far apart, and perpendicular to the direction for the motion; and is still more perfect if a printed word be fixed at the extremity of a vibrating wire, (as mentioned in the description of the Kaleidophone, in the Journal of Science, N.S., No. xxiii. p. 344). This experiment indicates that there is a faint production of colours at the limits of light and darkness.

From all the known facts, it may be inferred that luminous impressions, continued on the same part of the retina, are evanescent in proportion to their feebleness; and that there are two means by which weak objects may be rendered continuously visible: 1st, by shifting their positions on the retina, and 2ndly, by causing them to act intermittently on the same points of the retina.

Though these are obvious inferences from the collected observations above stated, some of the facts separately presented might appear to admit of other explanations. Thus Majendie and Desmoulins concluded, from the circum-stances noticed by them, 'that the sum of a certain number of impressions on different points of the retina in a given time may render a body visible, which would not be so were the interval of the impressions greater, or their number not sufficient.' This explanation would answer only for a limited number of the facts now brought together, and would exclude the experiments of Prévost, where the image is periodically presented to the same part of the retina.

There are various other optical, or rather visual phenomena which equally manifest the truth of the inferences above drawn; but as they are complicated with other circumstances foreign to the present purpose, viz., illustrating the explanation formerly given of the vascular figure of the retina, the consideration of them will be deferred to a future occasion.

4.6. Brewster with appendix by Wheatstone: "On the undulations excited in the retina by the action of luminous points and lines". *Report of the British Association, Transactions of the Sections*, 1832, 548–551.

In this communication the author considers a variety of cases when light affects other parts of the retina than those on which it directly falls, – either by rendering them more or less sensible to light and particular colours, or by altering the tints which are visible there, or by the excitement of undulations in the retina from the illuminated part. The following are the results of Sir D. Brewster's experiments on the last of these phænomena, as exhibited by the action of luminous points and lines.

1. If we look through a narrow aperture, about the $^1/_{50}$th of an inch wide, at a bright part of the sky, or at the flame of a candle, we shall observe the luminous ground covered with a great number of broken parallel lines alternately light and dark. These lines are always parallel to the narrow slit, and of course change their place as the slit is moved round before the eye. Through a number of parallel slits, such as between the teeth of a comb, the broken parallel lines are seen more distinctly; and if we give the comb the motion oblique to the direction of its teeth, the broken lines become more distinct, though less straight than before, and new black lines appear, lying in different directions, as if they were detached portions of a number of dark ramifications. All these phænomena are seen more distinctly when we look at homogeneous light. If we use two systems of narrow slits, and cross them at different angles, we shall perceive two systems of broken lines crossing each other at the same angles; and if when the lines of the two systems are parallel we give one of them a rapid alternating motion perpendicular to the direction of its slits, the parallel broken fringes are seen with peculiar distinctness.

2. Phænomena analogous to those now described may be seen by looking at a number of parallel black lines drawn upon white paper, such as those which represent the sea in an engraved map, or by looking at the luminous intervals in a number of parallel wires seen against the sky. If the eye looks at any of these objects steadily and continuously, the black lines soon lose their straightness and their parallelism, and inclose luminous spaces somewhat like the links of a number of broken chains. When this change takes place, the eye which sees it experiences a good deal of uneasiness, – an effect which is communicated also to the eye which is shut. When this dazzling effect takes place, the luminous spaces between the broken lines become coloured, some with yellow and others with green and blue light.

The phænomena produced in these two experiments are obviously owing to *rectilineal undulations propagated across the retina*; and the interference and crossing of the undulations, by which the dark lines are broken into detached portions, and by which the colours are produced, arise from the unsteadiness of the head or the hand, which causes a want of parallelism in the successive undulations.

3. The action of small and bright points of light upon the retina produces phænomena of a very interesting kind. If we look at the sun through a small aperture at a great distance from the eye, or if we look at the diminutive image of the sun formed by a convex lens or a concave mirror, or seen in a convex surface, the light which falls upon the retina does not form a sharp and definite image of the luminous point, but it sends out in all directions an infinity of radiations, covering in some cases almost the whole retina. These radiations are extremely bright, and are accompanied in some cases by mottled colours of great variety and beauty. The bright point of light propagates around it circular undulations, which are broken and coloured by interference, and which, being in constant motion from the centre of the retina in all directions, occasion the radiations which have been mentioned.

4. If we look at the radiant image just described through a narrow aperture, a very singular effect is produced. A vortex of circular rays appears on each side of the radiant point, and the rays have a rapid whirling motion. The line joining the centres of the two vortices is always perpendicular to the narrow aperture. This remarkable configuration of the rays is evidently produced by the union of a system of parallel undulations with a system of circular ones, the intersections of the parallel fringes and the diverging radiations forming the circular rays, as in the case of ordinary caustics.

The preceding phænomena, continues the author, whatever be their true cause, clearly prove that light incident upon the retina exerts an action on parts of it upon which it does not directly fall, and that the same action renders other parts of the retina insensible to the light which actually falls upon these parts.

Upon this principle the author explains the experiments of Mr. T. Smith of Fochabers, in which the same object appeared, under certain conditions of vision, of different colours to the different eyes, the colour observed by the one eye being complementary to that observed by the other. He also refers to the same general principle of undulations propagated across the retina, for an explanation of the remarkable experiment on the eye, first made known by Dr. Purkinje of Breslau.

In this experiment, if a candle be held before one eye, at about a foot distance, and in a direction deviating a little from the line of distinct vision, – that eye sees a general mass of reddish light around the candle, and in this light, as a ground, are seen the ramifying blood-vessels of the retina, the base of the optic nerve, and the *foramen centrale*. Sir D. Brewster states it to be the most prevalent opinion, that the light which surrounds the candle is reflected back upon the retina, either by the inner concave surface of the crystalline lens or of the cornea; and that the objects are, somehow or other, magnified by these concave surfaces. His own view of the subject is, that the light was propagated from the luminous image of the candle, and that though the retina, in contact with the blood-vessels, is sensible to direct light, it is insensible to propagated light, and therefore the blood-vessels must be delineated in obscure lines. As there is no retina across the *foramen centrale*, it will of course appear as a black spot; and, owing to the obtuse vision of the optic nerve, it will appear less luminous than the surrounding retina.

After the reading of Sir David Brewster's paper, Mr. Wheatstone said, that having been the first person to introduce Purkinje's beautiful experiment into this country, and having repeated it a great number of times under a variety of forms, he would take the opportunity of stating a few particulars respecting it, which appeared not to be generally known. – The experiment succeeds best in a dark room, when, one eye being excluded from the light, the flame of a candle is placed by the side of the unshaded eye, but so as not to occupy any of the central part of the field of view. So long as the flame of the candle remains stationary, nothing further occurs than a diminution of the sensibility of the retina to light; but after the flame has been moved upwards and downwards, through a small space, for a length of time, varying with the susceptibility of the individual on whom the experiment is tried, the phænomenon presents itself. The blood-vessels of the retina, with all their ramifications, exactly as represented in the engravings of Sœmmerring, are distinctly seen, apparently projected on a plane before the eye, and greatly magnified. The image continues only while the flame is in motion; directly, or soon after, the flame becomes stationary, it dissolves into fragments and disappears.

Mr. Wheatstone dissented from the ingenious explanation of this appearance offered by Sir David Brewster, and also from that opinion stated to be the generally received one; and begged to repeat the solution he had published, and which he had not since been induced to relinquish. Mr. W. observed, that there was no difficulty in accounting for the image; it evidently was a shadow resulting from the obstruction of light by the blood-vessels spread over the retina; the real difficulty was to explain why this shadow is not always visible. To account for this, Mr. W. adduced several facts, which tended to prove *that an object, either more or less luminous than the ground on which it is placed, when continuously presented to the same point of the retina, becomes invisible; and the rapidity of its disappearance is greater as the difference of luminous intensity between the object and the ground is less; but by continually shifting the place of the image of the object on the retina, or by making it act intermittently on the same point, the object may be rendered permanently visible.* To apply this explanation to the phænomenon in question, Mr. W. observed, that whenever the flame of the candle changes its place, the shadows of the vessels fall on different parts of the retina; which is evident from the motion of the figure while the eye remains still, which is always in a contrary direction to that of the flame. Hence the shadow, being thus made to change its place on the retina, remains, according to the law above stated, permanently visible; but instantly the flame is at rest, the shadow also becomes stationary, and consequently disappears.

Mr. Wheatstone then exhibited an instrument for showing an original variation of this experiment: it consisted of a circular plate of metal, about two inches in diameter, blackened at its outer side, and perforated at its centre with an aperture about as large as an ordinary gun-hole; to the inner face was fixed a similar plate of ground glass. On placing the aperture between the eye and the flame of a candle, and keeping the plate in motion, so as to displace continually the image of the aperture on the retina, the blood-vessels will be seen distributed as before, but will now appear brighter, and the spaces between the ramifications will be seen filled with innumerable minute vessels, anastomosing with each other in every direction, which were invisible in the former experiment. In the very centre of the field of vision there is a small circular space, in which no traces of these vessels appear. Mr. W. remarked, that the absence of these minute obstructions to light will probably account for the greater distinctness with which small objects are there seen, and also the difference of colour observed by anatomists in that spot of the retina.

4.7. Brewster: "Observations on the supposed vision of the blood-vessels of the eye". *London and Edinburgh Philosophical Magazine and Journal of Science*, 1834, **4**, 115–120.*

In the Number of this Journal for September 1832, I had occasion to refer to the remarkable experiment described by Dr. Punkinje of Breslau, in which the blood-vessels of the retina are supposed to be exhibited; and though I had in vain tried to see this phænomenon, yet it had been so accurately described to me by Mr. Potter that I ventured to give an opinion respecting its cause. The paper which contained this explanation was read at the Physical section of the British Association at Oxford in June 1832, and Mr. Wheatstone, who was present, favoured the Meeting with some excellent observations on the subject. These observations have been printed in the Report of the Association for 1832, in the form of an Appendix to the abstract of my paper; and as they are highly interesting, and will form the groundwork of the following observations, I shall give them *verbatim*.

> After the reading of Sir David Brewster's paper, Mr. Wheatstone said, that having been the first person to introduce Purkinje's beautiful experiment into this country,

* See Lond. and Edinb. Phil. Mag., last Number, p. 43, and also vol. i, p. 318.

and having repeated it a great number of times under a variety of forms, he would take the opportunity of stating a few particulars respecting it, which appeared not to be generally known. The experiment succeeds best in a dark room, when, one eye being excluded from the light, the flame of a candle is placed by the side of the unshaded eye, but so as not to occupy any of the central part of the field of view. So long as the flame of the candle remains stationary, nothing further occurs than a diminution of the sensibility of the retina to light; but after the flame has been moved upwards and downwards, through a small space, for a length of time, varying with the susceptibility of the individual on whom the experiment is tried, the phænomenon presents itself. The blood-vessels of the retina, with all their ramifications, exactly as represented in the engravings of Sœmmerring, are distinctly seen, apparently projected on a plane before the eye, and greatly magnified. The image continues only while the flame is in motion: directly, or soon after, the flame becomes stationary, it dissolves into fragments and disappears.

Mr. Wheatstone dissented from the ingenious explanation of this appearance offered by Sir David Brewster, and also from that opinion stated to be the generally received one; and begged to repeat the solution he had published, and which he had not since been induced to relinquish. Mr. W. observed, that there was no difficulty in accounting for the image; it evidently was a shadow resulting from the obstruction of light by the blood-vessels spread over the retina; the real difficulty was to explain why this shadow is not always visible. To account for this, Mr. W. adduced several facts, which tended to prove *that an object, either more or less luminous than the ground on which it is placed, when continuously presented to the same point of the retina, becomes invisible; and the rapidity of its disappearance is greater as the difference of luminous intensity between the object and the ground is less; but by continually shifting the place of the image of the object on the retina, or by making it act intermittently on the same point, the object may be rendered permanently visible.* To apply this explanation to the phænomenon in question, Mr. W. observed, that whenever the flame of the candle changes its place, the shadows of the vessels fall on different parts of the retina; which is evident from the motion of the figure while the eye remains still, which is always in a contrary direction to that of the flame. Hence the shadow, being thus made to change its place on the retina, remains, according to the law above stated, permanently visible; but instantly the flame is at rest, the shadow also becomes stationary, and consequently disappears.

Mr. Wheatstone then exhibited an instrument for showing an original variation of this experiment: it consisted of a circular plate of metal, about two inches in diameter, blackened at its outer side, and perforated at its centre with an aperture about as large as an ordinary gun-hole; to the inner face was fixed a similar plate of ground glass. On placing the aperture between the eye and the flame of a candle, and keeping the plate in motion, so as to displace continually the image of the aperture on the retina, the blood-vessels will be seen distributed as before, but will now appear brighter, and the spaces between the ramifications will be seen filled with innumerable minute vessels, anastomosing with each other in every direction, which were invisible in the former experiment. In the very centre of the field of vision there is a small circular space, in which no traces of these vessels appear. Mr. W. remarked, that the absence of these minute obstructions to light will probably account for the greater distinctness with which small objects are there seen, and also for the difference of colour observed by anatomists in that spot of the retina.

In this experiment Mr. Wheatstone has described, 1st, the common method of seeing the blood-vessels, and 2ndly, an original variation of the experiment by which the blood-vessels are seen much more distinctly and completely.

As Mr. Wheatstone was so kind as to lend me, when at Oxford, his plate of metal, &c., I was enabled to see the very phænomenon which he saw, and I have repeated the experiment fifty times since under many modifications. I have therefore no hesitation in asserting that the *ramifications* exhibited by Mr. Wheatstone's apparatus *are not blood-vessels*, but are nothing more than the ramifications described in my paper already referred to (Lond. and Edinb. Phil. Mag., vol. i. p. 170. §. 1.). If we throw aside the ground glass in Mr. Wheatstone's apparatus, and look at a luminous surface through the circular aperture when moved as he describes, the same phænomenon will be seen; and if we substitute a rectilineal aperture, and make the line of motion perpendicular, or nearly so, to its longest sides, the phænomena will be seen still more distinctly; and if we look through one or more narrow slits, as in my experiment, the effect will be the same. In short, the edges of the circular aperture in Mr. Wheatstone's apparatus perpendicular to the line in which the aperture is moved, perform the part of the rectilineal slit or slits in my experiment. Mr. Wheatstone will have no difficulty in recognising the perfect identity of the two experiments, and he will therefore see that the ramifications are nothing more than the new forms given to the luminous and dark parallel lines produced by the action of light upon the retina. In order to demonstrate this, let us use Mr. Wheatstone's own apparatus. The general direction of the ramifications is invariably perpendicular to the direction in which the aperture is moved. If we change this direction from a horizontal to a vertical line the ramifications change their direction also, so that we can give them any inclination we please. They cannot, therefore, be pictures or representations of any blood-vessels in the eye.

This unequivocal result would have induced me to believe that the ramifications seen by the common method had a similar origin, and were owing to the action of the rectilineal sides of the flame upon the retina, had I not succeeded in seeing this phænomenon with my own eyes. At the Observatory of Cambridge, last summer, Sir John Herschel pointed out to Mr. Airy and myself the method by which he saw the ramifications, and we were all successful in observing the same phænomenon. This method scarcely differed from that described by Mr. Wheatstone, but the ramifications which I saw were *toto cœlo* different from those produced by Mr. Wheatstone's apparatus: they had not, indeed, one property in common but that of *ramifying.* The one was seen with great difficulty and occasionally in the middle of a brownish red light, which *did not proceed directly from the candle*; while the other was distinctly and continuously seen in the middle of condensed light *proceeding directly* from the candle or other luminous body.

Regarding, therefore, the phænomenon as real, and the ramifications as occasioned by a blood-vessel of the retina, I shall proceed to examine the different explanations that have been given of it.

The explanation given by Mr. Wheatstone is exceedingly ingenious; and the principle which he lays down, and which is printed in Italics, is in every respect well founded. This property of the retina, by which it is unable to maintain the continued visibility of an object seen *obliquely*, or at a distance from the axis of vision, was communicated by me to the Royal Society of Edinburgh on the 19th of January 1818, and has since appeared in several elementary works on optics; and it is a necessary corollary from the law of oblique vision, that any movement of the object must restore its visibility by removing the cause of its disappearance, namely, the continued action of the light upon the retina.

So far, therefore, Mr. Wheatstone's explanation is unimpeachable; but when he states that the motion of the flame causes *the shadows of the vessels to fall on different parts of the retina*, we can no longer follow him. Unless the blood-vessel is placed at a certain distance *in front of the retina*, and consequently in the vitreous humour, it can have no *moving* shadow; and unless it is within the refracted cone of rays which proceed from the candle, it can have no shadow either moveable or stationary. If the shadow here referred to, be the shadow produced from the direct light of the candle, then the blood-vessel would appear across the visible flame of the candle, and not at the side of it in the reddish brown light. But independent of these objections to the application of the optical principle previously laid down, there are two facts which appear to be conclusive against the explanation: the one is, that the blood-vessels of the retina are not at a distance from it; and the other, that the ramifications may be seen distinctly when the candle is not in motion.* There is one objection more to this explanation, which appears to me a formidable one: the ramifications ought to be distinctly and readily seen when the light which forms the shadow is reduced to the same state of dilution, and the same colour, as the reddish brown light on which they appear. This experiment I have repeatedly made with light of all degrees of dilution and divergency, but I have never been able to see a trace of the ramifications.

If the ramifications in question are the representation of a blood-vessel, it becomes very interesting to ascertain the cause to which their visibility is owing. The first step in the inquiry is obviously to determine the origin of the reddish brown light in which the phænomenon is seen. It is quite clear that the brown

---

* The force of this last objection will depend on the circumstances of the case. Mr. Wheatstone says that the image "continues only while the flame is in motion," and that "directly, or soon after, the flame becomes stationary, it dissolves into fragments and disappears." Now if this is a phænomenon of oblique vision, the image ought not to disappear permanently. One part of it should disappear while another part remains visible, and the whole may for a short time continue invisible; but it will soon reappear, because it would require great steadiness, both in the hand and head of the observer, to keep the shadow on the same part of the retina, though even this would not ensure its permanent invisibility. If this, therefore, were a phænomenon of indirect vision, the difficulty would consist in losing sight of the ramifications, whereas the difficulty really consists in seeing them; and this difficulty is so great with me, that I have never been able to see them again since I saw them at Cambridge.

light is no part of the cone of refracted rays that proceed from the candle: it is equally clear that it is not produced by two or more reflections from the curved surfaces which bound any of the humours of the eye, because in this case it would be of the same colour with the light of the candle: and I have besides ascertained that it has no focus; for if it had, it would expand and contract by any variation in the distance of the candle. It cannot proceed from any imperfect transparency in any of the coats or humours of the eye, because it is seen in eyes that have the most pure and perfect vision. It must, therefore, be light produced by a physio-logical action, or light propagated from, or induced by, the direct image of the candle upon the retina; and if this is the case, the explanation which I formerly gave of the phænomenon is likely to be the true one. The blood-vessels touching the retina will deaden, as it were, the part of the retina which they touch, or make it less sensible to the propagated light, and hence the blood-vessels will appear delineated in a fainter light than that which surrounds them. The distinctness with which the ramifications will thus be seen will vary with the intensity of the brown light, with the ever changing sensibility of the retina, and with the varying pressure of the blood-vessels themselves. If I could command the vision of these ramifications as Mr. Wheatstone can, it would not be difficult to institute experiments by which the preceding explanation could be cross-examined; and I therefore hope that he will resume the subject in reference to the facts and views which I have ventured to state.

Before concluding this notice I may mention, as connected with the subject, some curious phænomena which appear when we throw a condensed beam of light upon the retina so as to fill the whole eye. This may be done by holding near the eye a convex lens, about an inch in diameter, and an inch or so in focal length, so as to see its whole area filled with the light of a candle or lamp. If we move the lens backwards and forwards quickly, looking steadily at one point of the field, we shall see on each side of the axis of vision the ramifications described in my former paper and in the preceding pages. There are none of them visible within a certain space round the axis of vision; but in the axis of vision there is an irregularly illuminated or shaded circular spot, obviously corresponding to the *foramen centrale* of the retina; and in this spot, and for some distance round it, is seen a sort of network pattern, delineated in dark lines. This pattern* has sometimes all the regularity of one formed geometrically, with dark spots in the centre of each area, and the ground on which the pattern is seen is generally of a faint purple colour. But, what is more remarkable, the luminous field is crossed by exceedingly faint bands of red and green light perpendicular to the direction of the motion.

When the eye has not been fatigued by light, the luminous ground on which

---

* The very same phænomenon is seen, though less distinctly, when we look steadily at the moving or *flaring* summit of the flame of a candle.

these phænomena are seen has a minutely granular appearance; and by the continued action of the light an apparent effervescence appears over the whole, as if each grain of light, or the minute spaces between the grains, were becoming more or less luminous in succession.

Belleville, Dec. 18, 1833.

4.8. Brewster: "On the effect of compression and dilatation upon the retina". *London and Edinburgh Philosophical Magazine and Journal of Science*, 1832, 1, 89–92.*

The production of light by a gentle pressure upon the eyeball, or by a sudden stroke upon the eye, is a fact which has been long known, but which, so far as I know, has never been carefully examined. In the sixteenth Query, at the end of his Optics, Sir Isaac Newton describes the fact, and reasons upon it in the following manner:

> When a man in the dark presses either corner of his eye with his finger, and turns his eye away from his finger, he will see a circle of colours like those in the feather of a peacock's tail. If the eye and the finger remain quiet these colours vanish in a second, but if the finger be moved with a quavering motion they appear again. Do not these colours arise from such motions excited in the bottom of the eye by the pressure and motion of the finger, as at other times are excited there by light for causing vision? And do not the motions once excited continue about a second of time before they cease? And when a man by a stroke upon his eye sees a flash of light, are not the like motions excited in the retina by the stroke? And when a coal of fire moved nimbly in the circumference of a circle makes the whole circumference appear like a circle of fire, is it not because the motions excited in the bottom of the eye by the rays of light are of a lasting nature, and continue till the coal of fire in going round returns to its former place? And, considering the lastingness of the motions excited in the bottom of the eye by light, are they not of a vibrating nature?

The circle of light referred to in this passage always appears opposite to the point of pressure, and its centre has the same visible direction as that of a ray of light incident on the centre of the compressed portion of the retina. The reason why the phænomenon is best seen by turning the eye away from the finger is, that the retina is thus brought under the point of pressure; for if the eye remains at rest, or is turned towards the finger, the luminous circle is either imperfectly seen or disappears altogether, because the finger then presses, either wholly or partly, upon a part of the eyeball beneath which the retina does not extend. Sir Isaac Newton is mistaken in saying, "that the colours vanish in a second when the eye and the finger remain quiet." They undoubtedly continue as long as the pressure

* Read before the British Association at Oxford, June 22, 1832.

is kept up; and in proof of this I may mention a case which I had occasion particularly to study, in which the patient constantly saw the luminous circle, in consequence of an excrescence on the inside of the eyelid, which produced a continued pressure on the eyeball.

Sir Isaac Newton has not named the colours which he saw in the luminous circle, any further than by saying that they are like those in the feather of a peacock's tail. Although I have made the experiment a thousand times, under all varieties of circumstances, I have never been able to observe any other circles but *black* and *white* ones, with the exception of a general *red* tinge which is seen when the eyelids are closed, and which is produced by the light which passes through them.

When a gentle pressure is first applied so as to compress slightly the fine pulpy substance of the retina, a circular spot of colourless light is produced, though the eye is in total darkness, and has not been exposed to light for many hours. If light is now admitted to the eye, the compressed part of the retina is more sensible to the light than any other part, and consequently appears more luminous. Hence it follows, *that a slight compression of the retina increases its sensibility to the light which falls upon it, and creates a sensation of light when the eye is in absolute darkness.*

If we now increase the pressure, the circular spot of light gradually becomes darker, and at last black, and is surrounded with a bright luminous ring of light. By augmenting the pressure still more, a luminous spot appears in the middle of the central dark one, and another luminous spot diametrically opposite, and beneath the point of pressure. Considering the eye as an elastic sphere filled with incompressible fluids, it is obvious that a ring of fluid will rise round the point depressed by the finger, and that its pressure from within outwards will *dilate* the part of the retina under the finger which was formerly compressed, and will compress all that part of the retina in contact with the elevated ring. An increase of pressure will be resisted by the opposite part of the retina, and will thus produce a compression at both extremities of the axis of pressure, occasioning the diametrically opposite spot of light, and also the luminous spot in the middle of the circular black space. Hence we conclude, *that when the retina is dilated under exposure to light it becomes absolutely blind, or insensible to all luminous impressions.*

These properties of the retina often exhibit themselves involuntarily when the body is in a state of perfect health. When we move the eyeball by the action of its own muscles, the retina is affected beneath the place where the muscles pull the eyeball; and there may be seen opposite each eye and towards the nose two semicircles or crescents of light; and other two extremely faint towards the temples. At particular times when the retina is more sensible than at others, these crescents become complete circles or rings of light. From the same cause, in the act of sneezing, gleams of light are emitted from each eye, during both the inhalation of the air and its subsequent expulsion; and in blowing air violently through the nostrils two patches of light appear above the axis of the eye, and in front of it; while other two luminous spots unite into one, and appear about the point of the nose, when the eyes are turned in that direction.

The phænomena which have been described are those produced by the parts of the retina which are most affected by any given pressure; but it is obvious that this pressure is propagated over the whole retina; – and it is a curious fact, that though this pressure is too weak to produce a luminous impression, it has yet power to modify other impressions previously made upon the membrane. If, from looking at the sun, the eye sees a *pinkish-brown* spectrum, a pressure upon another part of the retina will change it to a *green* spectrum; and when the pressure is removed it will again become *brown*. If the pressure is such as to diminish the sensibility of the retina, it will either diminish or entirely remove a weak spectral impression.

When the eye is pressed in front by putting the finger on the eyelid above the cornea, no luminous spectrum is seen; and I have not ventured to make the pressure sufficiently strong to make an impression on the back of the eye. I know a case, however, in which this effect was produced accidentally. A person, in a state of intense grief, had been sitting for some time with his hand pressed against his eye; – the moment the hand was removed and the eye opened, a black spot, the size of a sixpence, was seen in the axis of vision.

It is from pressures on the retina that those floating masses of light are produced, which appear in particular states of indisposition. In affections of the stomach the pressure of the blood-vessels upon the retina is shown in the dark by a faint blue light, floating before the eye and passing off at one side. As the pressure increases, the blue light becomes *green*, then *yellow*, and sometimes even *red*, all these colours being occasionally seen at the edge of the luminous mass.

The preceding observations on the influence of dilatation in making the retina insensible to light, render it extremely probable that the disease in that membrane, called *Amaurosis*, may sometimes arise from a general distention of the eyeball, arising from a superabundance of the fluids which it incloses. If this be the case, the removal of the pressure might be effected by puncturing the eyeball (where it can be done with safety), and letting out a portion of the aqueous humour. How far such an operation would be effectual when the disease has been of long standing can be determined only by experiment.

4.9. Brewster: "On the influence of successive impulses of light upon the retina". *London and Edinburgh Philosophical Magazine and Journal of Science*, 1834, 4, 241–245.

From the remarkable experiment of Mrs. Griffiths, described in a former Number,* it appears that the reticulated structure of the retina may be rendered

*See Lond. and Edinb. Phil. Mag., vol. iv. p. 43

visible by throwing light suddenly on the closed eye when in a state of repose, and especially in the morning, before the retina has been subjected to the action of any other light.

In repeating this experiment, I have found that a remarkable structure may be exhibited at any time, and whether the eyes are open or shut, by subjecting the retina to the action of successive impulses of light. If, when we are walking beside a high iron railing, we direct the closed eye to the sun so that his light shall be successively interrupted by the iron rails, a structure resembling a kaleidoscopic pattern, having the *foramen centrale* in its centre, will be rudely seen. The pattern is not formed in distinct lines, but by patches of reddish light of different degrees of intensity. When the sun's rays are powerful, and when their successive action has been kept up for a short time, the whole field of vision is filled with a brilliant pattern, as if it consisted of the brightest tartan, composed of red and green squares of dazzling brightness. The green colours prevail chiefly at the centre, corresponding to the *foramen centrale,* and here we observe the dark-lined *network* pattern which I have described in Number 20,* and which is totally distinct from the reticulated structure noticed by Mrs. Griffiths. The brilliancy of the spectrum thus produced, and the beauty of its colours, exceed any optical phænomenon which I have witnessed, and so dazzling is its effect that the eye is soon obliged to withdraw itself from its overpowering influence.

The very same phænomena may be seen by looking at the sun through the distended fingers when they are made to move backwards and forwards, or rather from right to left, and from left to right, in front of the eye.

The colours of the spectrum above described have their origin in the *red* light transmitted through the eyelids, and *green* tints being the accidental or complementary colour of the *red*; but the phænomenon may be seen in a great measure without colour by opening the eye, and interposing between the eye and the sun any white transparent ground, such as thin white paper or ground glass, or by directing the eye immediately to a bright sky, or to the ground when covered with snow. In these different forms of the experiment the effect varies greatly with the intensity of the light and the state of the eye, but the following general description of the phænomena will be found tolerably correct. In order to make the light produce a series of successive impulses on the retina, and on the same parts of it, I look through the openings of the revolving disc of the phenakistiscope with one eye, and fix it steadily upon the same point of the luminous ground.

When the disc revolves with great velocity, a very *faint* and uniform light is seen over the whole luminous surface. As the velocity diminishes, the light becomes less uniform, and a flickering or wavering motion commences. Patches of a *bluish-purple* colour appear in different parts of the field, forming a sort of network, the intersections between the meshes of which are of a faint *lemon-yellow* colour, the accidental colour of the bluish purple. The pattern of this

* *Ibid.* p. 119, *note.*

network is related to the centre or point on which the eye is fixed, and seems to belong either to a hexagonal or octagonal division of the circle. The centre of the pattern, corresponding to the *foramen centrale,* is a square or lozenge, one of whose diagonals is vertical; but as the differently coloured patches or elements of the pattern are constantly changing their colour, their intensity of light, and even their form, owing to the unsteadiness of the eye and the revolving disc, I have never been able to draw the pattern, or to trace how the patches or interstices of the net-work spring from the sides and angles of the central lozenge. That the reticulated structure is related to this central square or to the central foramen of the eye is unquestionable; and I have no doubt that observers who have younger eyes than mine, and who shall have the courage to repeat the experiments with the direct light of the sun, and with a disc having narrow slits, and revolving upon a fixed axis so as to have its velocity uniform, will be able to obtain an accurate representation of the pattern in question.

Within and around the central lozenge, is seen with great distinctness the dark-lined network pattern already mentioned, and apparently unconnected with the larger pattern. As the spaces, however, or patches, which compose the larger pattern diminish in size towards the centre, it is possible that the dark-lined network, with dark specks in the centre of the figures, and having all the regularity of a geometrical figure drawn with ink, may be the central part of the larger patterns seen more distinctly by direct vision; but I cannot admit this notion, because under favourable circumstances a similar dark-lined pattern, with extremely small spaces between the meshes, appears throughout the rest of the field of view, especially in the external part of it where it first begins to show itself.

The colours which appear in the principal pattern are chiefly *bluish purple,* and its complementary colour *lemon-yellow,* but as the former increases in depth or approaches to blackness, the latter becomes more white. These different colours sometimes appear in the different patches of the pattern, and sometimes they appear in succession over a considerable part of the field. They are, however, most distinctly seen in the central lozenge, the inner part being sometimes *purple* and then *yellow,* while the outer part of it is first *yellow* and then *purple.* The central lozenge is sometimes marked out by whitish, and sometimes by greenish light, and I have frequently seen in its centre a *blush-red* of a very rare tint. The succession of colours in the lozenge is very beautiful, each colour advancing to the centre, replacing that which preceded it, and then disappearing.

The cause of the colours themselves is obvious. The action of white light on the retina renders it first insensible to the *red* rays,* and consequently a white object or ground appears *bluish purple* or *blue* in solar light, and *green* in candle light, the colour varying with the intensity of the exciting light, and with the distance of the image of the white object from the excited point. The other colour which appears in the preceding experiments is a faint *lemon-yellow,* which is the complementary

* See Lond. and Edinb. Phil. Mag., vol. iii. p. 169.

colour of the *bluish purple*. It deserves also to be noticed that these colours are the very same as those produced by the action of light falling on the retina at a distance from the axis of vision. When we look, for example, indirectly, or rather obliquely, at a candle for some time, the image of the candle itself becomes *bluish purple* surrounded with a nebulosity of *yellow* light, the accidental colour being the invariable companion of the primitive one.

In order to explain why no colours appear during a very rapid rotation of the disc, and why the primitive and the accidental colour succeed each other in the pattern, let us call

$\quad$ T$\quad$ the time in which the disc revolves,
$\quad$ *n*$\quad$ the number of apertures in its margin,
$\quad$ D$\quad$ the duration of the impression of direct light, and
$\quad$ *d*$\quad$ the duration of its complementary colour.

It is obvious that $\frac{T}{n}$ will be the time which elapses between each consecutive impulse of light on the retina, or the time during which the eye has the opake part of the disc opposite the pupil. When $\frac{T}{n}$ is very small, or the velocity very great, or when $\frac{T}{n}$ is very much less than D, (D is = eight thirds, or nearly one eighth of a second,) the ground will be uniformly luminous, because the direct impression of the one aperture has not begun to fade away before the succeeding aperture makes a new impression. When $\frac{T}{n}$, however, is nearly equal to D, the impression of the direct light is nearly gone, and hence arises the flickering or wavering appearance of the luminous ground, which becomes a maximum when $\frac{T}{n} =$ D; for when this takes place the direct impression of the one aperture is just gone before the other aperture renews it. When $\frac{T}{n}$ is greater than D, the accidental colour of the direct impression begins to show itself; and when $\frac{T}{n} =$ D $+\frac{d}{2}$, the accidental colour will be about its brightest, and will be seen to succeed the direct impression, the latter being now *bluish purple,* and the former *lemon-yellow.* When $\frac{T}{n} =$ D $+ d$, the opake space between the apertures will begin to be visible, and the phænomena will disappear.

As the reticulated pattern is marked out by different colours, and even by the same colour in different states of intensity, it follows that different parts of the retina have different degrees of sensibility to light. The lines which form the network are probably thicker than the interstices between them, and consequently less susceptible to luminous impressions. In like manner the interstices nearest to the *foramen centrale* are probably thinner than those more remote, and hence it is easy to understand why they exhibit a greater sensibility and a more rapid change of colour. If these views are correct, we not only obtain a general explanation of the phænomena which we have described, but of many others which have hitherto perplexed the optical physiologist, and among these we may enumerate the phænomena of oblique vision, and the superior distinctness of objects when they are seen directly along the axis of the eye.

In a former paper I had occasion to mention a very remarkable fact, which I had long ago discovered, that the intensity of a given light may be increased physiologically by causing it to act upon the retina by successive impulses of a given duration. Those who may repeat the preceding experiments will obtain demonstration of the truth of this new property of light. The maximum physiological

intensity seems to take place when $\frac{T}{n}$ is nearly equal to $D + d$.

Belleville, Feb. 20. 1834.

4.10. Brewster: "On the optical phenomena, nature, and locality of muscae volitantes; with observations on the structure of the vitreous humour, and on the vision of objects placed within the eye". *Transactions of the Royal Society of Edinburgh*, 1844, **15**, 377–385.

Although some of the phenomena of *Muscæ volitantes* may be seen by persons of all ages, and with the best eyes; and though those which are more peculiarly entitled to the name are exceedingly common beyond the middle period of life; yet no account has been given of them that has even the slightest pretension to accuracy. M. de La Hire, in his *Differens accidens de la Vue*, describes these *Muscæ* as of *two* kinds; some permanent and fixed, which he ascribes to small drops of extravasated blood upon the retina; and others, as flying about, and changing their place, even though the eye be fixed. The *first* kind, he describes as like a dark spot upon a white ground; and the *second*, as like the knots of a deal board. Some parts of them, he says, are very clear, and surrounded with dark threads, and are accompanied with long fillets of irregular shapes, which are bright in the middle, and terminated on each side by parallel black threads.

In order to account for these knots and irregular fillets, de La Hire supposes that the aqueous humour is *sometimes* troubled with some little mothery ropy substance, some parts of which, by the figures of their little surfaces, or by refractive powers different from the humour itself, may cast their distinct images upon the retina. He supposes them in the *aqueous* humour rather than in the vitreous, because of its greater fluidity for a freedom of descent, and because they will then appear to descend, as being situated *before* the pupil, or, at least, *before* the place of intersection of the pencils.*

Dr Porterfield, who has given a very inaccurate drawing of the filamentous *muscæ*, considers them as produced by diaphanous particles and filaments, that swim in the *aqueous* humour before the crystalline; and he regards the distinct pictures of them upon the *retina* of *long-sighted* persons, as produced by the rays which pass *through* the dense particles, having suffered a greater refraction than those which pass *by* them, so as to be converged to *foci* upon the retina.†

The latest writer on this subject, Mr Mackenzie of Glasgow, describes the *muscæ* as resembling *minute, twisted, semi-transparent* tubes, partially filled with globules, which sometimes appear in motion; while another set are more opaque, or perfectly dark, and follow the motions of the eye. The latter he considers as "of a more dangerous character than the former, and as occasioned, generally, by a partial insensibility of the retina," either from the pressure of some "irregular projecting point or points of the choroid, or from some other cause." Mr Mackenzie regards the globules within the semi-transparent tubes, as probably "blood passing through the vessels of the retina, or of the vitreous humour;" and he remarks, "that neither these semi-transparent tubes themselves, nor any of the filamentous muscæ, or black spots (which are so frequently complained of), possess any real motion, independent of the general motion of the eyeball;" and hence he concludes that they "must be referred either to the retina itself – including, of course, the three laminæ of which it is composed, – or to the choroid coat." "The probability is," he adds, "that the semi-transparent muscæ, of a tubular form, are owing to dilatation of the branches of the *arteria centralis retinæ*.‡"

Such was the state of our information on the subject of *Muscæ volitantes*, when my attention was specially directed to it, in consequence of finding in my own eye a good example of the phenomenon; and, having carefully investigated the facts as observed by other persons in their own eyes, I trust I shall be able to lay before the Society a correct description, and a satisfactory explanation, of the general phenomena.

Although the bodies which are within the eyeball, and give rise to the phenomena under consideration, are often seen under ordinary circumstances, yet, in

---

* Smith's Optics, vol. ii. Rem. p. 5.   † Treatise on the Eye, vol. ii. p. 74–80.
‡ Practical Treatise on the Diseases of the Eye, 1830, pp. 748, 750.

order to see them with distinctness, we must look at the sky, or a luminous object, either through a very minute aperture, or, when the light is limited or feeble, through a lens or microscopic doublet, of very short focus, held close to the eye. By this means, we shall observe a luminous ground, covered, more or less, with transparent filaments or tubes, transparent circles, exceedingly minute, and (when they do exist) with *Muscæ*, or black spots like flies.

In examining the transparent filaments, I have observed them of *four* or *five* different sizes, the smallest of which are the most distinct. These distinct filaments are bounded by two sharp black lines, and the space between them is more luminous than the general ground on which they are seen. In the larger filaments, the black lines are coloured at their edges, and, on the outside of each of them, are one or more coloured fringes.

The minute transparent circles, when smallest, have a luminous centre, with a sharp black circle round it. In the larger ones, this circle is coloured at its edges; and, on the outside of it, are one or more circular coloured fringes. These spherical bodies sometimes exist singly, and sometimes in groups, partly connected by small filaments, and partly by an invisible film, to which they seem attached. They sometimes adhere to the outside of the filaments, and very frequently occur *within* the filaments, so as to prove that these filaments are *tubular.* These spherical bodies have, like the filaments, *four* or *five* different sizes.

In making observations on these spherical bodies, the observer will sometimes see luminous spots pass through the field; but as these arise from the state of the lubricating fluid on the outside of the cornea, they have no connection with the phenomena under our consideration.

The transparent filaments, already described, are seldom seen single. Two or three are united, like threads crossing one another; and sometimes a great number are united, like a loose heap of thread, in which case, obscure spots appear at the places where the crossings of the filaments are most numerous.

In some cases, a single long filament is once or twice doubled up upon itself, and sometimes a *knot* is, or appears to be, tied upon it, consisting of several folds, as it were, of the filament. This *knot* has several *very dark spots* at the places where the different portions of the filament are in contact; and this accumulation, as it were, of black specks, constitutes the real *muscæ*. In many, indeed in almost all of these *muscæ*, when distinct, a little bright yellow light accompanies the black specks.

All the bodies which we have now described have two different motions; one arising from the motion of the head or eyeball, and the other when the eyeball is absolutely fixed. By a toss of the head, they are thrown into different absolute and relative positions, sometimes ascending and descending in succession, sometimes oscillating between two limits, and generally with different velocities. When the eye is first applied to the lens or aperture, the field of view is tolerably free of these moving bodies; but the light seems to stir them up, as it were, and, to a certain extent, the longer we view them, the more numerous do they become.

If the centre of motion of the eyeball coincides with the centre of visible direction, the *Muscæ* will *ascend* when the eye looks *upward*, and *vice versa*, whether they are placed before or behind that common centre. If the eyeball remains fixed, the *Muscæ* in *front* of the above centre will have the *direction* of their *real* and *apparent* motions the same, and those *behind* that centre will have these two directions *different*. Hence the appearance of two opposite currents when the eyeball is turned quickly from one extreme of its range, either vertically or horizontally, to its mean position; and so rapid is their motion through the luminous field, that it seems covered with continuous lines parallel to the direction in which the eyeball has been moved, – an effect arising from the duration of the impression of light upon the retina.

If we mark individual filaments, or groups, or knots, we shall find that they change their shapes, one part of a filament doubling itself over another, and again resuming its elongated form. The minute spherical bodies separate and approach one another; but I have not been able to satisfy myself that those within the tubular filaments change their place. They often *appear* to do so; but as this *may* arise from the bending of the filament, or from the varying obliquity of different parts of it arising from its change of form or place, we are not entitled to consider them as moveable within the tube. It is certain, however, that they have no progressive motion, as supposed by Mr Mackenzie.

In order to obtain a correct knowledge of the phenomena of the real *Muscæ*, I confined my attention to one in my own eye, of which I first made a drawing in October 1838. It is represented in the annexed figure, and consists of four filaments, ABC, BDE, FGH, and AK. Between BC and BDE there is a sort of transparent web containing a great number of minute spherical specks, and something similar, though less extensive, below FGH. The real *Musca* exists at A,

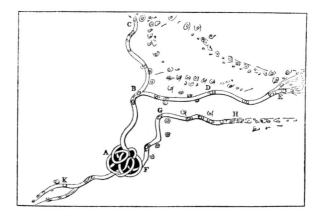

and has obviously been produced by the accidental overlapping of the different filaments which are united with it. In four and a half years, the *Musca* at A has perceptibly increased in size, and the length of the associated filaments has diminished. It is distinctly seen without any of its accompaniments in ordinary light, but is, in no respects, injurious to vision, as it is never stationary in the axis of the eye. When seen by means of the lens, the long branch FGH takes various positions, sometimes falling below the knot or *musca* A, and sometimes crossing the main branch AB, below B. The branch BDE has often a loop at D, and FGH another at G.

Having had occasion to study the phenomena of the diffraction of light, as produced by transparent fibres and films of different forms, I could not fail to observe that the phenomena above described were the shadows formed on the retina by divergent light passing by and through transparent filaments and particles placed within the eyeball. They are indeed perfectly identical, and may be accurately imitated in various ways. If we crush a crystalline lens in distilled water, or macerate some very thin laminæ of it, and dry a drop of the fluid on a piece of glass, we shall perceive, with a fine microscope a little out of focus, or with an ill adjusted illuminating apparatus, a number of minute fibres, single and in groups, and knots, with minute spherical particles, which display the very same phenomena as the analogous bodies within the eyeball.

Hence it follows, that the filaments and spherical particles, whose diffracted shadows have four or five different sizes, have the same magnitude, and are placed at four or five different distances from the retina; those which give the sharp, black, and minute shadows, being placed near the retina, and those which are large and ill defined at a distance from it. These various bodies, though they change their place, still preserve their general distance from the retina, thus clearly indicating that the vitreous humour is composed of cells within which the filaments and *muscæ* are lodged. That they do not exist in the aqueous humour is very obvious, because if they did, they would either rise to the top or sink to the bottom of the aqueous chamber when the eyeball was at rest, and thus withdraw themselves entirely from the field of view, which they never do.

In order to obtain farther information respecting these *muscæ*, I fixed the eyeball in different positions, and looking at a sheet of white paper, I marked upon it the various positions on the paper where the *Musca* rested. It never withdrew itself from the field of view, and suffered no sensible change in its size; but it rested in positions at different distances from the axis of vision. In one position of the head, I could bring the *musca* into the optic axis so as to obtain the most perfect vision of it, but in all other positions of the head, it rested at a distance from the optic axis; though in these it could, by a toss of the head, be made to cross the axis of vision. In making these experiments, we must recollect that, as the *musca* is generally seen by oblique vision, it will very frequently disappear, though it has not withdrawn itself from the field of view. In all positions of the head, the *musca* appears to descend, so that it must actually *ascend* in the vitreous humour, and be specifically lighter.

Now, it is obvious, that, if we determine the visible position of the *Musca* when at rest in different positions of the head, we determine the direction of lines passing from the centre of visible direction through the points in the vitreous humour where the musca rested, and thus obtain a general notion of the *form of the cell* in which it is contained. But we may go still farther, and determine with considerable accuracy the diameter of the *Musca* or its filaments, and also their distance from the retina, and thus obtain a knowledge of its locality, and of the form of the cavity by which its excursions are limited.

In order to do this, I place before the eye two bright sources of light, so as to obtain from them, by the method already described, two divergent beams of light, and I thus obtain double images on the retina of all objects placed within the eyeball. The filaments of *Muscæ* in the anterior part of the vitreous humour will have their double images very distant: those in the middle of it will have their double images much nearer: those near the retina will have their two images close or perhaps overlapping each other; while any object on the retina itself, any black spot arising from defective sensibility, will have only one image, as it were. Now, if we measure the distance of the two sources of light from each other, and also their distance from the centre of visible direction, when the two images of the filaments, &c., are just in contact, we may determine the size of the filament and its exact position, as well as its distance from the retina. In making this experiment, I first found that the angle of apparent magnitude of the shadow of the filament ABC was eight minutes, and consequently that it subtended this angle at the centre of visible direction.* Now, if we take the radius of the retina as 0.524 of an inch, the diameter of the shadow of the filament will be 0.00122, or $^1/_{820}$th of an inch, and its distance from the retina 0.0118, or $^1/_{85}$th part of an inch.

When we use a small aperture alone for producing a divergent pencil, the centre of divergency must necessarily be without the eyeball; but we may throw the centre of divergency within the eyeball, and place it at any distance from the retina, by using a lens of the proper focus. If we wish to place this centre near the retina, a lens of considerable focal length must be used, and as the light collected by it will be powerful, it will extinguish all the smaller filaments and minute spheres, and allow only the larger *Muscæ* to be seen. We must therefore reduce its aperture by looking through a pin-hole or other minute opening. When we wish to have a clear field of view for examining the larger *Muscæ*, we may extinguish all the smaller ones by increasing the luminosity of the field. If we wish to study the filaments or *Muscæ* that may be placed about the middle of the vitreous humour, we must use a lens of such an aperture as will obliterate all those more remote from the retina.

* This may be done by projecting it upon a luminous surface, and marking its apparent size; or by comparing it with the images of objects of known dimensions seen with a fine microscope.

It is very obvious, from the preceding observations that objects placed within the eyeball are not seen, as Dr Porterfield believes, by rays *which pass* through *dense particles having suffered a greater refraction than those which pass* by *them*. A fibre or particle of glass of nearly the same refractive power as the vitreous humour will be seen distinctly by means of its image formed on the retina by diffracted pencils. If the light is not sufficiently divergent, or is too intense to produce and exhibit the diffracted image, the object will be invisible, unless it be of such a size, and so near the retina, as to shew itself by its ordinary shadow. But in whatever way the image of the object is formed, the mind takes cognizance of it, or gives it an external locality, by means of the same law of visible direction which regulates the vision of objects placed without the eyeball.

While these results exhibit the true physical cause of all the optical phenomena and limited movements of the filaments and *Muscæ*, they lead also to some important and useful conclusion of a more general nature. It had been conjectured that the vitreous humour of animals was enclosed in separate bags or cells connected with the hyaloid membrane by which the vitreous mass is enveloped. The preceeding experiments not only appear to demonstrate that this is the structure of the vitreous humour in man, but to shew that there are at least *four* or *five* cells between the retina and the posterior surface of the crystalline lens. The limited motion of the *Muscæ* indicates that the cell in which they float is of very limited extent. When the vertical diameter of the eyeball, in its natural position, is placed, by the inclination of the head, 30° to the right hand of a vertical line, and the optic axis of the eye directed 20° below a horizontal line, the *Musca* is seen along the optic axis, and consequently in the most perfect manner. One point of its cell must therefore touch the optical axis.

I have endeavoured, with the assitance of my eminent colleague Dr Reid, to discover cells in the vitreous humour of quadrupeds and fishes by the aid of the microscope and other means, but we have not succeeded: and unless some chemical substance shall be found which acts differently upon the albuminous fluid and the membranous septa, it is not likely that they will be otherwise rendered visible.*

Mr Ware, in a paper on the *Muscæ Volitantes of nervous persons,*† describes some as "globules twisted together, and others as like the flue that is swept from bedrooms," and he considers it "probable that they depend on a steady pressure on one or more minute points of the retina which are situated near the axis of vision."‡ In the cases described by Mr Ware, the *Muscæ* were liable to great and

---

* The vitreous humour, when slowly dried, either by itself, or along with parts of the septa in which it may be contained, shoots into beautiful crystalline ramifications proceeding from the four angles of a quadrilateral crystal. Thin six-sided plates frequently occur, but they seem to exercise no action upon polarised light, probably on account of their thinness. The same effects were produced when the vitreous humour from a fresh eye was well washed in distilled water.

†Medico-Chirurgical Trans., 1814, vol. v., p. 255.

‡ Id. Id., p. 266.

sudden changes in intensity and number, particularly from causes affecting the nervous system, and hence they cannot be regarded as of the same character as the *Muscae* described in this paper, unless we suppose that *Muscae*, invisible under ordinary circumstances, become visible in consequence of an increased sensibility of the retina.

This supposition, however, is by no means probable, because the *Muscae* are not visible by any light of their own, and an increase of sensibility in the retina would affect equally the luminous field on which they are seen. But, as this point is of some importance both in a physiological and a medical aspect, I have submitted it to direct experiment. With this view, I examined the *Muscae* in the morning before the sensibility of the retina had been diminished by exposure to daylight, and found that they were neither increased in number or intensity. I varied this experiment by diminishing the sensibility of the retina. This was done by holding a bright gas flame close to the eye, and near the axis of vision, till the retina lost its sensibility to all the rays of the spectrum, except a few of the more refrangible ones.* In this case, too, the *Muscae* were as numerous and distinct as before, and we may therefore consider it as certain, that the *Muscae* described by Mr Ware, in so far as they were of the same character as those of the healthy eye, are not affected by any variation in the sensibility of the retina. I am disposed to think that they consisted of the ordinary *Muscae* seen simultaneously with others produced by the pressure of the bloodvessels on the retina, and that it was the latter only which underwent the variations which he describes.

It is not easy to form any rational conjecture respecting the cause and purpose of the numerous filaments by which the *Muscae* are produced; for as they exist in all eyes, whether young or old, they are neither the result of disease, nor do they indicate its approach. Were they fixed or regularly distributed, we might regard them as transparent vessels which supply the vitreous humour; but existing, as they do, in detached and floating portions, they resemble more the remains of some organic structure whose functions are no longer necessary. But though these filaments have no morbid character, they may nevertheless obstruct and even destroy vision. They certainly interfere with nice microscopical observations, and in observing the minute and almost imperceptible lines in the solar spectrum, I have found them to be occasionally injurious. It is quite possible that some of the cells near the retina and around the optic axis might be filled up with accumulated *Muscae*, and produce a considerable degree of blindness; but this is an effect of them which there is little occasion to apprehend.

Mr Mackenzie† informs us, "that few symptoms prove so alarming to persons of a nervous habit or constitution as *Muscae volitantes*, and they immediately suppose that they are about to lose their sight by cataract or amaurosis." Professor Plateau of Ghent, to whom I had communicated, at his own request, some of the

---

* Lond. and Edin. Phil. Mag., 1832, vol. i., p. 172, vol. ii., p. 168.
† Practical Treatise, &c., p. 751.

preceding results, mentions to me, that few physicians are able to distinguish between the *Muscæ* described above, and those appearances which indicate amaurosis, and that they often, without cause, alarm patients who consult them for the first time respecting such affections of the eye. He assures me that he has already been the means of freeing from alarm many persons with *Muscæ volitantes*, and that he had even done this to a distinguished physician.*

The details in the preceding pages may, therefore, be considered as establishing the important fact, that *Muscæ volitantes* have no connection whatever either with *Cataract* or *Amaurosis*, and that they are nearly altogether harmless. This result has been deduced by the aid of a recondite property of divergent light, which has only been developed in our own day, and which seems to have no bearing whatever of an utilitarian character. And this is but one of numerous proofs which the progress of knowledge is daily accumulating, that the most abstract and apparently transcendental truths in physical science will sooner or later add their tribute to supply human wants, and alleviate human sufferings. Nor has science performed one of the least important of her functions when she enables us, either in our own case, or in that of others, to dispel those anxieties and fears which are the necessary offspring of ignorance and error.

4.11. Brewster: "A notice explaining the cause of an optical phenomenon observed by the Rev. W. Selwyn". *Report of the British Association, Transactions of the Sections*, 1844, p. 8.

When a number of parallel black lines are intersected at right angles by other black lines, so as to inclose a number of squares or rectangles, a white spot appears at the intersections of all the lines. In order to discover the cause of this phænomenon, Sir David Brewster made the experiment with the broad opake bars of an old-fashioned window opposed to the light of the sky. Along all the bars he saw a whitish nebulous light, which was the complementary or accidental colour of the black bars seen simultaneously with the bars. The same luminosity was of course seen of equal intensity along all the bars, but at the crossings the intensity of its light was greatest, so as to produce the white spot already mentioned. Now this spot did not arise from any increased effect at the intersections, but from a *diminution* of the complementary luminosity at all other parts of the interesecting lines. This diminution of intensity arises from the action of the white squares or rectangles upon the retina tending to diminish the sensibility

* Professor Plateau mentions that he had been led to suppose that the *Muscæ* had their seat in the vitreous humour rather than in the aqueous; but that he had been stopped by the difficulty of reconciling this opinion with the viscosity of the vitreous humour. As the vitreous humour is *perfectly fluid* within each cell, the viscosity here supposed being only apparent, no longer presents any difficulty.

of that membrane along the parts corresponding to the black lines, and is always greatest by oblique vision. It is an action analogous to that which takes place when a strip of paper laid upon a green or any other coloured glass disappears when the eye is fixed upon a point an inch or two distant from the paper. Hence the luminous spots are brightest when not seen directly. [The phænomenon thus explained was communicated to Sir David Brewster by the Rev. W. Selwyn.]

4.12. Wheatstone: "On the singular effect of the juxtaposition of certain colours under particular circumstances". *Report of the British Association, Transactions of the Sections*, 1844, p. 10.

Having had his attention drawn to the fact, that a carpet worked with a small pattern in green and red, when illuminated with gas-light, if viewed carelessly, produced an effect upon the eye as if all the parts of the pattern were in motion, he was led to have several patterns worked in various contrasted pairs of colours; and he found that in many of them the motion was perceptible, but in none so remarkably as those in red and green; it appeared also to be necessary that the illumination should be gas-light, as the effect did not appear to manifest itself in daylight, at least in diffused daylight. He accounted for it by the eye retaining its sensibility for various colours during various lengths of time.

4.13. Brewster: "On the same subject". *Report of the British Association, Transactions of the Sections*, 1844, p. 10.

Sir David Brewster stated that he and Prof. Wheatstone had brought to York separate communications on this experiment, with specimens of the rug-work in which it is best exhibited. Having seen Prof. Wheatstone's specimens, he had been induced to limit his communication to a few observations on Prof. Wheatstone's paper. When Sir D. Brewster came to York, he was not aware of the phænomena taking place with any other colour but *red* and *green*. Prof. Wheatstone had, however, shown him that *red* and *blue* answered equally well; and he had received letters from two ladies in Scotland, who had not only found that *red* and *blue* exhibited the phænomenon, but had both given the probable explanation of their doing so, by ascribing it to the *blue* becoming *green* in the *yellow* light of the candle.

In order to give an explanation of what has been called by some the *fluttering hearts*, from one of the colours having the shape of hearts, Sir David Brewster mentioned an experiment for the purpose of showing that any fixed object will appear to move on the ground upon which it is fixed, when the light which illuminates it is constantly changing its position and intensity. This experiment consists in moving a candle rapidly in all directions, in front of a statue. The varying lights and shadows produce varying expressions, which give the appearance of life and motion to the features of the statue. Now, in the case of the vibrating hearts, the mixture of the *red* and *green*, whether seen as direct or as accidental impressions, produces successions of light and shadow which gave the appearance of motion to the figure upon the *red* or *green* ground. This effect is greatly increased by that remarkable property of oblique vision, in which the retina increases in sensibility as the point impressed is removed from the *foramen centrale*. Hence when we look fixedly at one of the vibrating hearts, it nearly ceases to vibrate, while the others, which are seen obliquely, vibrate with greater distinctness. The phænomenon has been stated to be invisible in daylight; but Sir David Brewster mentioned that he had, that morning, found that it took place in daylight, provided the coloured surface was illuminated from a small hole in the shutter of a dark room. The experiment, indeed, he found to fail even in candlelight, if the illumination proceeded from a great number of lights, or from a mass of light producing a *quaquaversus* illumination like that of the sky. He referred also to the effects produced by coloured glasses, and mentioned some facts regarding the unequal absorption of the two colours, which, in drawing conclusions from such experiments, required to be attended to.

4.14. Brewster: "Notice of two new properties of the retina". *Report of the British Association, Transactions of the Sections*, 1845, pp. 9–10.

One of these properties related to the inferior sensibility of the retina at that part of it which corresponds to the *Foramen centrale* of Soemmering, and which opens itself only when the eyes are directed to a faintly illuminated surface. The other property of the retina appeared after the observer's eye had been impressed with the luminous stripes seen by looking out of a railway carriage in rapid motion at the stones, or other white bodies lying near the rails. When the eye is quickly shut under this impression, a motion is perceived in a direction transverse to the real impression on the retina; and there is the appearance of lines complementary in the same transverse direction.

4.15. Brewster: "On the compensation of impressions moving over the retina". *Report of the British Association, Transactions of the Sections,* 1861, p. 29.

The author stated that when, in railway travelling, they looked at the lines which the stones or gravel or other objects formed in consequence of the durations of their impressions on the retina, and quickly transferred the eye to the same lines further back, where the velocity was slower, the stones or gravel or other objects would, for an instant, be distinctly seen, just as rapidly revolving objects are seen in the dark when they are illuminated by an electric flash or the light of an exploded copper cap. A similar, but not the same, phenomenon will be seen when we look at the moving lines through a slit and quickly look away from the slit, so that the lines may be seen by indirect vision on a part of the retina not previously impressed. This class of phenomena may be best studied with a rapidly revolving disc, by quickly transferring the eye from the lines on the marginal part of the disc to those near the centre of rotation, where the velocity is less. When the marginal velocity is greatest, the point of compensation is nearest the centre, as might have been expected from the experiment in a railway carriage; but what could not, he thought, have been anticipated, was that the point of compensation was not in the same radius as the point to which the eye was first directed. The author explained this statement by means of a diagram which was exhibited. He had not been able to see the point of compensation close to the centre of rotation, where it doubtless must be, with a certain velocity, so that its locus must be in a curve.

4.16. Brewster: "On the optical study of the retina". *Report of the British Association, Transactions of the Sections,* 1861, p. 29.

There were two structures in the retina (hexangular and quadrangular) that could be exhibited by optical means, the one by the successive impulses of light, and the other by the action of faint light entering the eye, or produced within it, either from the duration of a luminous impression, or from a local pressure upon the retina. The first of these structures was best seen by the light of a white cloud, through the slits or apertures of a revolving disc, placed midway between its circumference and its centre of rotation, in order to protect the eye from light which did not pass through the slits. When the disc revolved rapidly the field of view exhibited neither colour nor structure, but merely a diminution of light. When the velocity had reached a certain point, the field of vision became yellowish white, then yellow and bluish. Occasionally the yellow had the form of a rectangular cross, between the branches of which were four dark spaces. With a diminished velocity the whole field because uniformly blue, and was now covered with the hexagonal pattern formed by deep-black lines, the lines being darker at the place of the *foramen centrale*. As there are no fewer than eight different layers in the retina, it was of great importance to ascertain the functions which they individually performed in conveying visual impressions to the brain, and it was only by optical means that this inquiry could be conducted. The anatomist had ably performed his part with the aid of the microscope, and it was probably from the improvement of this instrument chiefly that we could expect any further discoveries, unless the morbid anatomy of the retina should connect certain imperfections of vision with the condition of certain layers of the membrane. When the eye was left in darkness, by the sudden extinction of a light, there were several points at the margin of the retina which retained the light longer than the rest. There could be no doubt that these effects were produced by structural differences. In the case of the *foramen* the difference had been recognized by the anatomist, and was proved by the remarkable phenomenon of Haidinger's brushes, and by other optical facts, such as the instability and superior brightness of oblique impressions on the retina. We had, consequently, an optical principle which enabled us to explain the quadrangular structure he had referred to. It was not improbable, when we looked at the complete structure of the retina, and even of its individual layers, that the structure of each of them might be exhibited optically.

4.17. Brewster: "On hemiopsy, or half-vision". *Transactions of the Royal Society of Edinburgh*, 1865, **24**, 15–18.

The affection of Half-vision, or Half-blindness as it has been called, was first distinctly described by Dr Wollaston, in a paper "On Semidecussation of the Optic Nerves," published in the Philosophical Transactions for 1824. "It is now more than twenty years," he says,

> since I was first affected with this peculiar state of vision, in consequence of violent exercise I had taken for two or three hours before. I suddenly found that I could see but half the face of a man whom I met, and it was the same with every object I looked at. In attempting to read the name Johnson over the door, I saw only SON, the commencement of the name being wholly obliterated from my view. In this instance, the loss of sight was towards my left, and was the same, whether I looked with my right eye or my left. This blindness was not so complete as to amount to absolute blackness, but was a shaded darkness, without definite outline. The complaint lasted only about a quarter of an hour.

In 1822, Dr Wollaston had another attack of hemiopsy, with this difference, that the blindness was to the right of the centre of vision, and he has referred to three other cases among his friends; but in these, the affection was accompanied with headache and indigestion.

In republishing Dr Wollaston's paper in the "*Annales de Chimie et Physique,*"* M. Arago says, that he knows *four* cases of hemiopsy, and that he himself had experienced three attacks of it, followed by headache above the right eye.

In the "Cyclopædia of Practical Surgery," published in 1841, Mr Tyrrell describes Hemiopsy as "Functional amaurosis from general disturbance." He informs us that "he has experienced this form of amaurosis several times," and that he has been consulted by several fellow-sufferers of both sexes. In all these cases the affection was attended with severe headache, giddiness, and gastric irritation, sometimes preceding, and sometimes following, the attack.

In the accounts which have been given of these different cases of hemiopsy, no attempt has been made to ascertain the optical condition of the eye when it is said to be half-blind, or to determine the locality and immediate cause of the complaint. Dr Wollaston describes the blindness as a shaded darkness without definite outline. M. Arago says nothing about darkness; and the insensibility of the retina, of which he speaks, must mean its insensibility to visual and not to luminous impressions. Mr Tyrrell, on the other hand, simply states, that the obscurity takes place in different portions of the retina, and varies in its extent at different times.

Having myself experienced several attacks of hemiopsy, I have been enabled to ascertain the optical condition of the retina when under its influence, and to determine the extent of the affection, and its immediate cause.

In reading the different cases of hemiopsy, we are led to infer that there is vision in one-half of the retina, and blindness in the other. But this is not the case. The blindness, or insensibility to distinct impressions, exists chiefly in a small portion of the retina to the right or left hand of the *foramen centrale*, and extends itself irregularly to other parts of the retina on the same side, in the neighbourhood of which the vision is uninjured. In some cases the upper half of the object is invisible, the part of the retina paralysed being a little below the *foramen centrale*. On some occasions, in absolute darkness, when a faint glow of light was produced by some uniform pressure upon the whole of the retina, I have observed a great number of black spots, corresponding to parts of the retina upon which no pressure was exerted.

In the case of ordinary hemiopsy, as observed by myself, there is neither darkness nor obscurity, the portion of the paper from which the letters disappear being as bright as those upon which they are seen. Now, this is a remarkable condition of the retina. While it is sensible to luminous impressions, it is insensible to the lines and shades of the pictures which it receives of external objects; or, in other words, the retina is in certain parts of it in such a state that the

* 1824, vol. xxvii. p. 109.

light which falls upon it is irradiated, or passes into the dark lines or shades of the pictures upon it, and obliterates them. This irradiation exists to a small degree, even when the vision is perfect at the *foramen centrale*, and it may be produced artificially in a sound eye, on parts of the retina remote from the foramen, and as completely, though temporarily, as in hemiopsy. In order to prove this, we have only to look obliquely at a narrow strip of paper placed upon a green cloth, that is, to fix the eye upon a point a little distant from the strip of paper. After a short time the strip of paper will disappear partially or wholly, and the space which it occupied will be green, or the colour of the ground upon which it is laid.*

This temporary insensibility of the retina in the part of it covered by the picture of the strip of paper, or its inability to maintain constant vision of it, can arise only from its being paralysed by the continued action of light, an effect not likely to be produced, and never observed, in the ordinary use of the eye.

The insensibility of the retina, in cases of hemiopsy, and the consequent irradiation of the light into the space occupied with the letters, or the objects which disappear, though a phenomenon of the same kind as that which takes place in oblique vision, has yet a very different origin. The parts which are in these cases affected extend irregularly from the *foramen centrale* to the margin of the retina, as if they were related to the distribution of its blood-vessels, and hence it was probable that the paralysis of the corresponding parts of the retina was produced by their pressure. This opinion might have long remained a reasonable explanation of hemiopsy, had not a phenomenon presented itself to me, which places it beyond a doubt. When I had a rather severe attack, which never took place unless I had been reading for a long time the small print of the *Times* newspaper, and which was never accompanied either with headache or gastric irritation, I went accidentally into a dark room, when I was surprised to observe that all the parts of the retina which were affected were slightly luminous, an effect invariably produced by pressure upon that membrane. If these views be correct, hemiopsy cannot be regarded as a case of amaurosis, or in any way connected, as has been supposed, with cerebral disturbance.

Dr Wollaston endeavoured to explain the phenomena of hemiopsy, and the fact of single vision with two eyes, by what he calls the semidecussation of the optic nerves, a doctrine which Sir Isaac Newton had suggested, and employed to account for single vision.† A fibre of the right-hand side of the optic nerve is supposed to decussate or divide itself into two fibres, sending *one* to the right side of the right eye, and *another* to the right side of the left eye, while a fibre on the left-hand side of the optic nerve also decussates, sending *one* fibre to the left side of the left eye, and *another* to the left side of the right eye. Hence, Sir Isaac Newton drew the conclusion, that an impression on each of the two half fibres would convey a single sensation to the brain; and hence, Dr Wollaston concluded

---

* Letters on Natural Magic. Let. II. p. 13.   † Optics, p. 320.

that hemiopsy in one eye must be accompanied with hemiopsy in the other.

Ingenious as these explanations are, the anatomical facts by which alone they could be supported have not been established. Dr Alison,* who has adopted the opinion of Newton, and reasoned upon it, admits that the anatomical evidence is still defective; and the late Mr Twining† has adduced nine cases of disease in the optic nerves and thalami, which stand in direct opposition to the hypothesis of semidecussation. Dr Mackenzie, too, adopting the same view of the subject as Mr Twining, distinctly asserts that "the great mass of facts in Pathology and Experimental Anatomy, touching this question, go to prove that injuries and diseases affecting one side of the brain, instead of *hemiopsia* in both eyes, produce amaurosis only in the opposite eye."

The two great facts of hemiopsy in both eyes, and of what is called single vision with two eyes, do not require the hypothesis of semidecussation to explain them. If hemiopsy is produced by the distended blood-vessels of the retina, these vessels must be similarly distributed in each eye, and similarly affected by any change in the system; and, consequently, must produce the same effect upon each retina, and upon the same part of it.

In explaining single vision with two eyes, we have no occasion to appeal to double fibres in the optic nerves, or to corresponding points on the retina. There is, in reality, no such thing as single vision, that is a single image seen by both eyes. With two sound eyes every object is seen double, and it appears single only when, by the law of visible position, the one image is placed above the other. But even in this case the object is seen double, by means of two dissimilar images of it which are not coincident. By shutting the right eye, we lose sight of a part on the right side of the double image, which is seen only by the right eye; and by shutting the left eye, we lose sight of a part on the left side of the double image, which is seen only by the left eye. If one eye gives a better picture than the other, the duplicity of the apparently single image is more easily seen. By shutting the good eye the imperfect picture is seen, and by shutting the bad eye we insulate the perfect picture. It is difficult to understand how opical writers and physiologists should have so long demanded a single sensation for the production of a single picture from the two pictures imprinted on the two retinas. If we had the hundred eyes of Argus, the production of an apparently single picture would have been the necessary result of the Law of Visible Position.

---

* Edinburgh Transactions, vol. xiii. p. 479.
† Trans. Med. Soc., Calcutta, vol. ii. p. 151 or, Edin. Journal of Science, July 1828, vol. ix. p. 143.

4.18. Brewster: "On a new property of the retina". *Transactions of the Royal Society of Edinburgh*, 1866, **24**, 327–329.

In a paper on Hemiopsy, published in the present volume of the Transactions (p. 15), I have mentioned the remarkable fact, that the parts of the retina which are insensible to visual, are sensible to luminous impressions, the light being occasioned by irradiation from the adjacent parts of the retina. The parts thus affected in hemiopsy extend irregularly from the *foramen centrale* to the margin of the retina; but the space which they occupy is so small, their distribution so irregular, and the time of their continuance so short, that it is difficult to make such observations upon them as would establish a general property of the retina.

Mr Airy, our distinguished Astronomer-Royal, who has had more than twenty attacks of hemiopsy, has been induced, by the perusal of my paper, to describe their character, and delineate the form of the parts insensible to visual impressions.* The hemiopsy, in his case, commences at the *foramen centrale* c, Fig. 1,

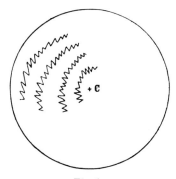

Fig. 1.

and extends outwards in a zig-zag curve line, the curve "being small at first, and gradually increasing in dimensions," as shown in the figure. It is accompanied with "tremor and boiling so oppressive, that if produced only in one eye, they may nearly extinguish the corresponding vision in the other," and it lasts from twenty to thirty minutes. It occurs sometimes on one side, and sometimes on the other side, of the foramen; and Mr Airy has "never been able to decide with certainty whether the disease really affects both eyes." On one occasion, when under its influence, he lost "his usual command of speech, and his memory failed so much that he did not know what he had said, or had attempted to say, and that he might be talking incoherently." He, therefore, entertained "no doubt that the seat of the disease was in the brain; that the disease is a species of paralysis; and that the ocular affection is only a secondary symptom."

* Philosophical Magazine, July 1865, vol. xxx. p. 19.

From these important facts, it will be seen that Mr Airy's case differs essentially from mine, in which the locality of the indistinctness occurs in irregular zig-zag lines proceeding, as in Fig. 2, from the foramen outwards, and not in a circular arch, as shown in Fig. 1. The "general obscuration," mentioned by Mr Airy, shows that the luminous impression on the affected parts is not so strong in his case as in mine, and that the retina is still sensible to light derived from the surrounding parts of irradiation. The severity of the affection in Mr Airy's case is remarkable. In mine the attack is little more than disagreeable, and I have never experienced the slightest effect either upon the speech or the memory. I have given this brief abstract of Mr Airy's interesting paper from the relation of hemiopsy to the permanent affection of the retina which I am about to describe.

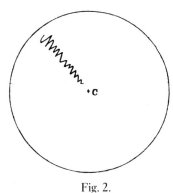

Fig. 2.

When without the hope of obtaining any precise information respecting the irradiation into the parts of the retina affected with hemiopsy, an accidental observation revealed to me the disagreeable fact that a considerable portion of the retina of my right eye was absolutely blind, or insensible to visual impressions; and I have thus been enabled, from the extent and permanence of the affection, to make whatever observations were necessary to ascertain the true character of the phenomenon.

The portion of the retina thus affected with what may be called *local amaurosis* is situated, in the field of vision, about 15° from the foramen, in a line to the left inclined 45° to the horizon. Its angular magnitude is about 6° in its greatest breadth, which corresponds to a space about the twenty-eighth of an inch on the retina.

When the image of a bright object covers the whole, or any part of this spot, it is invisible. If the image is the flame of a candle, or of the moon, or of the sun near the horizon, it is wholly invisible. The eye is therefore at this part of it absolutely insensible to light falling upon it from without. If we now direct the eye to the sky, to the white ceiling of a room, or to any extended white surface, no dark spot, even of the slightest shade, is seen in the field of vision. The portion of the retina, therefore, insensible to light incident upon it directly, or from without, has been illuminated by irradiation from the surrounding parts. But for this wise provision, an eye affected with local amaurosis would carry about with it a black spot, disfiguring the aspects of nature, and ever reminding the patient of his misfortune.

How long this condition of my retina has existed, I cannot discover. It may have existed for half a century, or more; and, but for a casual observation, its existence might never have been discovered. Whether it came on gradually, or was produced in some of the experiments in which the eye was exposed to the light of the sun, I have no means of ascertaining. If from the first of these causes, it is likely to extend itself; if from the second, it may remain as it is. Having observed it only for a year without noticing any enlargement, it is probable that it was produced by the strong action of light.

Owing to the compound structure of the retina, consisting of different layers and these layers composed of bodies of different shapes, it is very difficult to discover the part which each of them performs in the act of vision; but considering each element of the retina as a *rod*, the end of which next the vitreous humour is an expansion of the optic nerve, we know that distinct vision of external objects arises from the law of visible direction, by which every ray of light, at whatever angle it may fall, gives us vision of the point from which it proceeds, in a direction perpendicular to the part of the membrane on which it is incident. When this outer layer of the retina is insensible to the light of external objects, its luminosity, or the light which it exhibits, may be received from the surrounding parts of the expanded nerve by irradiation, or from the parts of the elemental rods behind it, if they were not paralysed, or if they are, by the action of the unparalysed rods around them.

Although in hemiopsy, and in the case of local amaurosis which I have described, the paralysed parts are still luminous, yet there are cases in which

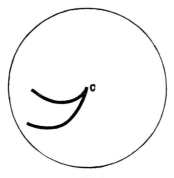

Fig. 3.

these parts are absolutely black, and into which no light is introduced by irradiation. An example of this fact presented itself to me in the morning of the 16th October 1837, and is represented in Fig. 3, where two black curved lines proceeded from the *foramen centrale* of the retina of the right eye. These lines were so black that, in the memorandum which I made at the time, I state that they were blacker than the black ink lines upon the paper. The lines continued only about *ten* minutes, and were probably produced by the pressure of blood-vessels, as I had, the day before, been subject to much giddiness. In this case, the elementary rods of the retina beneath these lines must have been paralysed throughout their length; and therefore, it is probable that the case of hemiopsy and local amaurosis, the paralysis affects only the end of the rods in contact with the vitreous humour, and formed by the expansion of the optic nerve.

In concluding this notice, I would suggest to philosophers and medical practitioners the importance of studying the manner in which sight and hearing are, in their own case, gradually impaired, for it is in the decay or decomposition of organic structures, as well as in their origin and growth, that valuable results may be presented to the physiologist; and facts of this kind have a peculiar value when the patient is himself a practised observer.

4.19. Wheatstone, cited in Airy: "On a distinct form of transient hemiopsia". *Philosophical Transactions of the Royal Society*, 1870, **160**, 253–254.

Very recently (1870, Jan 15) I have become acquainted, through the kindness of Professor Stokes, with the following description by Sir C. Wheatstone of a form of hemiopsia differing from my own in nothing but the total absence of colour. With the writer's permission I insert the whole.

I will here subjoin the note I made at the time I was first attacked with this affection.

Sept. 30th, 1849. – This evening I had a curious affection of vision. Whilst I was writing, characters near the centre of vision became invisible. Thus fixing my eyes on the figure 6 in the group $4^6/_7$, 4 and 7 were completely obliterated. On closing each eye alternately, I found precisely the same result. This did not arise from an ocular spectrum, for neither a black nor a coloured spot was projected on the paper, the disappearance was exactly that of an object when placed in the projection of the entrance of the optic nerve. After a short time the spot became larger, spreading towards the left in both eyes until it occupied a large oval space; objects at and near the centre of vision reappeared, but nearly the left half of each retina was blinded. The phenomenon in its later stages was accompanied by an effect like the motion of a luminous liquid. At the time the luminous mist entirely passed away, about half an hour after its commencement, a slight fainting sensation came over me.

I have frequently, though generally at very distant intervals, been subject to this affection. It has usually occurred whilst reading. It has always commenced near the centre of the retina, and ordinarily expanded towards the left. The zigzag luminous lines which border the spectrum externally do not commence until it has received some expansion, and they become brighter as it enlarges; before it disappears vision is restored to the central part of the retina, and when the zigzag lines arrive at the limit of the field of view, the entire vision becomes clear. On one occasion I drew with a pen the outline of the spot, a short time after its first development, as it appeared to each eye separately projected on the paper; both outlines exactly corresponded. I have never suffered any inconvenience after these attacks, and my vision, although I have at times tried my eyes severely with optical experiments, is I believe as good as ever, though I have been subject occasionally to this affection for more than twenty years. The only difference between the phenomena as they appear to me and as they are described by Dr. Airy is, that in my case they are always unaccompanied with colour.

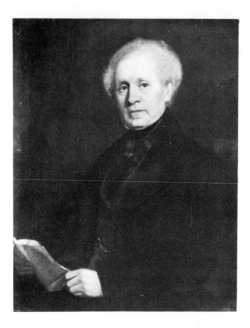

Brewster. An oil painting by James Wilson (1852). Reproduced by permission of the Hunterian Art Gallery, University of Glasgow.

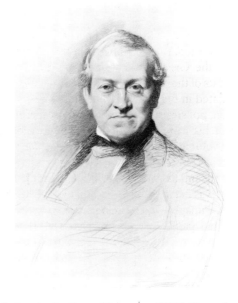

Wheatstone. A chalk drawing by Samuel Laurence (1868). Reproduced by permission of the National Portrait Gallery.

5. Assessment

5.1. Summary of Contributions

Neither Brewster nor Wheatstone were primarily concerned with research in vision. Rather, both were physicists and the majority of their published works were addressed to optics and electricity, respectively. In the obituaries, reprinted in Section 1.2, relatively little was said of their experiments in visual perception. None the less, Brewster and Wheatstone were the two most consistent students of vision writing in Britain during the period from about 1820 to 1860. It is also evident that their contributions to the study of perception were not confined to stereoscopic vision, but it is within this domain that their influence has been most profound.

Brewster's life-long interest was optics. This he defined in a broader manner than would be common today, because for him it incorporated sight as well as light. "Optics, from the Greek word which signifies *to see*, is that branch of knowledge which treats of the properties of *light* and of *vision*, as performed by the human eye" as he stated in the first sentence of his *Treatise on Optics* (Brewster, 1831, p. 1). It is, then, not surprising to find that his experiments on visual optics commenced early in his career. The long article on accidental colours (4.2) appeared in the first volume of his *Edinburgh Encyclopaedia*, the original edition of which was published in 1808. In the article he reported many experiments that he had conducted himself, and he concluded with reference to a further experimental series in which he was engaged while writing the article. Brewster retained an active interest in after-images, and he published several later papers (Brewster, 1834, 1839) addressed particularly to Plateau's (1834) theory of after-image fluctuations. These papers have not been reprinted in this collection because they would have proved difficult to follow without the inclusion of Plateau's article.

In the same year that saw the first volume of the *Edinburgh Encyclopaedia* James Wardrop, an Edinburgh eye surgeon and an acquaintance of Brewster, published his *Essays on the Morbid Anatomy of the Human Eye* (Wardrop, 1808). In it was the text of a letter from Brewster to Wardrop concerning the examination of a woman with keratoconus (conical cornea). In the examination Brewster used the variations in the size and form of the reflected images from a candle flame to determine the nature of the defect (see Levene, 1965, 1971). Wardrop noted in the second edition of his *Essays* that "Dr. Brewster has had occasion to examine a great variety of cases of conical cornea – and in all of them, without exception, he has detected inequalities in the superficial conformation of the cornea" (Wardrop, 1819, p. 134).

Brewster later suggested that the same technique could be used for determining the optical basis for ocular astigmatism. Thomas Young described the condition of astigmatism in 1801, but little notice was taken of his discovery. The condition was reported independently nearly 30 years later by George Biddell Airy, following his observation of its effect in his left eye. Airy's paper describing this "peculiar defect in the eye" was published initially in the *Transactions of the Cambridge Philosophical Society* of 1827, and reprinted in Brewster's *Edinburgh Journal of Science* in the same year. Airy did more than describe the defect – he also proposed how it could be corrected, with the use of a cylindrical lens before the eye. Following the article in Brewster's journal were some "Observations by the Editor", of which the following are the most pertinent:

> Mr. Airy does not seem to have ascertained in what part of the eye this curious defect exists – whether in the cornea or in the crystalline lens. By examining the image of a taper reflected from the outer surface of the cornea, he will readily discover whether its form is spherical or cylindrical. If it is spherical, there can be little doubt that the crystalline is at fault, and it will remain to be determined whether the differences of refraction in different planes arise from the lens having one or both of its surfaces cylindrical, or what is more probable, from a want of symmetry in the variation of its density – an effect which is very common at that period of life when the eye begins to feel the approach of age (Brewster, 1827, pp. 325–326).

According to Levene (1965, 1971) Brewster's technique, simple though it was, represented the first clinical use of corneal image reflections.

Brewster was also active in determining the structure of the crystalline lens. In 1816 he initiated a series of experiments for which he has recently been described as "surely one of the most able and innovative experimenters ever to work on the lens" (Duncan, in press). In the initial experiments Brewster (1816) used crossed polarizing methods to view the lens, and he observed dark vertical and horizontal lines against a light background. This was interpreted in terms of radially oriented structures in the lens that led to the birefringence. Similar fibrous structures had been proposed by earlier microscopists, but the issue was still much in contention. Some years later Brewster (1833b) supported this conclusion on the basis of diffraction microscopic experiments, and he even determined the dimensions of the repetitive structures within the lens. Brewster's work in this area has recently been confirmed using modern laser polarization techniques (see Duncan, in press, for a detailed description of Brewster's lens work).

Brewster's work on the structure of the lens was in striking contrast to his deliberations on its function.

> There is no part of the physiology of the eye which has excited more discussion than the power by which it accommodates itself to different distances. Although the most distinguished philosophers have contributed their optical skill, and the most acute anatomists their anatomical knowledge, yet, notwithstanding all this combination of science, the subject is as little understood at the present moment as it was in the days of Kepler, who first attempted the solution of the problem (Brewster, 1824, p. 77).

The candidate mechanisms for accommodation were the lengthening or shortening of the axis of the eye, variations in curvature of the lens, forward or backward movement of the lens, and variations in pupil size. Thomas Young's (1801) support for the second of these hypotheses was by no means universally accepted, despite the fact that it was sustained "with all the ingenuity that might be expected from his profound knowledge of Optics and Physiology" (Brewster, 1824, p. 78). The reason for Brewster's reluctance to accept it was the belief that the refractive index of the crystalline lens differed little from its surrounding fluid, in which case variations in its curvature would have had only a marginal focusing effect. Brewster confirmed the observation that the pupil contracted when viewing near objects, but he demonstrated that the focusing was not a consequence of the reduction in the aperture size.

> It appears to me impossible to avoid the conclusion, that the power of adjusting the eye depends on the mechanism which contracts and dilates the pupil; and, since this adjustment is independent of the variation of its aperture, it must be effected by the parts which are in immediate contact with the base of the iris (1824, p. 81),

that is, the ciliary muscles. Of the possibilities Brewster entertained, two methods of producing the adjustment seemed most consistent with the known characteristics of the eye: changes in the convexity of the capsule of the lens and increasing the distance of the crystalline lens from the retina. The first

> depending on a supposed alteration in curvature of the capsule of the lens, cannot produce the effect, because the *liquor morgagni*, in which the lens floats, has nearly the same refractive power as the acqueous humour, and therefore no change in the curvature of the membrane which separates them, could produce a perceptible deviation in the transmitted rays. The last hypothesis, therefore, remains as the only probable one, namely, the removal of the lens from the retina by the contraction of the pupil, the eye being adjusted to objects at the remote limit of its range when in a state of perfect repose (1824, p. 82).

Although Brewster's reasoning was impeccable he reached the wrong conclusion because the available evidence regarding the refractive indices of the ocular structures was wanting. His views did not change, and were repeated 20 years later, "although he must admit that he could not as yet satisfy his own mind with any of the explanations which he had given" (Brewster, 1844b, p. 11). It was left to Helmholtz (1856) to vindicate the crystalline curvature hypothesis initially proposed by Descartes, and so ingeniously supported by Young.

Despite these forays into physiological and visual optics, Brewster's early researches were devoted primarily to experiments in physical optics. Indeed, the decade from 1808 has been considered his most productive research phase (Cochran, 1981). He published many papers on the polarization of light in the *Transactions of the Royal Society* (1813b, 1814, 1815) which formed the basis of the law bearing his name, and for which he received the Royal Society's Copley medal, followed three years later by the award of the Rumford medal. He was elected a fellow of the Royal Society in 1815. He published his first book, a *Treatise on New Philosophical Instruments* in 1813, and he invented the kaleidoscope in 1816.

Brewster continued to investigate the polarization of light and to measure the optical characteristics of numerous crystals for the rest of his life, but his influence in the field of optics declined after this productive decade. In fact, with his middle and advancing years his approach to optics seemed to become more and more anachronistic to his contemporaries. Brewster's optics were experimental rather than theoretical. He remained as close to his observations as was possible, and he thought of broader theorizing as speculation. This was particularly the case with regard to the growing support for the wave theory of light and the mathematical tools that assisted in its analysis. The new mathematically based optics was championed in Britain by the trinity of Airy, Whewell* and Hamilton† (at Trinity Colleges, Cambridge and Dublin), and their clashes with Brewster became a recurrent theme of British Association meetings in the 1830s and 1840s (see Cantor, 1978; Morrell and Thackray, 1981). While accepting the phenomenon of interference and its interpretation in terms of wave theory, Brewster did not consider this to be evidence for the undulatory nature of light itself (Cantor, 1983; Olson, 1975).

Brewster's researches into visual phenomena accelerated from the 1820s. He did present a paper to the Royal Society of Edinburgh in 1818 on an affection of the eye (the disappearance of peripherally viewed targets), but only an abstract of

---

* William Whewell (1794–1866) spent all his academic life at Trinity College, Cambridge, and held two professorships as well as holding the post of Master from 1841 until his death. His disagreements with Brewster were not confined to optics. Whewell published an anonymous essay *Of the Plurality of Worlds*, in 1853. Brewster was asked to review it for the North British Review; his rebuttal expanded into a book *More Worlds than One, the Creed of the Philosopher, and the Hope of the Christian* (1854). It is Whewell we must thank for the introduction of many novel and succinct appellations, like scientist and physicist.

† William Rowan Hamilton (1805–1860) was the Professor of Astronomy at Trinity College, Dublin, and Astronomer Royal for Ireland. He met Brewster at the Oxford Observatory during the 1832 B.A. meeting. He wrote afterwards: "As to Brewster, though he and I are as nearly opposite as two persons can well be, whom the world would class together, yet I found it a very tolerable, and even not unpleasant thing, to spend a week in his society" (Graves, 1882, p. 573).

this was published (Brewster, 1818). The major impetus for further enquiries appears to have been his entry on *Optics* for Volume XV of his *Edinburgh Encyclopaedia* (Brewster, 1822, 1830b). This article formed the basis for his *Treatise on Optics* published nine years later, and it contained a section *On Vision*. It was his definition of visible direction as "the direction coinciding with the last portion of the ray" striking the retina that was challenged by Charles Bell (1823) and which Brewster (Article 2.2 and 1826b) so staunchly defended. Brewster's conception of visible direction belonged essentially to the eighteenth century. It was advocated by Smith (1738) and Porterfield (1759), although it was openly challenged by Wells (1792) on the basis of experiments on visible direction in monocular and binocular vision. Brewster was not swayed by Wells's arguments, and visible direction remained a cornerstone of his approach to vision. Not only was it used in Brewster's analysis of monocular and binocular vision, but it also enabled him to dispose of the problem of erect vision from an inverted retinal image: "The lines of visible direction necessarily cross each other at the centre of visible direction, so that those from the lower part of the image go to the upper part of the object, and those from the upper part of the image to the lower part of the object" (Brewster, 1831a, p. 295). Moreover, his definition of visible direction remained unchanged throughout his life. In the last of his articles reprinted here (4.18), which was published two years before his death, we find an equivalent description of the concept:

> we know that distinct vision of external objects arises from the law of visible direction by which every ray of light, at whatever angle it may fall, gives us vision of the point from which it proceeds, in a direction perpendicular to the part of the membrane on which it is incident.

The combined observations of Wells, Bell and Wheatstone did little to shake Brewster's belief in this "law".

In the 1820s and 1830s Brewster's studies were addressed mainly to subjective visual phenomena, similar to those examined independently by Purkinje. Brewster's observations were concerned with the perceptual fading of peripherally viewed objects, subjective colours from stationary and moving achromatic stimuli, distortions of geometrically periodic patterns, pressure images, entoptical phenomena, and the "fluttering hearts". All were related, where possible, to the known characteristics of the retina, or to variations in the image projected onto the retina. His work in these areas has largely been disregarded or forgotten. There appear to be several reasons for this. One concerns Brewster's writing style, which makes few concessions to the reader, who is generally assumed to be familiar with the body of Brewster's earlier work. Another relates to the titles given to his articles on vision; they were often vague or general, so that the phenomena under study were not readily evident. This stands in stark contrast to his articles in physical optics, which were precisely titled. A further basis for the neglect lies in Brewster's commitment to his "law of visible direction" as an explanatory device. His conception of visible direction was relatively unfashionable in his own day, but it was transformed soon after his death as a consequence of Hering's (1868) and Helmholtz's (1925) studies.

One of the areas of Brewster's research that has not been forgotten is that on the constitution of the solar spectrum. In 1831 he proposed "a new analysis of solar light indicating three primary colours, forming coincident spectra of equal length". That is, he argued that light was composed of red, yellow and blue "spaces". Each colour space extended over the whole spectrum, but predominated in that region corresponding to its colour (see Fig. 1). The primaries

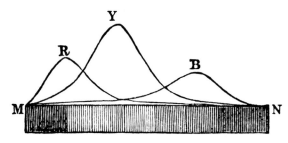

Fig. 1. The triple spectrum, as illustrated in Brewster's *Treatise on Optics* (1853, p. 80).

of red, yellow and blue were derived from absorption experiments using differently coloured filters. Only glasses of these three colours were required in combination to absorb all the light in the spectrum. The belief in the triple spectrum, stated initially in 1831 and repeated several times (Brewster, 1847, 1855b), derived from experiments in which prismatically separated sunlight was passed through variously coloured substances, and analysed. Brewster found that prismatic light of a given refraction changed colour when passed through a coloured filter. According to Newtonian theory the colour could be attenuated or removed but never changed in hue. The theory of the triple spectrum was strongly challenged by Brewster's contemporaries, particularly by Airy (1847). However, it was Helmholtz (1852) who finally laid it to rest. Helmholtz was able to reproduce Brewster's results:

> A careful repetition of at least the most important of his experiments, carried out in exact accordance with his method, and with every precaution hitherto deemed necessary, has indeed taught me that the facts which he affirms to have observed are described with perfect accuracy; indeed nothing else could be expected from so skillful an observer (Helmholtz, 1852, p. 403).

Helmholtz went on to demonstrate that certain other precautions were in fact necessary, which resulted in observations different from Brewster's, and in accordance with the Newtonian theory. These additional precautions consisted mainly of excluding the possibility of residual stray light or dispersion within the optical system, and in avoiding problems of perceived colour confusions at low levels of illumination. (See Sherman, 1981, for a more detailed discussion of Brewster's analysis of solar light and the reactions to it.)

Brewster's theory of the triple spectrum is probably remembered because it now seems so obviously wrong. Boring (1942) referred to it as "incorrect and sterile". It is easy for us to see it so, and dismiss it lightly. It says much, however, about Brewster. He would not wilfully have proposed any theory that challenged one advanced by his hero, Newton. The experimental results, though, were clear and repeatable, and could not be interpreted by him in any other way. This is yet another instance of Brewster, the scientist, who was prepared to follow the path that his experiments led regardless of the consequences. The fact that he refused to modify his views following Helmholtz's refutation says much about Brewster, the man. In 1855 Brewster presented a defence of his triple spectrum, addressed mainly to Helmholtz. More emphasis was placed on Helmholtz's replication of the earlier experiments than his failure to do so with more refined procedures. The suggestion that Brewster might have reported inaccurately the colours he saw was treated with scorn.

> The changes of colour by absorption which I have described I have distinctly seen, and seen as correctly as Newton saw his seven colours in the spectrum, and Hooke his composite tints in the soap-bubble; and, now that my eyes have nearly finished their work, I cannot mistrust, without reason, such good and faithful servants (Brewster, 1855b, p. 8).

Brewster also addressed himself to the problems of colour blindness, although some of his initial remarks were made anonymously (Brewster, 1822, 1826a, 1844a). He preferred the term colour blindness to Daltonism, particularly popular with the French, because "no person wishes to be immortalized by his imperfection. We cannot but regard it as degrading to the venerable name which it misapplies, as one of the worst examples of vicious nomenclature" (Brewster, 1844a, pp. 139–140). Of the many alternatives extant, the worst of which was considered to be *Chromatometablepsie*, Brewster used the term colour blindness "because it indicates simply blindness to one or more colours" (1844a, p. 140). Brewster had, in fact, examined the state of Dalton's* vision and found that he saw distinctly in the red extremity of the spectrum, but did not experience colour there. Dalton believed that his own colour blindness was due to having a blue

---

* John Dalton (1766–1844) first noticed his colour blindness when comparing botanical specimens of flowers. His own colour descriptions did not agree with those of his friends. He frequently surprised his fellow Quakers by attending prayer meetings in purple rather than black raiments. When he and Brewster attended the Oxford meeting of the British Association in 1832 "Dalton was the only one of the group who wore his scarlet robe all through the week, and two years later he attracted general attention by appearing in the same gay colouring at a Court levee" (Gordon, 1870, p. 173). Dalton remained a humble Quaker philosopher, teaching pupils in Manchester, even though his atomic theory of chemical combination had brought him universal recognition. Brewster held Dalton in very high regard, and as a memorial stated "among the great men who have illustrated the passing century, there is no brighter name than that of John Dalton" (Gordon, 1870, p. 172).

vitreous humour, which would have absorbed the red rays. Brewster considered that this was the only hypothesis for colour blindness capable of being proved or disproved. As it happens it was disproved – "after the death of Mr. Dalton the vitreous humour of his eyes was found to be perfectly colourless" (Brewster, 1853, p. 440). Brewster's theory was, of course, retinal. He believed that the retina was insensible to certain colours at the extreme ends of the spectrum. He drew the analogy between the "artificial colour blindness" that occurred when the normal eye lost its sensibility for a particular colour, and the loss of sensibility occurring in colour blindness. In the former, the red end of the spectrum "first becomes insensible"; in the latter, the majority of cases then known involved red blindness. Brewster saw little to distinguish his theory from Young's, which attributed colour blindness to "the absence or paralysis of those fibres of the retina which are calculated to perceive red" or from Herschel's, which proposed "a defect in the sensorium". "All these theories, indeed, are mere conjectures" (Brewster, 1844a, p. 135). Although Brewster saw no ready means of proving his own retinal theory he had even less confidence that those involving some more neural component could ever be addressed. Indeed, his comments on these theories are most illuminating, as they epitomize his approach to perception generally: "As I know nothing about the *sensorium*, or about its connexion with, or mode of operation upon, the nerves of sensation, I shall leave the merits of the new theory to those who feel themselves qualified for so arduous a task" (1844a, p. 135).

It was essentially this same issue that distinguished the theories of Brewster and Wheatstone with respect to stereoscopic vision. Wheatstone's first paper on the stereoscope (2.4) was the stimulus to Brewster's interests in binocular vision, in the 1840s. He had commented on binocular vision in the *Edinburgh Encyclo-paedia* article on optics, but only in a most peremptory manner, "When an object, therefore, is seen single with two eyes, it is in reality double, but the two images coincide so accurately, that they appear only as one, and having twice the brightness of the image formed by either eye alone" (1830b, p. 615). The implications of Wheatstone's experiments for these views, and for the "law of visible direction" were profound. For Brewster monocular vision was of paramount importance, and any aspects of binocular vision would require to conform to the monocular laws. The optical projection to a single eye could be defined with precision, and this determined the perception of space – accepting the law of visible direction. Equivalent optical projection to two eyes could be accounted for in the manner of the definition above: it would matter little which of the two monocular projections was used. Different optical projections to each eye posed problems: one object could not have two different monocular directions. Brewster's solution to this problem was Keplerian. Because there was only one point at which the two visible directions coincided, where the monocular directions intersected, then this must be the visible direction in binocular vision.

The German physiologists Vieth and Müller had sought to account for binocular single vision by going inwards, to propose retinally equivalent or corresponding points (see Müller, 1842). Müller (1826a) was aware of retinal disparity, but he considered that it was too small to be detected. Brewster's solution was to resort to geometrical optics, and to define the binocular centre at the intersection of the two visible directions. How this could be determined within the eyes was not discussed. It was taken to be a fact, as it offered the only means of reconciling the phenomenon of stereoscopic depth with the law of visible direction. In this sense, Brewster was the first projection theorist to address stereoscopic vision. Paradoxically, he was more closely akin to suppression theory (Porta, 1593) in accounting for binocular single vision.

Brewster's approach to binocular depth perception has not, however, been considered in these terms. Largely because of his use of the term convergence to define the binocular centre, it has been assumed that he meant convergence of the optic axes or convergent eye movements. Brewster is himself to blame, in part, for this misunderstanding because he did not apply the term with adequate precision and because he often referred to convergent eye movements in the same context. He did, however, make the difference explicit: "Hence we must draw a marked distinction between the vision of a solid (as an optical fact) when the eyes are fixed upon one point of it, and the resultant perception of its figure arising from the union of all the separate sensations received by the two eyes" (see p. 107). Brewster argued that eye movements assisted stereoscopic vision because the distinctness of vision was greatest near the visual axis. The whole figure would be seen with greater clarity following convergent eye movements over its surface. A second factor that has resulted in Brewster being classified as an eye movement theorist is that he did demonstrate a novel depth phenomenon that was dependent on convergence of the eyes – the wallpaper illusion (Article 2.7). "The successive convergency of the optic axes upon two points of an object at different distances exhibits to us the difference of distance when we have no other possible means of perceiving it" (Brewster, 1856, pp. 50–51). Under normal circumstances there are other means available, and the means proposed by Brewster was in terms of the positions of the binocular centres of the rays striking the eyes.

In the Appendix to article 2.7 Brewster mentioned the ease with which a friend saw the wallpaper illusion "having taken too much wine". On repeating this experiment recently not only did the depth effect present itself vividly but one of the observers saw it for the first time in this state, despite many previous sober inspections! There is also mention in the Appendix of another report of the illusion communicated by a Professor Christison. The fashions in wallpaper seem to have conspired to produce a crop of such sightings. An American, John Locke, described his many independent observations on the wallpaper illusion and related phenomena in 1849, which corresponded closely with Brewster's.

Again in the Appendix there is the report of Brewster's wine-drinking friend seeing the same phenomenon when viewing a cane-bottomed chair from above. The opposite effect (namely viewing the ceiling from beneath a cane-bottomed chair) with the same perceptual outcome was reported, independently, by a Rev. J. Maynard, of the Cape of Good Hope in 1866. For reasons that are by no means clear, he "performed 1000 experiments in this direction", and he reported the apparent size changes that accompanied the changes in apparent distance.

The late 1840s saw the announcement of Brewster's lenticular stereoscope and his binocular camera. Neither of these were used to further his theories of binocular vision. Indeed, in the 1850s he added little other than polemic to matters binocular. In 1856 his treatise on *The Stereoscope* was published, as were the acrimonious letters to *The Times* regarding the invention of the stereoscope. More will be said of the public dispute with Wheatstone in Section 5.2.

Brewster continued to write intermittently on subjective visual phenomena. One that had been of especial interest was Haidinger's brushes, because of its dependence on polarized light. Haidinger (1844) had shown that yellowish coloured brushes or sectors could be seen fleetingly when plane polarized light entered the eye; the brushes could be rendered visible for longer periods if the plane of polarization was continuously changing. Brewster addressed himself to this issue at the Edinburgh meeting of the British Association in 1850, over which he presided. He believed that the brushes were due to some polarizing structure existing in the cornea and crystalline lens, as well as in the tissues which lie in front of the sensitive layer of the retina (Brewster, 1850). Following his delivery "a beardless stripling" rose to dispute the interpretation, and suggested, in its stead, its basis in the macula lutea or yellow spot. This young man of nineteen, who challenged "the formidable Sir David Brewster" was James Clerk Maxwell.* His experiments on Haidinger's brushes were published six years later (Maxwell, 1856), and his conclusions were supported by Helmholtz (1924). Maxwell commenced his colour experiments using various versions of his colour top in the early 1850s; it was exhibited during the Glasgow meeting of the British Association in 1855, at the house of a Professor Ramsey. Brewster had been invited to attend, but did not. Maxwell's results and interpretations of colour and colour vision were at variance with Brewster's, supporting the primaries red, green and blue, as proposed earlier by Thomas Young (see Maxwell, 1890). He also gave

* James Clerk Maxwell (1831–1879) developed an early interest in vision. After reading the report of the 1849 British Association meeting he wrote to Lewis Campbell "This is Wheatstone's Stereoscope, which Sir David Brewster has taken up of late with much violence at the Brightish Association. (The violence consists in making two lenses out of one by breaking it)" (Campbell and Garnett, 1882, p. 125). Maxwell made a "Real Image Stereoscope" and demonstrated it at the Dundee meeting of the B.A. in 1867. It was essentially like Claudet's stereomonoscope, and consisted of a large magnifying glass separated from the stereoscopic pictures by two short focal length lenses. Unlike the stereomonoscope there was no ground glass surface on which the focused images were projected (see Gill, 1969). Maxwell's main impact on vision has been through his experiments on colour mixing. Important as these were, he is best known for his work on electromagnetic radiation.

detailed equations for colour specification, based upon experiments with the top and using variable sectors of coloured paper.

It is clear that Brewster could count amongst his adversaries the leading physicists of the nineteenth century.

While Brewster is remembered by his law, Wheatstone is immortalized by way of an instrument, his bridge for measuring resistances in electrical circuits. Wheatstone's genius was essentially instrumental – he displayed his ingenuity by devising contrivances for the precise measurements of phenomena, be they electrical or optical. His initial endeavours were also instrumental in the more conventional sense. Musical instrument manufacture was the business started in London by his father early in the century. Charles had a keen interest in both instruments and their means of propagating sound, particularly in the case of wind instruments. Indeed, one of the first ripples Wheatstone made on a wider public scene was the exhibition, in his father's shop, of the Enchanted Lyre. This consisted of a lyre suspended from the ceiling and controlled by unseen players in the room above (see Bowers, 1975). Of the various instruments Wheatstone invented the most popular has been the concertina – patented in 1829. However, it was the scientific rather than the commercial side of the family business that exacted most of Wheatstone's attention.

His early exhibitions of the Enchanted Lyre attracted the attention of a visiting Danish physicist, Oersted,* who subsequently corresponded with Wheatstone about their various experiments on sound, particularly regarding the Chladni figures. Wheatstone's first scientific paper, on "New experiments in sound" was published with Oersted's encouragement (see Wheatstone, 1823). Chladni's experiments were improved upon by using a thin layer of water on the plate, which enabled Wheatstone to detect more minute vibrations than was possible with sand. These experiments in turn led to the kaleidophone (Article 3.3).

Thomas Young (1800) had also been impressed by the Chladni figures. He had observed similar patterns by winding a silvered wire around a piano string, vibrating the string, and observing the reflected light with the aid of a microscope. Wheatstone's method dispensed with the need of a microscope, as the travel of his kaleidophone rods was much more extensive, but the figures so produced were similar using both techniques. Although the kaleidophone was designed to exhibit acoustical principles, they were expressed visually. Wheatstone was attracted to the visual phenomena that enabled the kaleidophone to produce such beautiful forms – the duration of the visual impression. The other novel contrivance described at the end of the article represented the operation of visual persistence in the opposite sense to its expression in the kaleidophone: by

---

* Hans Christian Oersted (1777–1851) demonstrated a relationship between electricity and magnetism for the first time in 1820. This occurred during a public lecture in Copenhagen, when the passage of an electric current through a wire produced a minute deflection of a compass needle. Oersted described these experiments in an article on Thermo-electricity for Brewster's *Edinburgh Encyclopaedia*.

successive exposures of fragments of a stationary pattern the whole is rendered visible.

Wheatstone's article on the kaleidophone was published in 1827. By this time he had made acquaintance with Michael Faraday, and in the next year Faraday gave the first of his many Friday evening lectures to the Royal Institution on Wheatstone's behalf (see Bowers, 1975). Faraday was sufficiently interested in visual phenomena similar to those initially examined by Wheatstone to write an article on certain "optical deceptions" seen with moving patterns (Faraday, 1831). This article proved to be the stimulus for the independent invention of several devices for synthesizing visual movement (see Article 3.1).

Thus was Wheatstone's interest in vision initiated. Indeed, in 1826 he wrote to Oersted describing the kaleidophone and stating that he had a paper on vision in preparation. This could have referred to the first of his anonymous articles on "Contributions to the physiology of vision" (4.4). Purkinje's book, which Wheatstone translated and précised, appeared in 1823. The basis for Wheatstone's title to his paper is not given. However, it may be of significance that the title given to Purkinje's book in Article 4.4 is *Essay on Subjective Phenomena of Vision*. This was actually the *subtitle* of the book. Its main title was *Observations and Experiments on the Physiology of the Senses*. Moreover, the words "Physiology of the Senses" were printed far more prominently than any others on the title page. A further factor could relate to the inclusion of Müller in the list of continental authors whose discoveries were to be translated. Johannes Müller wrote two books in 1826, the more important of which bore the title *On the Comparative Physiology of Vision in Man and Animals*. Whatever the origins of the descriptive phrase, it must have appealed to Wheatstone because he retained it for his two stereoscopic memoirs, despite the fact that they contained nothing of direct physiological import.

The introductory section to 4.4, the first of Wheatstone's specifically visual papers, makes it evident that he was familiar with the major writers on visual phenomena, both ancient and modern. He noted the range of disciplines brought to bear on the topic – "metaphysicians, physiologists, natural philosophers, and artists" – and appreciated that the attraction was that "vision has a peculiar claim on the attention of philosophers, as presenting some of those links which connect physical and mental phenomena" (4.4). What distinguished Wheatstone from the many other students of vision was his encyclopaedic knowledge and his linguistic skills. "His bibliographic knowledge was almost incredible. He seemed to know every book that was written and every fact recorded, and anyone in doubt had only to go to Wheatstone to get what he wanted" said Sir William Preece, an acquaintance of Wheatstone's (Bowers, 1975, p. 216).

Wheatstone wished to remove the ignorance of continental literature on vision he considered prevailed in Britain by translating the major contemporary works. He did not state why Purkinje's book was chosen for the first such treatment, but his summary remains the most complete account of Purkinje's observations in

English to this day. In the course of the translation Wheatstone must have tried to reproduce most of the phenomena described by Purkinje. The one singled out for detailed scrutiny by Wheatstone was that of rendering the retinal blood vessels visible. The simplicity of his apparatus contrasted with the sophistication of his thought. Using only a candle and a moving annular disc he proposed the basis for the visibility of the vessels, as shadows, and then formulated general principles of continuous visibility from the conditions of their visibility. Wheatstone amplified these principles following the paper delivered by Brewster at the 1832 meeting of the British Association (2.6). Wheatstone is introduced as "having been the first person to introduce Purkinje's beautiful experiment into this country, and having repeated it a great number of times under a variety of forms".

Purkinje's work is returned to in the second of the anonymous articles (4.5), but this is both shorter than the first, and not of the manner anticipated for the proposed series. At this time, in the early 1830s, Wheatstone was primarily involved in experiments on acoustics. His active involvement in acoustics was not to last much longer, although he maintained his family connection with musical instrument manufacture. His interests in vision were developing and those in electricity were stirring. He was also to become an academic, with his appointment to the Chair of Experimental Philosophy at King's College, London in 1834.

The connection between the kaleidophone and the measurement of the velocity of electricity was closer than would at first appear. The kaleidophone stimulated Wheatstone's experiments on visual persistence. Some of these experiments were demonstrated to a Friday evening meeting at the Royal Institution on 8 March, 1833. It is evident from the report in *The Athenaeum* that he had developed a novel device which consisted of a wheel which could be set in rapid motion "by means of a train of wheels immediately connected to it".* A similar arrangement was used for controlling the rapidly rotating mirrors used to reflect the images of sparks conducted through half a mile of insulated copper wire (see Bowers, 1975).

Wheatstone must have been cogitating upon phenomena of binocular vision in the very early 1830s. His interest was initiated by a chance observation, as he described in section 8 of Article 2.4. The light of a candle reflected from a lathe-turned metal plate appeared as a line standing beneath and above its surface. This only occurred during binocular observation. "It is curious, that an effect like this, which must have been seen thousands of times, should never have attracted sufficient attention to have been made the subject of philosophic observation. It was one of the earliest facts which drew my attention to the subject I am now treating" (p. 76). By the latter part of 1832 he had commissioned from the

---

* These experiments do not appear to have been published elsewhere, despite the hope expressed in Brewster's *Philosophical Magazine* (1833, p. 314) that the content of the lecture would soon appear in that journal.

opticians Murray and Heath stereoscopes "both of reflecting mirrors and refracting prisms" (Article 2.12). In November the same year he wrote to Brewster
that he was planning to present a paper on binocular vision to the Royal Society
"in which I shall describe a series of very curious optical illusions, which I believe
to be perfectly original" (Article 2.12). This suggests that he was in an advanced
stage with his experiments, although they were not published until 1838. During
this intervening period he was deflected from vision by his electrical researches –
both regarding its measurement and its practical application. As he stated in his
public dispute with Brewster:

> If any justification of the delay in publishing any complete results, after I had
> announced the general facts, be necessary, it may be found in the following
> circumstances. Between the periods referred to, I published, in 1833, my memoir
> "on the figures at vibrating surfaces," and, in 1834, my memoir "on the velocity of
> electricity and the duration of electric light," which gained for me admission to the
> French Academy of Sciences; from 1834 to 1838 I was engrossingly engaged in
> those experiments relating to electrical phenomena to which my last investigations
> had led me, and from which resulted all my inventions regarding the electric
> telegraph. It is not much to be wondered at, that, during this interval I was obliged to
> defer to a future time the consideration of subjects of less immediate interest
> (p. 181).

The memoir of 1838 described the problems of binocular vision from a
theoretical position – of perspective – rather than from the phenomenal observation that triggered his interest. This probably reflected his fascination with the
history of science, and he found a most apposite quotation from Leonardo da
Vinci with which to commence his more detailed deliberations. This he followed
with a cunundrum of his own:

> Had Leonardo da Vinci taken, instead of a sphere, a less simple figure for the
> purpose of his illustration, a cube for instance, he would not only have observed that
> the object obscured from each eye a different part of the more distant field of view,
> but the fact would also perhaps have forced itself upon his attention, that the object
> itself presented a different appearance to each eye (p. 67).

The insertion of the "perhaps" speaks volumes. Wheatstone concluded

> He failed to do this, and no subsequent writer within my knowledge has supplied the
> omission; the projection of two obviously dissimilar pictures on the two retinae when
> a single object is viewed, while the optic axes converge, must therefore be regarded
> as a new fact in the theory of vision (p. 67).

This new fact was pursued with all Wheatstone's instrumental ingenuity, and
culminated in his stereoscopes – although he only described the reflecting model
in his first memoir. The wonder at first seeing relief in two flat perspective
drawings mounted in the stereoscope can be recalled by all who have experienced

it. Wheatstone's wonder must have been infinitely greater because of its original-ity and of the uncertainty associated with it. Wheatstone not only described the depth seen in paired outline drawings, but he also reversed the depth by reversing the disparity, varied the magnitudes and inclinations of the paired figures and demonstrated binocular contour rivalry with different forms presented to each eye. These are only a few of the remarkable observations he made in this article. The impression of relief when viewing dissimilar pictures posed problems for all the received views of binocular combination, and Wheatstone addressed these in turn.

"Part the first" was not intended to provide all Wheatstone's observations and interpretations of binocular phenomena. Indeed, it could not have been con-sidered otherwise from the title alone. When his first memoir was written further experiments must have been either under way or anticipated, but there is little in the text to indicate the direction they would take; nor is there any suggestion of the time that would elapse before the appearance of the second memoir.

The stereoscope was demonstrated at the Newcastle meeting of the British Association in 1838, and Wheatstone delivered a paper "On binocular vision; and on the stereoscope, an instrument for illustrating its phenomena". This brief report was soon translated into French and German, as was the longer "Con-tributions" article. As William James was to note at the end of the century

> This essay . . . contains the germ of almost all the methods applied since to the study of optical perception. It seems a pity that England, leading off so brilliantly the modern epoch of this study, should so quickly have dropped out of the field. Almost all subsequent progress has been made in Germany, Holland, and, *longo intervallo*, America (James, 1890, pp. 226–227).

The fourteen years that spanned Wheatstone's two memoirs on binocular vision were active ones, but not for his visual researches. Electricity and tele-graphy demanded most of his energies. He delivered the first of his Bakerian lectures to the Royal Society, in which the "Wheatstone" bridge was first announced (Wheatstone, 1843). He improved the electric telegraph and developed submarine telegraphy, as well as designing the electromagnetic chronoscope (Article 3.4). However, there was a brief visual interlude. At the York meeting of the British Association, in 1844, he described a "singular effect of the juxtaposition of certain colours under particular circumstances" (4.12) – the apparent motion of contrasted colours, especially reds and greens, when viewed under gas-light. In the following paper (4.13). Brewster called this the fluttering hearts, by which term it is still known. Neither claim credit for the original observations, and do not state how their attention was drawn to it. Wheatstone had gone to the lengths of having samples of rug-work made up in different colours so that their efficacy at inducing motion could be determined. His interpretation of the phenomenon in terms of the eye "retaining its sensibility for various colours during various lengths of time" was also adopted by Helmholtz (1924).

This article represented one of Wheatstone's few sorties into either the physics or perception of colour. In 1835 he presented a brief report to the British Association on the prismatic spectrum produced by the light of an electric spark. From the lines in the spectrum he concluded that the light resulted from the volatization of the conductor material. According to Bowers (1975), Wheatstone continued working on spectrum analysis, although he did not publish any more papers on this topic.

The second "Contributions to the Physiology of Vision" was Wheatstone's second Bakerian lecture. The period between 1838 and 1852 had witnessed the publication of Daguerre's and of Talbot's photographic discoveries. Indeed, these were made public very shortly after the appearance of the first memoir, and huge advances in the techniques of photography were made in the 1840s. Shortly before the publication of Wheatstone's second memoir Frederick Scott Archer announced his collodion wet-plate process, which combined the sharpness of images, found in Daguerreotypes, with the reproducability of Talbot's negative process. Wheatstone was clearly instrumental in having the first photographs taken for the stereoscope. Buildings and statues were ideal subjects. Portraits posed more problems, as is evident from Henry Collen's comments sometime later:

> In 1841, when I was one of the very few who undertook to make use of Mr. Talbot's process, Mr. Wheatstone not only had the idea of making photographic portraits for the stereoscope, but at his request, and under his direction, in August of that year, I made a pair of stereoscopic portraits of Mr. Babbage, in whose possession they still remain; and if I remember rightly Mr. Wheatstone had previously obtained some daguerreotype portraits from Mr. Beard for the stereoscope. Successful as the portraits of Mr. Babbage were then considered, I did not pursue the subject, on account of the comparatively long time, at that period, required for the consecutive sittings for two pictures, without any movement on the part of the sitter (Collen, 1854, p. 200).

Wheatstone appreciated that with increasing distance from an object the dissimilarity of the pictures decreases. Accordingly, photographs taken with a separation of 2½ inches equivalent to the interocular distance would be almost identical for far objects. Under these circumstances an exaggerated separation was recommended: "I find an excellent effect when the axes are nearly parallel by pictures taken at an inclination of 7° or 8°, and even a difference of 16° or 17° has no decidedly bad effect" (see p. 158). Needless to say, Wheatstone did not restrict himself to the pictorial pleasures of stereoscopic photography; he also put them to good empirical use. By varying the angular separations of photographs and then viewing them with a fixed degree of convergence he was able to dissociate the cue of disparity from that of convergence.

In order to dissociate accommodation from convergence Wheatstone modified his mirror stereoscope, so that the arms could rotate about a common axis. He also presented illustrations of his prism and portable reflecting stereoscopes. The major novel contrivance described in the article is the pseudoscope, and he gave a lengthy description of the visual effects attendant upon using it. These were in turn related to the conversions of relief visible without any optical device. It is upon this point that the article ends, taking up some minor disagreement with Brewster on conversions of relief in binocular vision.

This abrupt ending is in many ways puzzling. No attempt was made to summarize his observations, no general theoretical statement was given and no directions for future pursuits were suggested. It is almost as though he tired of the topic. The general theoretical issues treated in the first memoir are virtually ignored in the second. He reported insightful experiments, ingenious inventions and graphic descriptions of the various novel phenomena, but these are not related to theories of binocular vision in the manner of the first memoir. His empiricism had become entirely experimental rather than being theoretical as well. Taken in isolation Wheatstone's second memoir remains a major work in vision research. However, it is cited rarely in comparison with the first paper, and if it is known it is usually because of the pseudoscope.

"Part the second" does not fulfil the expectations of it based upon "Part the First", and perhaps Wheatstone's realization of this was a factor in delaying its appearance. None the less, Wheatstone's two "Contributions to the Physiology of Vision" remain the classical articles on stereoscopic vision and richly reward reading. The first represents a more youthful and vigorous Wheatstone, alive to all the empirical and theoretical avenues opened by his brilliant invention; the second reflects a more secure experimentalist, who has spent much of his intellectual energy in other pursuits.

Wheatstone's only other publication on stereoscopic vision was the historical note on binocular microscopes (2.11), and in fact this is his last article on vision generally, even though he lived another 20 years. He did, of course, engage Brewster in combat across the pages of *The Times* in 1856, but that battle was not of his making. It is to the issue of the conflicts between Brewster and Wheatstone that we now turn.

Binocular rivalry.

5.2. The Brewster–Wheatstone Controversies

When Brewster and Wheatstone joined battle over the invention of the stereo-scope, in 1856, neither was a stranger to academic combat. Brewster had experienced numerous forays in the publication of the *Edinburgh Encyclopaedia,* and major confrontations with optical wave theorists both verbally, at British Association meetings, and in print. Wheatstone had quarrelled with his collaborator in telegraphy, William Cooke, over the contributions each had made to its invention, and the dispute was decided by formal arbitration (see Bowers, 1975). Thus, they were both well-versed in the arts of intellectual warfare. Indeed, this was a skill essential to any Victorian scientist of note, as such disputes were not infrequent. However, seldom have two contemporaries contributed so much to vision research, and harboured so much personal resentment. The obvious parallel is with Helmholtz and Hering, as they shared the animosities displayed by Brewster and Wheatstone. In fact, the parallels are more than superficial, because Helmholtz shared the empiricist views of Wheatstone, and Hering posited the processes of perception in the retina, as did Brewster, particularly for stereoscopic vision. Helmholtz and Hering also had major disagreements regarding visual direction.

The correspondence over the invention of the stereoscope in *The Times* (2.12) seems, in retrospect, petty. Brewster initially claimed that Mr Elliot had been the first to invent the ocular stereoscope, in 1834, although he did not make one until 1839. Taking the most charitable view possible, Brewster might have been right. For him, an ocular stereoscope was one that did not employ any optical devices, like mirrors, prisms or lenses, to separate the images to the two eyes. Although it seems highly probable that Wheatstone constructed his "ocular" devices before conceiving the idea of the reflecting stereoscope, there is no independent evidence of this. To pursue this point, however, is absurd.

The real purpose of Brewster's letters was not so much to cast doubt on the originality of Wheatstone's stereoscope as on his vision. As a leading authority of optics, and on the structure and function of the eye, Brewster would have been expected to invent a stereoscope rather than someone whose previous interests had been in sound. That it was not so must have been a constant irritation to Brewster. It is evident from his meagre considerations of binocular vision prior to Wheatstone's memoirs that his views of it were primitive even by the standards of the early nineteenth century. Having seen the honour of first demonstrating the nature of stereoscopic vision bestowed upon Wheatstone, Brewster tried to wrest it from him and by crediting it to the ancients. Brewster's knowledge of the classical texts on optics was extensive, as was his ability to read into them features which had not been seen by any earlier scholars. Such unusual scholarship might have had more sway but for Wheatstone's compendious intellect. The attribution of stereoscopic principles to the ancients could not be sustained.

The seeds of this controversy were sown much earlier. In 1832, at the Oxford meeting of the British Association, they clashed over their interpretations of the visibility of the retinal blood vessels. The dispute was not between equals, with regard to their reputations. The British Association owed its very existence, in considerable measure, to Brewster, who had long complained of Government neglect of science and scientists and had championed such a forum for the exchange of scientific intelligence. He had recently been knighted for his endeavours in this sphere, and was highly regarded as an international authority on optics. Wheatstone, on the other hand, was relatively unknown, and much younger. His scientific reputation was based upon a few papers published on sound; his article on the kaleidophone represented his only known contact with vision, because his translations (4.4 and 4.5) were published anonymously. None the less, this difference of opinion led to their first meeting, and the initiation of correspondence on their optical researches. It was in one of the early letters that Wheatstone mentioned his plans for a paper on binocular vision (see Article 2.12).

Brewster attended the annual gatherings of the British Association fairly regularly, Wheatstone less frequently. Wheatstone's reputation, however, was waxing, mainly as a consequence of his electrical experiments, whereas Brewster's was waning. As has been mentioned in Section 2.1, both were guests of W. H. F. Talbot prior to the Bristol meeting of the British Association in 1836. Among Talbot's other distinguished guests were Babbage, Whewell, and Roget. Brewster and Wheatstone would have had the opportunity to become acquainted on more intimate terms than was possible through the formal sessions of the B.A. Moreover, they shared a fascination in the experiments Talbot was conducting on fixing images formed in a camera obscura. There is no evidence of any residual animosity from the 1832 dispute; rather the reverse, as is indicated in a letter written by Brewster to his wife from Laycock Abbey: "Our party was increased last night by Dr. Roget, Mr. Babbage and Professor Wheatstone, so that we have all the elements of spending an agreeable week here" (Gordon, 1870, p. 165).

Brewster was so taken by the demonstration of Wheatstone's reflecting stereoscope at the Newcastle meeting of the British Association, in 1838, that he purchased a model for his own use. It led to the eventual realization that his consideration of binocular vision had been woefully inadequate, and that his "law of visible direction" was seriously challenged by the stereoscopic phenomena visible with Wheatstone's contrivance. Ironically, his resolution of these theoretical difficulties, in terms of the binocular centre where the monocular directions coincided, resulted in a greater similarity between his position and Wheatstone's than is generally realized. For representations of objects, either in three dimensions or as two two-dimensional pictures, both predict that depth will be seen. Wheatstone argued that the dissimilarity in the pictures on the retinae determined the perceived depth. Brewster believed that the projected dissimilarities were the same whether produced by objects or their equivalent two-dimensional representations: for both the binocular centres were located in the appropriate depth planes.

Wheatstone was not concerned only with reflecting the conditions that typically obtain in binocular vision, but in a different guise via the stereoscope. He wished to derive general principles. One such was that dissimilarities in the retinal images induce the appearance of depth, and it mattered not how the dissimilarities were determined. Accordingly, he presented two classes of dissimilarity that would not normally correspond to natural patterns of stimulation. One concerned the binocular combination of pictures having different monocular magnitudes, although he stated that this would occur naturally when viewing any object away from the median plane of the head. He did note that the differences in the sizes of the images could not be too great, otherwise binocular coincidence would not result. "It appears that if the inequality of the pictures be greater than the difference which exists between the two projections of the same object when seen in the most oblique position of the eyes (*i.e.* both turned to the extreme right or to the extreme left), ordinarily employed, they do not coalesce" (see p. 83). Brewster should have found little in this to dispute, but he did. "These extraordinary results are obviously subversive of the established laws of vision, but especially of the law of visible direction" (p. 101).

Wheatstone's second class of dissimilarity involved a configuration in which the stimulation of corresponding points resulted in their double vision. He reported that a thick vertical line in one eye will combine with a thick inclined line in the other, rather than a thin vertical (see Fig. 23, p. 83). Moreover, the thick line will appear in relief and the thin one will retain its vertical appearance. Brewster adopted the same approach to the second class that he had applied to the first, namely, that ocular equivocation (binocular rivalry) prevented the visibility of one or other half image:

> I have no hesitation in affirming that the phenomenon described by Mr. Wheatstone is an illusion, arising from the actual disappearance of one or more parts, or even the whole of one of the lines, and from the difficulty of observing the separation or superimposition of images in the circumstances under which the experiment is made (p. 103).

Brewster presented many variations of these configurations, including those corresponding to the pattern of stimulation produced by real three-dimensional objects.

Wheatstone's figure 23 (Article 2.4, p. 83) could not actually correspond to the pattern of stimulation produced by a line in depth intersecting a single vertical line. If the inclined line was nearer than the vertical in one half, it would be farther away in the other – in which case it would be partially obscured by the thin line. This has proved to be one of the few observations described by Wheatstone that has not been easy to repeat (see Helmholtz, 1925).

Brewster's arguments regarding the intersecting monocular directions have fared quite well with respect to stereoscopic phenomena. They applied to those situations in which the dissimilar pictures corresponded precisely to the projections produced by solid objects. They had to do so, because Brewster was essentially redescribing the conditions for which stereoscopic vision obtains. As Howard and Templeton (1966, p. 15) put it: "projection theories are at best a geometrical description of the optics of vision, they are not theories of how information is coded physiologically". Brewster said virtually nothing about physiology nor about mechanisms, because he considered that such deliberations were beyond the realm of experimental investigation. Eye movements, however, were not, and he did argue that successive convergent eye movements assisted stereoscopic vision (although Wheatstone had amply demonstrated that eye movements alone were not sufficient to induce stereoscopic depth).

Wheatstone was prepared to entertain the general proposition of disparity determining depth because he believed that the "seat of vision" was in the brain rather than the eye. Brewster, of course, thought otherwise. There is a paradox here, too, because Wheatstone, the empiricist, would have been hard pressed to explain how a pattern of stimulation never before encountered (because it does not correspond to an actual object) could be related to one's past experience of stimulation.

Wheatstone's appeal to the sensorium, to cognitive rather than optical considerations, was to have more and more influence throughout the remaining decades of the nineteenth century. It was espoused by Helmholtz, who elaborated upon it, and coined the phrase *unconscious inference.* Helmholtz's debt to Wheatstone was plainly stated in the introduction to the third volume of his Handbook: "From the empirical side it was Wheatstone especially who, by inventing the stereoscope, gave a powerful incentive to the investigation of the influence of experience on our visual apperceptions" (1925, p. 36).

Wheatstone's more cognitive approach also gave him the freedom to entertain possibilities that Brewster considered literally unnatural. One such was that the separations used for taking stereoscopic photographs could, and should for distant objects, exceed the interocular separation. Brewster's binocular camera allowed no such possibility – the lenses were fixed 2½ inches apart. The fact that the two images of distant objects are virtually identical would not have deterred Brewster, for so they are when normally viewed.

It would have been most appropriate to examine this issue by recourse to stereoscopic portraits taken of these great men from different separations. Alas, no records of such pictures are available. As a pale imitation of this the following paired photographs of Brewster's statue were taken (see Fig. 1). The upper pair

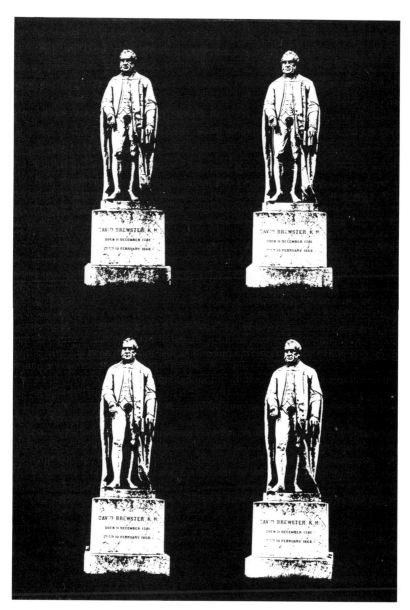

Fig. 1. Stereoscopic photographs of William Brodie's (1871) statue of Brewster, which stands outside the Chemistry Department, King's Buildings, University of Edinburgh. Unseen from these camera angles is a small stereoscope protruding beneath Brewster's robes. The photographs were taken from a distance of 6 m. The upper pair had a separation between the lenses of about 7 cm, whereas the separation was approximately 1 m for the lower pair.

were taken following Brewster's preference, with a separation of the camera approximating the interocular distance. The lower pair were taken with a separation of about 10°, which Wheatstone suggested produced an excellent effect. I leave it to the reader to determine whether they should best be viewed in a reflecting or a lenticular stereoscope!

The Brewster–Wheatstone controversy was clearly distasteful to Wheatstone. Brewster, by contrast, seemed to thrive on it, and he pursued it to great lengths via the Chimenti pictures. In the 1860's, when Brewster was writing on this last topic he was the Principal of Edinburgh University. This was perhaps the most tranquil period of his active life, and it could be said that he eventually mellowed a little. At least, he was then reconciled with Wheatstone. Both attended the Dundee meeting of the British Association in 1867. This was the last public function Brewster attended before his death, early in the next year. At the meeting Brewster went to Wheatstone and said "We have had much disagreeable discussion together, but I hope it is all forgotten" after which it is said they shook hands cordially. Following Brewster's previous inconsistencies in behaviour, Wheatstone was understandably a little wary. On repeating the anecdote to a friend Wheatstone said, "Do you really think he was sincere!" (see Gordon, 1870, p. 389).

5.3. Conclusions

A century after Wheatstone's death his life was chronicled with great affection by Bowers (1975). Wheatstone's (incomplete) scientific papers were republished, in 1879, shortly after his death. Brewster has not been accorded either a biography or a volume of scientific papers (selective though these would need to be). This is, perhaps, as he would have liked it. On his death bed he was asked if he wanted anyone to take charge of his scientific papers, to which he replied "No; I have done what every scientific man should do, viz., published almost all my observations of any value, just as they occurred" (Gordon, 1970, p. 412). None the less, some two centuries after his birth, a symposium on his life was held in Edinburgh (see Morrison-Low and Christie, 1983), though very little was said of his visual researches. It is hoped that the material incorporated in the present collection will make evident his contributions to visual science. The intention has also been to make more widely known the breadth of Wheatstone's researches in vision.

It seems unlikely that Brewster will find a biographer now. His character was not such as to evince the sympathy and affection necessary for so arduous a task. Indeed, one of the recurrent themes of the Brewster Bicentenary Symposium was the irrascibility of the man: he seemed to irritate most of those with whom he

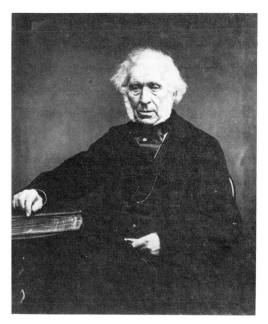

Brewster. Photograph taken, most probably, by Thomas Rodger of St. Andrews. Reproduced by kind permission of the University of St. Andrews.

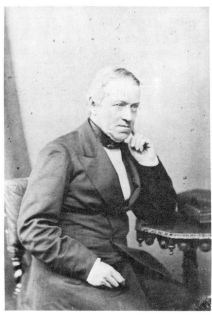

Wheatstone. Photograph taken for the London Stereoscopic Company. Reproduced by permission of the National Portrait Gallery.

came into contact. However, it is all too easy to dwell on the negative aspects of his personality and to overlook his achievements in science. Another theme of the Symposium was to remind us how much Brewster is forgotten. Professor William Cochran, who delivered the opening address, entitled a paper in the *New Scientist* "Who remembers David Brewster?" (Cochran, 1981). Earlier, Westfall, in editing Brewster's biography of Newton, reprinted in 1965, asked "Why has a figure who once strode so prominently upon the stage been so largely forgotten?" (Westfall, 1965, p. *x*). Indeed, Westfall considered that "If Sir David Brewster is known at all to the twentieth century, he is probably known through his biography of Newton" (p. *ix*). This is not the case in visual science, because his name is still popularly linked with his stereoscope. Many other aspects of his visual researches have been forgotten. If more words of my commentary have been addressed to Brewster, it is for this reason. Posterity has treated Wheatstone more kindly than Brewster. I have tried to redress the balance a little, without wishing to deny the greater import of Wheatstone's experimental work in vision.

Brewster's optics, both physical and visual, were related, and his work on them followed a similar general pattern. Early in his career, in the second decade of the nineteenth century, he enjoyed a period of great productivity. The concepts that were formulated then remained with him for life. It was this reluctance to modify his theoretical ideas, in the face of mounting evidence against them, that has fostered the subsequent neglect of his work. It can be argued that this neglect might be warranted in physical optics, where the pace of change has been rapid. In visual science the pace is more measured.

What Brewster and Wheatstone saw, we should be able to see, too. However, we no longer look in the way they did. We are far more dependent upon, and distracted by, the sophisticated machinery that fills our laboratories. By comparison the equipment they used was primitive. Hence they relied on instruments that we tend to neglect – highly refined observational skills. It is the corpus of their observations that warrants recall.

In the first half of the nineteenth century, sharply defined boundaries around specialized areas of scientific endeavour were rare. To write on visual phenomena required only eyes and insight regarding what was of interest. The latter placed strict demands on the writer – namely, a knowledge of what had been seen before and interpretations given to the observations. Both Brewster and Wheatstone were well-versed in the history of science generally, and of vision in particular. Both were scholars of a high order, with command of classical as well as modern languages. Wheatstone's historical scholarship was displayed indirectly in the substance of his papers. Brewster's was expressed in his numerous encyclopaedia entries, his reviews and in his books. In addition to the historical material in his treatises on the kaleidoscope, the stereoscope, optics and natural magic, he wrote biographies of the metaphorical *Martyrs of Science* (Galileo, Brahe and Kepler), and his life of Newton. This last is referred to as a masterpiece by Newton's most recent biographer (Westfall, 1980).

The factor that distinguished Brewster from Wheatstone was the direction from which this history should be viewed. Brewster looked backwards, whereas Wheatstone looked to the future. Brewster's theories were rooted in the previous century, whereas Wheatstone's inferential theories were influential then and now. They can be stated with little change in terminology today. However, we should not forget Brewster's strictures against speculation – for they, too, apply equally today. We know little of the sensorium, despite the fact that we frequently seduce ourselves with the contrary belief. Moreover, the modern projection theorists should note the logical consistency with which Brewster pursued his interpretations. To amplify a point made above: our observational repertoire is enlarged by occasional advances in technology; our theories of vision change less.

Despite these theoretical alignments of Brewster and Wheatstone, they were both essentially experimentalists. They were happier conducting experiments than interpreting them in a broader theoretical framework. Both were more concerned with the consequences of their vision than with their visions. Their differences have been with regard to the latter; with respect to the former they were in closer correspondence.

Of the many overlaps and coincidences in Brewster's and Wheatstone's researches on vision that have emerged from this collection, the following seems a suitable one with which to close. In the second, enlarged edition *The Kaleido-scope*, beneath Brewster's name and a long (but selective) list of his scientific honours, was the following inscription "*Nihil tangit quod non ornat*". Bowers (1975) opened his biography with the same statement, addressed to Wheastone by Faraday: "There was nothing he touched that he did not adorn".

Bibliography

Aepinus, F. De coloribus accidentalibus. *Novum Commentare*, 1769, **10**, 215.

Aguilonius, F. *Opticorum libri sex philosophis juxta ac mathematicis utiles*. Antwerp: 1613.

Airy, G. B. On a peculiar defect in the eye and a mode of correcting it. *Edinburgh Journal of Science*, 1827, **7**, 322–325.

Airy, G. B. The Astronomer Royal on Sir David Brewster's New Analysis of Solar Light. *London, Edinburgh and Dublin Philosophical Magazine and Journal of Science*, 1847, **30**, 73–76.

Airy, G. B. The Astronomer Royal on hemiopsy. *London, Edinburgh and Dublin Philosophical Magazine and Journal of Science*, 1865, **30**, 19–21.

Airy, H. On a distinct form of transient hemiopsia. *Philosophical Transactions of the Royal Society*, 1870, **160**, 247–264.

D'Alembert, J. le R. *Opuscules Mathematique; ou, mémoires sur différens sujets de géométrie, de méchanique, d'optique, d'astronomie, etc.*, 8 volumes, Paris, 1761–1780.

D'Alembert, J. le R. Nouvelles Recherche sur les verres optique; pour servir de suite a la théorie qui en et été donnée dans le Volume III des Opuscules Mathematiques. *Mémoires de l'Académie des Science*, 1765, pp. 53–105.

Alison, W. P. On single and correct vision by means of double and inverted images on the retinae. *Transactions of the Royal Society of Edinburgh*, 1836, **13**, 472–493.

Anderson, R. Brewster and the Reform of the Scottish Universities. In A. D. Morrison-Low and J. R. R. Christie (Eds.) *"Martyr of Science": Sir David Brewster, 1781–1868*. Edinburgh: HMSO, 1983.

D'Arcy, Chevalier. Mémoire sur la durée de la sensation de la vue. *Mémoires de l'Académie des Science*, 1765, pp. 439–451.

Arnold, H. J. P. *William Henry Fox Talbot. Pioneer of Photography and Man of Science*. London: Hutchinson Benham, 1977.

Athenaeum, 16 March, 1833, pp. 170–171. (Mr. Wheatstone on the duration of luminous impressions on the organ of vision).

Athenaeum, 8 September, 1838, p. 650. (Report of the Eighth B. A. Meeting).

Babbage, C. *Reflections on the Decline of Science in England, and on some of its Causes*. London: Fellowes, 1830.

Babbage, C. *Passages from the Life of a Philosopher*. London: Longman, Green, Longman, Roberts & Green, 1864.

Bacon, F. *Sylva Sylvarum: or a Naturall Historie*. London: W. Rawley, 1627.

Ballentyne, D. W. G. and Lovett, D. R. *A Dictionary of Named Effects and Laws*. London: Chapman Hall, 3rd Edition, 1970.

Bartels, C. M. N. *Beitrage zur Physiologie der Gesichtssinnes*. Berlin, 1834.

Bell, C. *The Anatomy of the Human Body*, Volume 3. London: Longman, Rees, Cadell and Davies, 1803.

Bell, C. *Idea of a New Anatomy of the Brain*, printed privately, 1811; reprinted in G. Gordon-Taylor and E. W. Walls, *Sir Charles Bell. His Life and Times*. Edinburgh: Livingstone, 1956, pp. 218–231.

Bell, C. On the motions of the eye, in illustration of the uses of the muscles and of the orbit. *Philosophical Transactions of the Royal Society*, 1823, **113**, 166–186.

Bell, C. *The Hand, Its Mechanism and Vital Endowments, as evincing Design. Bridgewater Treatise IV*. London: William Pickering, 1833.

Berkeley, G. *An Essay towards a New Theory of Vision*. Dublin, 1709.

Berkeley, G. *The Works of George Berkeley*. London: Thomas Tegg, 1843.

Birch, T. *The History of the Royal Society of London for Improving of Natural Knowledge*, 4 volumes. London: Royal Society, 1756.

Blackwood's Magazine, 1842, **51**, 812–830. Berkeley and Idealism. (Anonymous review.)

Boring, E. G. *Sensation and Perception in the History of Experimental Psychology*. New York: Appleton-Century, 1942.

Bouguer, P. Sur la grandeur apparente des objets. *Mémoires de l'Académie des Science de Paris*. 1755, pp. 99–112.

Bowers, B. *Sir Charles Wheatstone F.R.S. 1802–1875*. London: HMSO, 1975.

Bradley, R. *New Improvements in Planting and Gardening, both Philosophical and Practical*. London: W. Mears. 1717. (The Sixth Edition (London: E. L. Simmons, 1818) includes a section "Description and use of the instrument now called a kaleidoscope, as published by its original inventor, R. Bradley.")

Breguet, M. Télégraphic électrique. *Comptes Rendus de l'Académie des Sciences*. 1845, **21**, 760–763.

Brewster, D. *Treatise on New Philosophical Instruments for various Purposes in the Arts and Sciences. With Experiments on Light and Colours*. Edinburgh: W. Blackwood, 1813a.

Brewster, D. On some properties of light. *Philosophical Transactions of the Royal Society*, 1813b, **103**, 101–109.

Brewster, D. On the polarization of light by oblique transmission through all bodies, whether crystallized or uncrystallized. *Philosophical Transactions of the Royal Society*, 1814, **104**, 219–230.

Brewster D. On the laws which regulate the polarization of light by reflection from transparent bodies. *Philosophical Transactions of the Royal Society*, 1815, **105**, 125–159.

Brewster, D. On a singular affection of the eye in the healthy state, in consequence of which it loses the power of seeing objects within the sphere of distinct vision. (Abstract) *Annals of Philosophy*, 1818, **11**, 151.

Brewster, D. *A Treatise on the Kaleidoscope*. Edinburgh: A. Constable, 1819.

Brewster, D. Observations on the preceding paper. *Edinburgh Philosophical Journal*, 1822, **6**, 140–141. (The preceding paper is: Butter, J. Remarks on the insensibility of the eye to certain colours, pp. 135–140.)

Brewster, D. On the accommodation of the eye to different distances. *Edinburgh Journal of Science*, 1824, **1**, 77–83.

Brewster, D. Contributions to popular science. No. V. On the invisibility of certain colours to certain eyes. *Edinburgh Journal of Science*, 1826a, **4**, 85–87. (Published anonymously.)

Brewster, D. Farther observations on the supposed optical and physiological discoveries of Mr. Charles Bell. *Edinburgh Journal of Science*, 1826b, **5**, 259–268. (Published anonymously.)

Brewster, D. Observations by the Editor. *Edinburgh Journal of Science*, 1827, **7**, 325–326. (See Airy, 1827.)

Brewster, D. Preface to *Edinburgh Encyclopaedia*, Volume 1. Edinburgh: Blackwoods, 1830a.

Brewster, D. Optics, in *Edinburgh Encyclopaedia*, Volume XV, 1830b, pp. 460–662. (Originally published in 1822.)

Brewster, D. Review of 'Decline of Science in England'. *Quarterly Review*, 1830c, **43**, 305–342.

Brewster, D. *A Treatise on Optics*. London: Longman, Rees, Orme, Brown, Green and Taylor, 1831a. (In the series of Lardner's *Cabinet Cyclopaedia*.)

Brewster, D. Experiments on ocular spectra produced by the action of the sun's light on the retina. By Sir Isaac Newton. *Edinburgh Journal of Science*, 1831b, **4**, 75–77. (Published anonymously.)

Brewster, D. On a new analysis of solar light indicating three primary colours, forming coincident spectra of equal length. *Edinburgh Journal of Science*, 1831c, **5**, 197–206.

Brewster, D. *Letters on Natural Magic Addressed to Sir Walter Scott, Bart.* London: John Murray, 1832a.

Brewster, D. On the undulations excited in the retina by the action of luminous points and lines. *London and Edinburgh Philosophical Magazine and Journal of Science*, 1832b, **1**, 169–174.

Brewster, D. Report on the recent progress of optics. *Report of the British Association for the Advancement of Science*, 1832c, pp. 308–322.

Brewster, D. Observations on the action of light upon the retina; with an examination of the phenomenon described by Mr. Smith of Fochabers. *London and Edinburgh Philosophical Magazine and Journal of Science*, 1833a, **2**, 168–175.

Brewster, D. On the anatomical and optical structure of the crystalline lenses of animals, particularly of the cod. *Philosophical Transactions of the Royal Society*, 1833b, **123**, 323–332.

Brewster. D. Account of two experiments on accidental colours, with observations on their theory. *London and Edinburgh Philosophical Magazine and Journal of Science*, 1834, **4**, 574–575.

Brewster, D. On an ocular parallax in vision, and on the law of visible direction. *Report of the British Association, Transactions of the Sections*, 1838, pp. 7–9.

Brewster, D. Observations on Professor Plateau's defence of his theory of accidental colours. *London and Edinburgh Philosophical Magazine and Journal of Science*, 1839, **15**, 435–441.

Brewster, D. *The Martyrs of Science; or, the Lives of Galileo, Tycho Brahe, and Kepler.* London: John Murray, 1841.

Brewster, D. Review of four books on photography. *Edinburgh Review*, 1843, **76**, 309–344. (Published anonymously.)

Brewster, D. Observations on colour-blindness, or insensibility to the impressions of certain colours. *London, Edinburgh and Dublin Philosophical Magazine and Journal of Science*, 1844a, **25**, 134–141.

Brewster, D. On the accommodation of the eye to various distances. *Report of the British Association. Transactions of the Sections*, 1844b, pp. 10–11.

Brewster, D. On the new analysis of solar light. *London, Edinburgh and Dublin Philosophical Magazine and Journal of Science*, 1847a, **30**, 305–318.

Brewster, D. Review of seven books on photography. *North British Review*, 1847b, **7**, 465–504. (Published anonymously.)

Brewster, D. Description of a binocular camera. *Report of the British Association, Transactions of the Sections*, 1849, p. 5.

Brewster, D. On the polarizing structure of the eye. *Report of the British Association. Transactions of the Sections*. 1850, pp. 5–6.

Brewster, D. Binocular vision and the stereoscope. *North British Review*, 1852, 33, 165–204. (Published anonymously.)

Brewster, D. *A Treatise on Optics*, Revised Edition. London: Longman, Brown, Green and Longman, 1853.

Brewster, D. *More Worlds than One, the Creed of the Philosopher and the Hope of the Christian*. London: John Murray, 1854.

Brewster, D. *Memoirs of the Life, Writings, and Discoveries of Sir Isaac Newton*, 2 volumes. Edinburgh: Thomas Constable, 1855a. (Reprinted in 1965. Edited by R. S. Westfall.)

Brewster, D. On the triple spectrum. *Report of the British Association. Transactions of the Sections*, 1855b, pp. 7–9.

Brewster, D. *The Stereoscope. Its History, Theory, and Construction*. London: John Murray, 1856.

Brewster, D. *The Kaleidoscope. Its History, Theory, and Construction*. London: John Murray, 1858, Second Edition.

Brewster, D. On the coloured houppes or sectors of Haidinger. *London, Edinburgh and Dublin Philosophical Magazine and Journal of Science*, 1859, **17**, 323–326.

Brewster, D. On binocular lustre. *Report of the British Association. Transactions of the Sections*, 1861, pp. 29–31.

Briggs, W. *Ophthalmo-graphia, sive oculi ejusque partium descriptio anatomica, nec non, ejusdem nova visionis theoria*. London, 1686.

Bruce, D. *Sun Pictures. The Hill-Adamson Calotypes*. London: Studio Vista, 1973.

Brücke, E. Über die stereoskopischen Erscheinungen und Wheatstone's Angriff auf die Lehre von den identischen Stellen der Netzhäute. *Müller's Archiv für Anatomie und Physiologie*, 1841, pp. 459–476.

Buffon, N. Dissertation sur les couleurs accidentelles. *Mémoires de l'Académie des Sciences de Paris*, 1743, pp. 147–158.

Buffon, N. *Oeuvres complètes de Buffon*. Paris: Pilon, 1749.

Campbell, L. and Garnett, W. *The Life of James Clarke Maxwell*. London: Macmillan, 1882.

Cantor, G. N. The historiography of Georgian optics. *History of Science*, 1978, **16**, 1–21.

Cantor, G. N. Brewster on the nature of light. In A. D. Morrison-Low and J. R. R. Christie (Eds.) *"Martyr of Science"; Sir David Brewster 1781–1868*. Edinburgh: HMSO, 1983.

Carpenter, W. B. *The Microscope: and its Revelations*. London: Churchill, 1856.

Cherubin d'Orleans. *La Vision parfaite, ou les Concours des deux Axes de la Vision, en un seul point de l'Objet*. Paris, 1677.

Chevreul, M. E. *De la Loi du Contraste Simultané des Couleurs*. Paris, 1839.

Chladni, E. F. F. *Traité d'Acoustique*. Paris, 1809.

Claudet, A. The stereoscope and its photographic applications. *Journal of the Society of Arts*, 1853, pp. 97–99.

Clay, R. S. The stereoscope. *Transactions of the Optical Society*, 1927–28, **29**, 149–166.

Cochran, W. Who remembers David Brewster? *New Scientist*, 1981, **92**, 815–817.

Coe, B. *Cameras. From Daguerreotypes to Instant Pictures*. London: Marshall Cavendish, 1978.

Cohen, J. and Gordon, D. A. The Prevost-Fechner-Benham subjective colours. *Psychological Bulletin*, 1949, **46**, 97–133.

Collen, H. Earliest stereoscopic portraits. *Journal of the Photographic Society*, 1854, **1**, 200.

Daguerre, L. J. M. *Historique et description des procédés du Daguerréotype et du Diorama*. Paris, 1839.

Dalton, J. Extraordinary facts relating to the vision of colours. *Memoirs of the Manchester Literary and Philosophical Society*, 1798, **5**, 28–45.

Dancer, J. B. John Benjamin Dancer, F.R.A.S. 1812–1887. An autobiographical sketch, with some letters. *Memoirs and Proceedings of the Manchester Literary and Philosophical Society*, 1964–65, **107**, 115–142.

Darwin, R. W. New experiments on the ocular spectra of lights and colours. *Philosophical Transactions of the Royal Society*, 1786, **76**, 313–348.

Day, R. H. and Power, R. P. Apparent reversal (oscillation) of rotary motion in depth: An investigation and a general theory. *Psychological Review*, 1965, **72**, 117–127.

DeChales, C. F. Milliet. *Cursus seu mundus mathematicus*. Lyon, 1674.

Delambre, J. B. J. *Analyse des Travaux de la Classe des Sciences Mathématiques et Physiques de l'Institut Royal de France*. Paris, 1815.

Dove, H. W. Beschreibung mehrerer Prismenstereoskope und eines einfachen Spiegel-stereoskops. *Poggendorff's Annalen der Physik und Chemie*, 1851, **83**, 183–189.

Duncan, G. Structural order in the lens. In H. Davson (Ed.) *The Eye*, Volume 3. London: Academic Press, in press.

Dudley, L. P. *Stereoptics*. London: MacDonald, 1951.

Edgell, B. and Symes, W. L. The Wheatstone-Hipp chronoscope. Its adjustments, accuracy, and control. *British Journal of Psychology*, 1906–1908, **2**, 58–87.

Edinburgh Encyclopaedia. Volumes 1–18. Edinburgh: Blackwoods. (Reprinted, 1830.)

Elliot, J. The Stereoscope. *London, Edinburgh and Dublin Philosophical Magazine and Journal of Science*, 1852, **3**, 397.

Emerson, E. On the perception of relief. *American Journal of Science and Arts*, 1862, **34**, 312–316. (Reprinted in *The London, Edinburgh and Dublin Philosophical Magazine and Journal of Science*, 1863, **26**, 125–130.)

Emerson, E. The Chimenti pictures: A reply to Sir David Brewster. *The British Journal of Photography*, 1864a, 111–112, 1864b, 132–133, 1864c, 167–169, 1864d, 202–204.

Faraday, M. On a peculiar class of optical deceptions. *Journal of the Royal Institution*, 1831, **1**, 205–223.

Faye, M. Sur un nouveau système de stéréoscope. *Compte Rendu des Seances de L'Académie des Sciences*, 1856, 6 October, pp. 673–674. (Also published in *Cosmos*, 1856, **9**, 374–375.)

Fechner, G. T. *Elemente der Psychophysik*. Leipzig, 1860.

Galen, *De usu partium corporis humani*, 1550.

Gall, J. F. and Spurzheim, G. *Anatomie et Physiologie du système nerveux*. Paris, 1819.

Gassendi, P. *Opera Omnia*. Lugduni. 1658.

Gill, A. T., Antoine François Jean Claudet (1797–1867). *The Photographic Journal*, 1967, **107**, 405–409.

Gill, A. T. Early stereoscopes. *The Photographic Journal*, 1969, **109**, 546–559, 606–614, 641–651.

Gmelin, P. F. De fallaci visione per microscopia composita notata. *Philosophical Transactions of the Royal Society*, 1744, p. 382.

Goethe, J. W. von. *Zur Farbenlehre*. Tübingen: Cotta, 1810.

Gordon, Mrs. *The Home Life of Sir David Brewster*. Edinburgh: Edmonston and Douglas, 1869. Second edition, 1870.

Graves, R. P. *Life of Sir William Rowan Hamilton*. Dublin: Hodges, Figgis, 1882, Volume 1.

Gregory, R. L. The 4th dimension of 3-D. *Perception*, 1980, **9**, 613–616.

Gregory, R. L. The 4th dimension of 3-D (2). *Perception*, 1981a, **10**, 1–4.

Gregory, R. L. *Mind in Science*. London: Weidenfeld and Nicolson, 1981b, p. 410.

Griffiths, Mrs. Observations on the vision of the retina. *London and Edinburgh Philosophical Magazine and Journal of Science*, 1834, **4**, 43–46.

Gulick, W. L. and Lawson, R. B. *Human Stereopsis: A Psychophysical Approach*. Oxford: Oxford University Press, 1976.

Haidinger, W. Ueber das directe Erkennen des polarisirten Lichts und der Lage der Polarisationsebene. *Annalen der Physik und Chemie*, 1844, **63**, 29–39.

Hartley, D. *Observations on Man, his Frame, his Duty, and his Expectations*. London, 1749.

Hawksbee, F. Apparatus for making experiments on the refraction of fluids. *Philosophical Transactions of the Royal Society*, 1710, p. 204.

Hay, D. M. *The Natural Principles and Analogy of the Harmony of Form*. Edinburgh, 1842.

Helmholtz, H. On Sir David Brewster's new analysis of solar light. *London, Edinburgh and Dublin Philosophical Magazine and Journal of Science*, 1852, **4**, 401–416.

Helmholtz, H. *Handbuch der physiologischen Optik*. Erster Band. Leipzig: Voss, 1856.

Helmholtz, H. *Handbuch der physiologischen Optik*. Zweiter Band. Leipzig: Voss, 1860.

Helmholtz, H. *Handbuch der physiologischen Optik*. Dritte Band. Leipzig: Voss, 1866.

Helmholtz, H. *Physiological Optics*. (English translation by J. P. C. Southall. New York: Optical Society of America.) Volumes 1 and 2, 1924, Volume 3, 1925.

Helmholtz, H. *Popular Lectures on Scientific Subjects*. (English translation by E. Atkinson.) London: Longmans, Green, 1873.

Hering, E. *Die Lehre vom binocularen Sehen*. Leipzig: Engelmann, 1868.

Hermann, L. Eine Erscheinung simultanen Contrastes. *Pflügers Archiv für die gesamte Physiologie des Menschen und der Tiere*, 1870, **3**, 13–15.

Herschel, J. F. W. and South, J. Observations of the apparent distances and position of 380 double and triple stars, made in the years 1821, 1822, and 1823, and compared with those of other astronomers. *Philosophical Transactions of the Royal Society*, 1824, **114**, 1.

Hibbert, S. *Sketches of the Philosophy of Apparitions*. Edinburgh, 1824.

De la Hire, M. Dissertation sur les differens accidens de la vue. *Mémoires de l'Académie Royale des Sciences. Depuis 1666 jusqu'à 1699*, (dated 1730), **9**, 530–634. (Also referred to as "Oeuvres diverses de M. de la Hire".)

Hogg, J. *The Microscope: Its History, Construction, and Applications*. London: The Illustrated London Library and W. S. Orr, 1854.

Horner, W. G. On the properties of the daedeleum, a new instrument of optical illusion. *London and Edinburgh Philosophical Magazine and Journal of Science*, 1834, **4**, 36–41.

Howard, I. P. *Human Visual Orientation*. Chichester: Wiley, 1982.

Howard, I. P. and Templeton, W. B. *Human Spatial Orientation*. London: Wiley, 1966.

James, W. *Principles of Psychology*, Vol. 2. London: Macmillan, 1890.

Janin. *Mémoires et Observations sur l'Oeil*. Lyon, 1772.

Julesz, B. *Foundations of Cyclopean Perception*. Chicago: University of Chicago Press, 1971.

Jurin, J. *An Essay upon distinct and indistinct vision*. In Smith's *Opticks*, Volume II, 1738, pp. 115–171.

Kaufman, L. *Sight and Mind*. Oxford: Oxford University Press, 1974.

Kircher, A. *Ars Magna Lucis et Umbrae*. Rome, 1646.

Knox, R. On the discovery of the foramen centrale of the retina in the eyes of reptiles. *Edinburgh Philosophical Journal*, 1823, **9**, 358.

La Place P. S. in Haüy, R. J. *An Elementary Treatise on Natural Philosophy*. (Translated by O. Gregory.) London: Kearsley, 1807.

Lehot, M. *Nouvelle Théorie de la Vision*. Paris, 1823.

Leonardo da Vinci. *Trattato della Pittura*. Parigi: Giacomo Langlois, 1651.

Leonardo da Vinci. *A Treatise of Painting*. London: Taylor, 1721.

Levene, J. R. The true inventors of the keratoscope and photo-keratoscope. *British Journal for the History of Science*, 1965, **2**, 324–343.

Levene, J. R. Sir David Brewster (1781–1868) and the clinical detection of corneal anomalies. *XIIᵉ Congrès International d'Histoire des Sciences*. Paris: Albert Blanchard, 1971, pp. 105–109.

Locke, J. *An Essay Concerning Human Understanding*. London: Basset, 1690.

Locke, J. On single and double vision produced by viewing objects with both eyes: and on an optical illusion with regard to the distance of objects. *American Journal of Science and Arts*, 1849, **7**, 68–74.

MacKenzie, W. *Practical Treatise on the Diseases of the Eye*. London: Longman, 1830.

Magendie, F. and Desmoulins, A. *Anatomie des Systèmes Nerveux des Animaux à vertèbres*. Paris, 1825.

Malebranche, N. *De la Recherche de la Verité*. Paris, 1674.

Mariotte, E. Nouvelle decouverte touchant de la vue, contenue en plusiers lettres écrites par Messrs. Mariotte, Pecquet, et Perrault, in *Oeuvres de Mariotte*. Paris: La Haye, 1740.

Maxwell, J. C. On the unequal sensitivity of the *Foramen Centrale* to light of different colours. *Report of the British Association. Transactions of the Sections*, 1856, p. 12.

Maxwell, J. C. On a real image stereoscope. *Report of the British Association. Transactions of the Sections*, 1867, p. 11.

Maxwell, J. C. *The Scientific Papers of James Clerk Maxwell*, 2 volumes. Edited by W. D. Niven. Paris: Libraire Scientific, J. Hermann, 1890.

Maynard, G. (Theophilus). Letter in *Toronto Royal Standard*, 1836, Nov. 28, pp. 2–3.

Maynard, J. Note on binocular vision. *Quarterly Journal of the Microscopical Society*, 1866, **6**, 50–52.

Mayo, H. *Outlines of Human Physiology*, 3rd Edition. London, 1833.

Millar, A. H. *James Bowman Lindsay and other Pioneers of Invention*. Dundee: MacLeod, 1925, pp. 83–94.

Monge, G. *Géométrie Descriptive*. Paris, 1798.

Morrell, J. and Thackray, A. *Gentlemen of Science*. Oxford: Clarendon Press, 1981.

Morrison-Low, A. D. Brewster and scientific instruments. In A. D. Morrison-Low and J. R. R. Christie (Eds) *"Martyr of Science": Sir David Brewster, 1781–1868*. Edinburgh, HMSO, 1983.

Morrison-Low, A. D. and Christie, J. R. R. (Eds). *"Martyr of Science": Sir David Brewster 1781–1868*. Edinburgh: HMSO, 1983.

Moser, L. Über das Auge. *Dove's Repertorium der Physik. Band V*. Berlin, 1844.

Müller, J. *Zur Vergleichenden Physiologie des Gesichtssinnes des Menschen und der Thiere, nebst einen Versuch über die Bewegungen der Augen und über den menschlichen Blick*. Leipzig: Cnobloch, 1826a.

Müller, J. *Über die phantastischen Gesichtserscheinungen*. Coblenz: Hölscher, 1826b.

Müller, J. *Elements of Physiology*. Vol. II. (English translation by W. Baly.) London: Taylor and Walton, 1842.

Necker, L. A. Observations on some remarkable phenomena seen in Switzerland; and an optical phenomenon which occurs on viewing a figure of a crystal or geometrical solid. *London and Edinburgh Philosophical Magazine and Journal of Science*, 1832, **1**, 329–337.

Newton, I. *Opticks: or, a Treatise of the Reflections, Refractions, Inflections and Colours of Light*. London: Innys, 1718, 2nd Edition.

Niépce, N. Notice sur l'Héliographie. In L. J. M. Daguerre *Histoire et description des procédés du Daguerréotype*. Paris, 1839.

Oliphant, Mrs. *William Blackwood and his Sons. Their Magazine and Friends*. Edinburgh: Blackwood, 1907.

Olson, R. *Scottish Philosophy and British Physics 1750–1880*. Princeton, New Jersey: Princeton University Press, 1975, pp. 177–188.

Ono, H. On Wells's (1792) law of visual direction. *Perception and Psychophysics*, 1981, **30**, 403–406.

Paris, J. A. *Philosophy in Sport made Science in Earnest! Being an attempt to illustrate the first principles of Natural Philosophy*. London, 1827.

Pepper, J. H. *Cyclopaedic Science Simplified*. London: Frederick Warne, 1869.

Du Petit, F. P. Mémoire sur les yeux gelés, dans lequel on détermine la grandeur des chambres qui renferment l'humeur aqueuse. *Mémoires de l'Académie des Science de Paris*, 1725, p. 48.

Plateau, J. H. F. Sur un nouveau genre d'illusions optiques. *Correspondance mathematique et physique de l'Observatoire de Bruxelles*, 1832, **7**, 365–368. (The communication is dated January 20, 1833.)

Plateau, J. Essai d'une théorie générale comprenant ensemble des apparences visuelles qui succèdent à la contemplation des objets colorées, et de celles qui accompagnent cette contemplation. *Mémoires de l'Académie Royale de Belgique*, 1834, **8**, 1–68.

Plateau, J. Betrachtungen über ein von Herrn Talbot vorgeschlagenes photometrisches Princip, *Annalen der Physik und Chemie*, 1835, **111**, 457–468.

Porta, G. B. *Magia Naturalis*. Naples: M. Cancer, 1558.

Porta, G. B. *De Refractione Optices Parte*. Naples, 1593.

Porterfield, W. *A Treatise on the Eye, the Manner and Phenomena of Vision*. Edinburgh: Hamilton and Balfour, 1759.

Prévost, A. P. *Essai sur la théorie de la Vision binoculaire*. Geneva, 1843.

Prévost, B. Sur une apparence de décomposition de la lumière blanche par le mouvement du corps qui la réfléchit. *Mémoires de la Société de Physique et d'Histoire Naturelle*, 1826, **3**, 121.

Purkinje, J. *Beobachtungen und Versuche zur Physiologie der Sinne. Beiträge zur Kenntniss des Sehens in subjecktiver Hinsicht*. Erstes Bändchen. Prague: Calve, 1823.

Purkinje, J. *Beobachtungen und Versuche zur Physiologie der Sinne. Neue Beiträge zur Kenntniss des Sehens in subjecktiver Hinsicht*. Zweites Bändchen. Berlin: Reimer, 1825.

Raspail, F. P. *Nouveau Système de Chimie Organique*. Paris, 1833.

Reade, J. B. The Chimenti pictures. *The Photographic Journal*, 1862, **8**, 29–30.

Reid, T. *Enquiry into the Human Mind on the Principles of Common Sense*. Edinburgh, 1764.

Richards, W. The fortification illusions of migraines. *Scientific American*, 1971, **224** (5), 88–96.

Riddell, J. L. Notice of a binocular microscope. *American Journal of Science and Arts*, 1853, **15**, 68.

Rittenhouse, D. Explanation of an optical deception. *Transactions of the American Philosophical Society*, 1786, **2**, 37–42.

de la Rive, A. *A Treatise on Electricity in Theory and Practice*. 3 Volumes. London, 1853–1858.

Rogers, W. B. Observations on binocular vision. *American Journal of Science and Arts*, 1856, **21**, 80–95.

Roget, P. M. On the Kaleidoscope. *Annals of Philosophy*, 1818, **11**, 375–378.

Roget, P. M. Kaleidoscope in *Encyclopaedia Britannica*. Supplement to the 4th, 5th and 6th Editions. Edinburgh: Archibald Constable, 1824, pp. 163–171.

Roget, P. M. Explanation of an optical deception in the appearance of the spokes of a wheel seen through vertical apertures. *Philosophical Transactions of the Royal Society*, 1825, **115**, 131–140.

Roget, P. M. *Animal and Vegetable Physiology Considered with Reference to Natural Theology*. *Bridgewater Treatise V*, Volume II. London: William Pickering, 1834.

Rohault, J. *Traité de physique*. Paris, 1671.

Rood, O. N. *Modern Chromatics, with Applications to Art and Industry*. New York: Appleton, 1879.

Scherffer, C. *Dissertatione de Coloribus accidentalibus*. Vienna, 1761.

Schiff, W. *Perception: An Applied Approach*. Boston: Houghton Mifflin, 1980, p. 261.

Serre, M. Note sur la persistance des impressions sur la retine. *Annales d'Oculiste*, 1839, **1**, 291.

Shairp, J. C., Tait, P. G. and Adams-Reilly, A. *Life and Letters of James David Forbes, F. R. S.* London: MacMillan, 1873.

Sherman, P. D. *Colour Vision in the Nineteenth Century*. Bristol: Hilger, 1981.

Smith, R. *A compleat System of Opticks in Four Books*. Cambridge: published by the author, 1738.

Smith, T. Account of a singular phenomenon in vision. *Edinburgh Journal of Science*, 1826, **5**, 52–54.

Smith, T. Investigation of certain remarkable and unexplained phænomena of vision, in which they are traced to functional actions of the brain. *London and Edinburgh Philosophical Magazine and Journal of Science*, 1832, **1**, 249–258 and 343–349.

Smythies, J. R. A preliminary analysis of the stroboscopic patterns. *Nature*, 1957, **179**, 523–524.

Soemmerring, S. T. *Abbildungen des menschlichen Auges*. Frankfurt: Varrentrapp und Wenner, 1804.

Stampfer, S. *Die stroboskopischen Scheiben oder optische Zauberscheiben, deren Theorie und Wissenschaftliche Anwendung*. Vienna, 1833.

Steinbuch, J. G. *Beytrag zur Physiologie der Sinne*. Nürnberg, 1811.

Tacquet, A. *Opera Mathematica*. Antwerp: Meursium, 1669.

Talbot, W. H. F. Proposed philosophical experiments. *London and Edinburgh Philosophical Magazine and Journal of Science*, 1833, **3**, 81–82.

Talbot, W. H. F. Experiments on light. *London and Edinburgh Philosophical Magazine and Journal of Science*, 1834, **5**, 321–334.

Talbot, W. H. F. Some account of the art of photogenic drawing, or the process by which natural objects may be made to delineate themselves without the aid of the artist's pencil. Paper read to the Royal Society, January 31, 1839. Abstract in *Abstracts of The Papers Printed in the Philosophical Transactions of the Royal Society of London*, Vol. 4, 1837–1843, pp. 120–121.

Talbot, W. H. F. The process of calotype photogenic drawing. *Proceedings of the Royal Society*, 1841, **4**, 12–16.

Theophilus (G. Maynard). Letter in the *Toronto Royal Standard*, Nov. 28, 1836, pp. 2–3.

Thomas, D. B. *The First Negatives*. London: HMSO, 1964.

Tortual, J. *Die Sinne des Menschen*. Münster, 1827.

Du Tour, E. F. Mémoire pour établir que le point visible est vu dans le rayon qui va de ce point à l'oeil. *Mémoires de savans Etrangé*, 1784, **6**, 241.

Troxler, D. Über das Verschwinden gegebener Gegenstände innerhalb unsers Gesichtskreises. *Ophthalmologisches Bibliothek*, 1804, **2**, 1–53.

Twining, W. On single vision and the union of the optic nerves. *Edinburgh Journal of Science*, 1828, **9**, 143–153.

Tyndall, J. *Der Schall. Acht Vorlesungen Gehalten in der Royal Institution von Gross-Britannien*. Braunschweig: Vieweg, 1869.

Tyrrell, F. *Practical Work on the Diseases of the Eye and their Treatment Medically, Topically, and by Operation*. London: Churchill, 1840.

Tyrrell, F. *Cyclopaedia of Practical Surgery*, 1841.

Vallée, L. L. *Traité de la Science du Dessein*. Paris: Courcier, 1821.

Varignon. Lignes suivant lesquelles des arbres doivent être plantés pour être vues deux à deux aux extrémités de chaque ordonnée à ces lignes sous des angles de sinus données. *Mémoire de l'Académie des Sciences de Paris*, 1717.

Volkmann, A. W. *Neue Beiträge zur Physiologie des Gesichtssines*. Leipzig, 1837.

Wade, N. J. A note on the discovery of subjective colours. *Vision Research*, 1977a, **17**, 671–672.

Wade, N. J. Distortions and disappearances of geometrical patterns. *Perception*, 1977b, **6**, 407–433.

Wade, N. J. Sir Charles Bell on visual direction. *Perception*, 1978a, **7**, 359–362.

Wade, N. J. Why do patterned afterimages fluctuate in visibility? *Psychological Bulletin*, 1978b, **85**, 338–352.

Wallace, W. Clay. *The Structure of the Eye with Reference to Natural Theology*. New York: Wiley and Long, 1836.

Wardrop, J. *Essays on the Morbid Anatomy of the Human Eye*, Volume 1. Edinburgh: Archibald Constable, 1808.

Wardrop, J. *Essays on the Morbid Anatomy of the Human Eye*, Volume 1, 2nd Edition. London: Archibald Constable, 1819.

Ware, J. Muscae volitantes of nervous persons. *Medico-Chirurgical Transactions*, 1814, **5**, 255.

Wells, W. C. *An Essay on Single Vision with Two Eyes; Together with Experiments and Observations on several other Subjects in Optics*. London: Cadell, 1792.

Wenham, F. H. On the application of binocular vision to the microscope. *Transactions of the Microscopical Society of London*, 1854, **2**, 1–13.

Westfall, R. S. Introduction to *Memoirs of the Life, Writings, and Discoveries of Sir Isaac Newton* by D. Brewster. New York: Johnson Reprint Corp., 1965, pp. *ix–xlv*.

Westfall, R. S. *Never at Rest. A Biography of Isaac Newton*. Cambridge: Cambridge University Press, 1980.

Wheatstone, C. New Experiments on sound. *Annals of Philosophy*, 1823, **6**, 81–90.

Wheatstone, C. On the duration of luminous impressions on the organ of vision. *Athenaeum*, 1833a, 16 March, 170–171.

Wheatstone, C. Remarks on one of Mr. Talbot's proposed philosophical experiments. *London and Edinburgh Philosophical Magazine and Journal of Science*, 1833b, **3**, 204–205.

Wheatstone, C. An account of some experiments to measure the velocity of electricity and the duration of electric light. *Philosophical Transactions of the Royal Society*, 1834, **124**, 583–591.

Wheatstone, C. On the prismatic decomposition of electric light. *Report of the British Association, Transactions of the Sections*, 1835, pp. 11–12.

Wheatstone, C. On binocular vision; and on the stereoscope, an instrument for illustrating its phenomena. *Report of the British Association, Transactions of the Sections*, 1838a, pp. 16–17.

Wheatstone, C. De la vision binoculaire et du stéréoscope. *Bibliothèque Universelle de Genève*, 1838b, **17**, 174–175.

Wheatstone, C. Ueber das Sehen mit zwei Augen und das Stereoskop. *Poggendorff's Annalen der Physik und Chemie*, 1839, **47**, 625–627.

Wheatstone, C. Description of the electromagnetic clock. *Proceedings of the Royal Society*, 1840a, **4**, 249–250.

Wheatstone, C. Account of an electro-magnetic telegraph. *Annals of Electricity*, 1840b, **5**, 337–349.

Wheatstone, C. Sur la physiologie de la vision (1). *Annales de Chimie et de Physique*, 1841, **2**, 330–370.

Wheatstone, C. Beiträge zur Physiologie des Gesichtssinnes. Erster Theil. *Poggendorff's Annalen der Physik und Chemie*, 1842, Supplementary volume 1, 1–48.

Wheatstone, C. An account of several new instruments and processes for determining the constants of a voltaic circuit. *Philosophical Transactions of the Royal Society*, 1843, **133**, 303–327.

Wheatstone, C. Note sur le Chronoscope électromagnétique. *Comptes Rendus*, 1845, **20**, 1554–1561.

Wheatstone, C. On a means of determining the apparent solar time by the diurnal changes of the plane of polarization at the North Pole of the sky. *Report of the British Association, Transactions of the Sections*, 1848, pp. 10–12.

Wheatstone, C. Invention of the stereoscope. *London, Edinburgh and Dublin Philosophical Magazine and Journal of Science*, 1852, **3**, 478.

Wheatstone, C. Experiments on the successive polarization of light, with the description of a new polarizing apparatus. *Proceedings of the Royal Society*, 1871, **19**, 381–389.

Wheatstone, C. *The Scientific Papers of Sir Charles Wheatstone, D.C.L., F.R.S.* London: Physical Society of London, 1879.

Whewell, W. *The Philosophy of the Inductive Sciences.* London: Parker, 1840.

Whewell, W. *Of the Plurality of Worlds. An Essay*, 1853.

Williams, L. P. *Michael Faraday.* London: Chapman and Hall, 1965.

Wolff, J. *Journal of Rev. J. Wolff in a Series of Letters to Sir T. Baring, Bart.; Containing an Account of his Missionary Labours from the years 1827 to 1831; and from the years 1835 to 1838.* London, 1839.

Wollaston, W. H. On the semi-decussation of the optic nerves. *Philosophical Transactions of the Royal Society*, 1824, **114**, 222. (Reprinted in *Annales de Chimie et Physique*, 1824, **27**, 109.)

Wyld, R. S. *The Philosophy of the Senses: or, Man in Connexion with the Material World.* Edinburgh: Oliver and Boyd, 1852.

Young, T. Outlines of experiments and enquiries respecting sound and light. *Philosophical Transactions of the Royal Society*, 1800, **90**, 106–150.

Young, T. On the mechanism of the eye. *Philosophical Transactions of the Royal Society*, 1801, **91**, 23–88.

Young, T. *A Course of Lectures on Natural Philosophy and the Mechanical Arts.* London: J. Johnson, 1807.

Name Index

Subject Index